Infectious Diseases: A Global Outlook

Infectious Diseases:
A Global Outlook

Edited by **Daniel Enger**

New Jersey

Published by Foster Academics,
61 Van Reypen Street,
Jersey City, NJ 07306, USA
www.fosteracademics.com

Infectious Diseases: A Global Outlook
Edited by Daniel Enger

International Standard Book Number: 978-1-63242-244-6 (Hardback)

Printed in the United States of America.

Contents

Preface

Infectious diseases and similar problems have been one of the unavoidable outcomes of war throughout the world. This book provides a comprehensive analysis of the pathogenesis of infectious disease. Numerous valuable and well-illustrated descriptions are included in this book as it covers the evolution of such diseases to their advancement. The contents of the book are divided into two sections namely: 'General Epidemics and Its Control through Mathematical Approach' and 'Immuno-Kinetics and Vaccination'. The book would serve as a useful source to the researchers and scientists working in this discipline.

This book has been the outcome of endless efforts put in by authors and researchers on various issues and topics within the field. The book is a comprehensive collection of significant researches that are addressed in a variety of chapters. It will surely enhance the knowledge of the field among readers across the globe.

It is indeed an immense pleasure to thank our researchers and authors for their efforts to submit their piece of writing before the deadlines. Finally in the end, I would like to thank my family and colleagues who have been a great source of inspiration and support.

Editor

Part 1

General Epidemics and Its Control
Through Mathematical Approach

Biomedical Importance of Host Genetic Factors in Infectious Diseases

Farrukh Jamal[1], Tabish Qidwai[2] and Sangram Singh[1]

[1]Department of Biochemistry, Dr. Ram Manohar Lohia Avadh University, Faizabad, U.P.
[2]Department of Biotechnology, Faculty of Engineering and Technology, R.B.S. College, Agra, U.P., India

1. Introduction

Tuberculosis, human immunodeficiency virus/acquired immunodeficiency syndrome and malaria are the three most profound cause of death worldwide. In developing country tuberculosis is a serious problem. It is estimated that one third of the world's population is infected with *M. tuberculosis*; however, only a minority (10%) of those infected ever develop clinical disease (Corbett et al., 2003). Such clinical diversity suggests that factors other than bacterial infection alone determine disease development. Tuberculosis (TB) is a significant disease affecting both humans and animals. Susceptibility to *Mycobacterium tuberculosis* is relatively higher in humans than other primates and guinea pigs. Cattle, rabbits and cats are susceptible to *M. bovis* and are quite resistant to *M. tuberculosis*.

Each year, 8.8 million patients are newly diagnosed with active TB and 1.6 million patients die of TB. The rapid spread of the human immunodeficiency virus has fueled the TB epidemic, especially in sub-Saharan Africa, where 28% of TB patients are HIV positive (WHO 2007). The current first-line treatment for TB is a multidrug regimen consisting of rifampin, isoniazid, pyrazinamide, and ethambutol (RIZE). Several major problems are associated with the currently available TB treatment. There is an increasing incidence of multidrug-resistant (MDR; resistance to at least rifampin and isoniazid) and extensively drug-resistant (XDR; MDR resistance plus resistance to a fluoroquinolone and an aminoglycoside) which is creating an alarming situation as far as treatment of the disease is concerned.

1.1 Causes of drug resistance

The emergence of drug resistance in *M. tuberculosis* in India has been associated with a variety of management, health provider and patient-related factors. These include, deficient or deteriorating TB control programs resulting in inadequate administration of effective treatment; poor case holding, administration of sub-standard drugs, inadequate or irregular drug supply and lack of supervision; ignorance of health care workers in epidemiology, treatment and control; improper prescription of regimens; interruption of chemotherapy due to side effects; non-adherence of patients to the prescribed drug therapy; availability of anti-TB drugs across the counter, without prescription; massive bacillary load; illiteracy and low socio-economic status of the patients; the epidemic of HIV infection; laboratory delays in identification and susceptibility testing of M. tuberculosis isolates; use of non-standardized laboratory techniques, poor quality drug powders and lack of quality control measures; use of anti-TB drugs for indications other than tuberculosis.

1.2 Initial drug resistance in India

Indian Council of Medical Research (ICMR) undertook drug resistance studies during 1965-67 in nine urban areas of the country. However, this exercise was not a surveillance study and did not use strict sampling techniques, the centres being selected more for logistic considerations than for epidemiological reasons. Sputum specimens collected from all patients attending chest clinics were tested for drug susceptibility to streptomycin, Isoniazid, para amino salicyctic acid (PAS) and thioacetazone. The first study was on patients who had denied any history of previous treatment, while in the second study, patients with and without previous chemotherapy was included. The results showed that in the first study resistance to Isoniazid ranged from 11-20 per cent, to streptomycin from 8-20 per cent and to both drugs from 4-11 per cent. The second study showed resistance to Isoniazid to range from 15-69 per cent, to streptomycin from 12-63 per cent and to both drugs from 5-58 per cent. Further, the level of drug resistance was proportional to the duration of previous treatment.

1.3 Multi drug resistance in other countries

Resistance towards the responsible pathogens are also seen in developed countries. The situation has worsened often due to limited resource available to investigate and provide reliable susceptibility data on which rational treatments can be based as well as means to optimize the use of antimicrobial agents. The emergence of multi-drug-resistant isolates in tuberculosis, acute respiratory infections and diarrhea, often referred to as diseases of poverty, has had its greatest toll in developing countries. The epidemic of HIV/AIDS, with over 30 million cases in developing countries, has greatly enlarged the population of immuno compromised patients. The disease has left these patients at great risk of numerous infections and even greater risks of acquiring highly resistant organisms during long periods of hospitalization. This article discusses antimicrobial resistance in developing countries and the associated risk factors. Magnitude of resistance by regions Africa, America, Eastern Mediterranean, European, South East Asian, Western Pacific region has shown greater diversity in TB.

2. Symptoms

Symptoms of tuberculosis include: a bad cough that lasts 3 weeks or longer, pain in the chest, coughing up blood or sputum (phlegm from deep inside the lungs). Other symptoms of active TB disease are weakness or fatigue, weight loss, no appetite, chills, fever and sweating at night.

3. Spread

TB spreads through the air from one person to another. The bacteria are put into the air when a person with active TB disease of the lungs or throat coughs or sneezes. People nearby may breathe in these bacteria and get infected. When a person breathes in TB bacteria, which may settle in the lungs and begin to grow. From there, they can move through the blood to other parts of the body, such as the kidney, spine, and brain. TB in the lungs or throat can be infectious. This means that the bacteria can spread to other people. TB in other parts of the body, such as the kidney or spine, is usually not infectious.People with active TB disease are most likely to spread it to people they spend time with every day. This includes family members, friends, and coworkers.

4. Diagnoses

4.1 Molecular diagnosis of *Mycobacterium*

During the past several years, many molecular methods have been developed for direct detection, species identification, and drug susceptibility testing of mycobacteria.

4.1.1 Direct detection of mycobacteria from specimens

Many mycobacterial species, including *M. tuberculosis*, grow extremely slowly in the laboratory and require 3–8 weeks of incubation on solid medium or at least 2 weeks in a radiometric liquid culture system (BACTEC). This slow growth often leads to delay in TB diagnosis. Nucleic acid amplification (NAA) methods allow for detection of mycobacterial DNA or RNA directly from the specimens before the culture results are available. The Food and Drug Administration (FDA) has approved two NAA tests for direct detection of *M. tuberculosis* from clinical specimens. These are the Enhanced *Mycobacterium tuberculosis* Direct Test (E-MTD; Gen-Probe, San Diego, CA) and the Amplicor *Mycobacterium tuberculosis* Test (Amplicor; Roche Diagnostic Systems, Inc., Branchburg, NJ).

4.1.2 Amplicor test

Based on PCR assay, Mycobacterium is amplified. After amplification, the amplicons are denatured to form single strands and added to a microtiter plate containing a bound, *M. tuberculosis* complex-specific oligonucleotide probe. An avidin-horseradish peroxidase conjugate then binds to the bound, biotin-labeled amplicons. The conjugate reacts with peroxide and 3, 39, 5, 59-tetramethylbenzidine in dimethylformamide to form a color complex. The results are measured with a photometer.

4.1.3 E-MTD

The E-MTD test is based on the transcription-mediated amplification system developed by Kwoh et al. (1989). In this assay, rRNA is released from the target cells by sonication, and a promoter-primer binds to the rRNA target. Reverse transcriptase is then used to copy rRNA to a cDNA-RNA hybrid. The initial RNA strand is degraded, and a second primer binds to the cDNA and is extended, leading to the formation of double-stranded cDNA, which is then transcribed by DNA-directed RNA polymerase to produce more rRNA molecules. The new transcripts serve as templates for reverse transcription and further amplification. The

RNA amplicons are detected with an acridinium ester-labeled DNA probe in a solution hybridization assay.

4.1.4 DNA probes

Commercial DNA probes are available for detection of mycobacterium. These are based on species-specific DNA probes that hybridize with rRNA released from bacteria. The probes are labeled with acridinium ester, and results are measured with a luminometer.

4.1.5 Line-probe assay

The Line Probe assay (LiPA; Inno-Genetics N.V., Zwijndrecht, Belgium) has been developed for rapid detection of RIF resistance. The test is based on the reverse hybridization method, and it consists of PCR amplification of a segment of the *rpoB* gene and denaturation and hybridization of the biotinylated PCR amplicons to capture probes bound to a nitrocellulose strip. The bound amplicons are then detected with alkaline phosphatase-conjugated streptavidin and BCIP/NBT chromogen, producing a color reaction.

4.2 TB skin test

The TB skin test may be used to find out if you have TB infection. You can get a skin test at any pathology laboratory. A technician will inject a small amount of testing fluid (called tuberculin or PPD) just under the skin on the under side of the forearm. After 48 hours, you must return to have your skin test read by the laboratory technician. You may have a swelling where the tuberculin was injected. The technician will measure this swelling and tell you if your reaction to the test is positive or negative. A positive reaction usually means that you have been infected by someone with active TB.

5. National and international status

Tuberculosis (TB) is a major, global public health problem, particularly in sub-Saharan Africa, where the prevalence of TB is increasing dramatically with the rise of the HIV pandemic. One third of the world is infected by Mtb (*Mycobacterium tuberculosis*). (Raviglione et al., 1995). According to the World Health Organization, almost 8 million new cases of TB occur annually, with 2 million deaths attributed to the disease each year. There were globally an estimated 9.27 million new cases of tuberculosis (TB) and 1.3 million deaths in 2007 (WHO, 2009).

Uganda is one of the world's 22 highest burden countries with TB, with an estimated annual risk of tuberculosis infection of 3% and an annual incidence of new smear positive TB cases of 9.2 per 1000 in an urban setting (Guwatudde et al., 2003). Pakistan ranks 7th globally in terms of tuberculosis (TB) disease burden (Ansari et al., 2009).

TB is one of the leading causes of mortality in India killing more than 300,000 people every year. The Human Immunodeficiency Virus (HIV, the virus that causes AIDS) is the strongest risk factor for tuberculosis among adults. Tuberculosis is one of the earliest opportunistic diseases to develop amongst persons infected with HIV. HIV debilitates the immune system increasing the vulnerability to TB and enhancing the risk of progression from TB infection to TB disease. An HIV positive person is six times (50-60% life time risk) more likely of developing TB disease once infected with TB bacilli, as compared to an HIV negative person, who has a 10% life-time risk. Since 1993, the Government of India has been implementing the WHO-recommended DOTS strategy via the Revised National Tuberculosis Control Programme (RNTCP). The revised strategy was pilot-tested in 1993 and launched as a national programme in 1997. By March 2006, the programme was implemented nationwide in 633 districts, covering 1114 million (100%) population.

India accounts for one fifth of the world's incident TB cases. The reported incidence in 2003 was 168 per 100,000 and in 2006 is nearly 175 per 100,000. Every year, nearly 2 million people die in India, and nearly 1 million cases are smear positive; An estimated 40% of the Indian population is latently infected with *M. tuberculosis*. A number of factors - cultural, social, political, economic and technical - have determined the nature of society's response to TB. It has been shown that most of the infectious TB cases in a rural community in South India. About three-fourths of them are worried about their sickness; and, about half of them actively seek treatment for their symptoms at rural medical hospital. The existing facilities deal with only a very small fraction of even these patients who are actively seeking treatment. The various study report carried out in India has shown increase in TB and MDR-TB . India is classified along with the sub-Saharan African countries to be among those with a high burden of TB.

5.1 Epidemiology

The aim of epidemiology is the determination of natural history of disease and measurement of its frequency.

5.1.1 Aims of epidemiology

- Describe the trends of disease.
- Evaluation of intervention
- Define the risk group
- Frequency, distribution, time, place and person

6. Available drugs

6.1 Fluoroquinolone- fluoroquinolone is a promising class of drugs for the treatment of TB

6.1.1 Moxifloxacin- Moxifloxacin is a broad-spectrum 8-methoxy fluoroquinolone with activity against both gram-positive and gram-negative bacteria, including anaerobes. It inhibits bacterial DNA gyrase, an enzyme that is essential for the maintenance of DNA supercoils.

6.1.2 Gatifloxacin: Like the other fluoroquinolones, gatifloxacin blocks the bacterial DNA gyrase, thereby preventing chromosomal replication.

6.2 Diarylquinolines. Diarylquinolines have been identified in a process of screening various compounds for potential anti-TB activity.

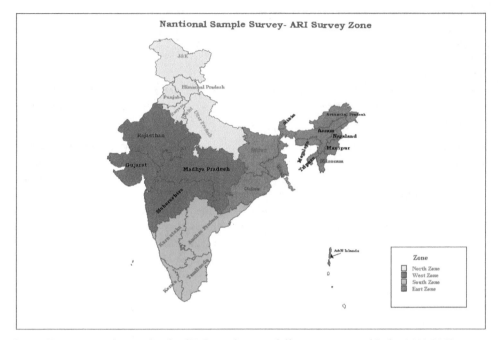

Fig. 1. Estimation of annual risk of Tuberculosis in different regions of India 2000-2003 (From National TB Institute Bangalore).

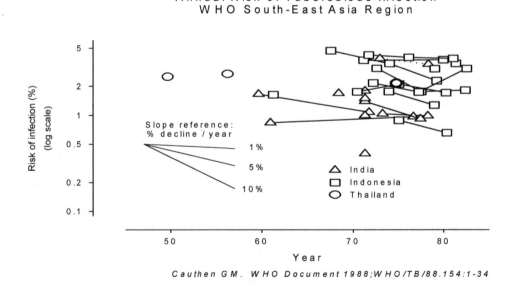

Fig. 2. Annual risk of Tuberculosis infection in South East Asia region.

A Model for the Epidemiology of Tuberculosis

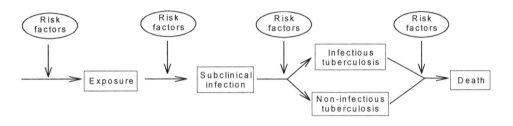

Rieder HL. Infection 1995;23:1-4

Fig. 3. Model of epidemiology of Tuberculosis.

6.2.1 TMC207: it inhibits the mycobacterial ATP synthase enzyme

6.2.2 PA-824. Activated: PA-824 inhibits the synthesis of proteins and cell wall lipids.

6.3 Nitroimidazopyrans: Nitroimidazopyrans have been derived from the bicyclic nitroimidazofurans that were originally developed for cancer chemotherapy but also exhibited activity against tuberculosis.

6.3.1 OPC-67683: OPC-67683 is a mycolic acid biosynthesis inhibitor.

6.4 Diamines

6.4.1 SQ109: SQ109 inhibits mycobacterial cell wall synthesis.

6.5 Pyrroles: In the search for compounds with activity against mycobacteria and fungi, several pyrrole derivatives have been developed.

7. Genetic polymorphisms and tuberculosis

The genetic contribution of the host plays a significant role in determining susceptibility to developing the active form of tuberculosis and severity of infection (Comstock, 1978; Schurr, 2007). Several genes of host immune response appear to play role in tuberculosis. Genetic polymorphisms and tuberculosis have been identified in several genes of host. A number of genes have been identified that play important role in tuberculosis (Fernando & Britton, 2006; Hoal, 2002). Several candidate gene studies and genome-wide linkage association studies (Bellamy et al., 2000; Jamieson et al., 2004; Miller et al., 2004; Cooke et al., 2008; Berrington & Hawn, 2007) have been performed for investigation of their role in disease risk.

Infectious disease has profound impact on human evolution. Tuberculosis is a multifactorial disorder in which the environment interacts with host-related factors, contributing to the overall phenotype. Improved understanding of the individuals balance between degrees of exposure and inherited genetic susceptibility to infection, as well as the respective effects of environmental and host-related factors will improve the understanding in the development of disease. Several host genes have been proven to contribute to active tuberculosis (TB) (Pesut, 2009). In human genome different types of variations are reported such as copy number variations (CNV), microsatellite repeats (SSR) and single nucleotide polymorphisms (SNP). Among these SNPs is the most common type of variations. Presence of polymorphisms affects either structure or level of gene products.

SNP description alone will not be sufficient to describe susceptibility to tuberculosis in a broad diverse population, and thus, functional gene studies need to be done. A real challenge is to associate candidate genes with a biologically plausible mechanism that explains the epidemiological data for tuberculosis in which only 10% of the infected individuals will develop tuberculosis. Lienhardt et al., (2002) stated that host-related and environmental factors for tuberculosis have usually been investigated separately using different study designs. Joint investigation of the genetic, immunologic, and environmental factors at play in susceptibility to tuberculosis represents an innovative goal for obtaining a better understanding of the pathogenesis of the disease. Host genetic susceptibility has been suggested as one of the most important explanations for inter-individual differences in tuberculosis (TB) risk. Multi-drug-resistant tuberculosis (MDR TB) is caused by strains of the tuberculosis bacteria resistant to the two most effective anti-tuberculosis drugs available-isoniazid and rifampicin. MDR TB can only be diagnosed in a specialized laboratory.

8. Genetic polymorphisms in tuberculosis pathogenesis

8.1 Tumor necrosis factor-alpha (TNF-α) polymorphisms

The host genetic factor plays a significant role in determining susceptibility to developing the active form of tuberculosis (Schurr, 2007). Several host immune response genes appear to play role in tuberculosis. Tumor necrosis factor-α (TNF-α) and lymphotoxin-α (LT-α), genes located within the MHC III region of chromosome 6, shows close linkage to the HLA class I (HLA-B) and class II (HLA-DR) genes (Nedwin et al., 1985) and play role in the pathogenesis of tuberculosis due to its role in the formation and maintenance of granulomas. It also plays a major role in host defense to *M. tuberculosis* by its synergistic action with interferon-γ (IFN-γ) to activate macrophages and thereby affects disease perpetuation (Mohan et al., 2001). Elevated serum TNF-α (sTNF-α) levels have been reported in advanced tuberculosis patients compared to those with mild tuberculosis and healthy controls. Several promoter polymorphisms region of TNF-α and the intron-1 polymorphism of LT-α, have been associated with altered levels of TNF-α (Sharma et al., 2008; 2010). Some of these polymorphisms have also been studied in several ethnic groups. Correa Paula et al. (2005) detected TNF-α gene polymorphisms (-308 and -238) in controls and patients of several diseases [systemic lupus erythematosus (SLE), rheumatoid arthritis (RA), primary Sjogren's syndrome (SS), and tuberculosis (TB)]. TNF -308G was associated with TB and -308 GG genotype was protective for autoimmunity. TNF-238A allele was protective for autoimmunity but a susceptibility factor for TB. Haplotype -308A-238G have been reported as a protective factor for TB, but susceptibility factor for RA, SLE, and primary SS; opposite association of TNF polymorphism with autoimmunity and TB, suggested that autoimmune diseases are a consequence of natural selection for enhanced TB resistance. Ates et al., (2008), detected TNF-α (-308 G/A, -238 G/A, -376 G/A) and IL10 (-1,082 G/A, -819 C/T, -592 C/A) polymorphisms in patients with TB and healthy controls. A significant association was found between TB and -1,082 G allele. Significant difference was observed in IL10 GCC and ACC haplotypes distribution between TB and controls. No significant association was found between IL-10 -819 C/T, TNF-α, 308 G/A, -238 G/A, -376 G/A polymorphisms and Tuberculosis. Sharma et al. 2010, performed a case control study including TNF-α gene (-1031, -863, -857, -308,-238) and LT-α gene (+252) polymorphisms in North-Indian population. No significant differences of the allele frequencies between the tuberculosis patients and controls have been reported. All the polymorphisms included in this study did not give a significant association with any of the patient sub-groups but a significant difference in the serum TNF-α level in the patients and the controls have been reported.

8.2 ALOX5 polymorphisms

ALOX5 gene encodes 5-lipoxygenase (5-LO) that play a key role in the biosynthesis of LTs and LXs from arachidonic acid. Leukotrienes (LTs) and lipoxins (LXs) are play a role in the generation of appropriate responses to inflammatory disease (Parkinson, 2006) and are involved in the regulation of immune cells and cytokine release. Phagocytosis of microorganisms by alveolar macrophages and polymorphonuclear leukocytes PMN was shown to be dependent on LTB_4, class of LXs (Bailie, 1996; Mancuso et al., 2001). A T-helper cell type 1 immune response is supported by enhanced production of interferon (IFN)- γ and interleukin (IL)-12 (Aliberti et al., 2002). The anti-inflammatory properties of LXs antagonize those of LTs in innate immunity by inhibiting PMN and NK cell functions, suppressing IL-12 release and modulating the immune response by stimulation of IL-4 production (Hachicha et al., 1999), while blocking IL-5 and IL-13 and inhibiting eosinophil effector functions (Bandeira-Melo et al., 2000). A case control study was performed by Herb et al. 2008 including a variable number of tandem repeats (VNTR) in promoter and an exonic non-synonymous variant g.760G>A polymorphisms in TB patients and controls from Ghana. Carriers of one variant and one wild-type VNTR allele ($n = 5$) or of the exonic allele g.760A had a higher risk of TB. The strongest association with TB was for the 'non-5/760A' haplotype as compared to the 'non-5/760G' haplotype.

8.3 CD209 polymorphism

CD209 on chromosome 19p13.3, encodes dendritic Cell-Specific ICAM3-Grabbing Non-integrin (DC-SIGN), is a C-type lectin, expressed on subsets of dendritic cells (DCs) and alveolar macrophages (Soilleux, 2000; Tailleux, 2003). DC-SIGN has ability to bind a variety of ligands (Gordon, 2002), endogenous ligands include endothelial cells through ICAM-2, T-lymphocytes through ICAM-3, neutrophils through MAC-1 and various endogenous glycosylated structures (Gordon, 2002; Van Kyook et al., 2003), exogenous ligands such as glycosylated moieties on *M. leprae, M. tuberculosis,* Bacillus Calmette-Guérin (BCG), *H. pylori, K. pneumoniae, S. pneumoniae,* HIV-1, HIV-2, SIV-1, Dengue virus, Ebola Virus, Cytomegalovirus, Hepatitis C virus, *S. mansoni, L. pifanoi and C. albicans* (Alvarez et al., 2002;

Tassaneetrithep et al., 2003). The contribution of *CD209* polymorphisms in human susceptibility to infectious diseases including *M. tuberculosis* and *M. leprae*, HIV-1, and Dengue is important (Barreiro et al., 2006). CD209 -336A/G (rs4804803) promoter polymorphism have shown an association with infectious disease susceptibility or protection in *M. leprae* case-control study. Martin et al. (2004) demonstrated that the -336G allele was associated with susceptibility to parenteral but not mucosal HIV-1 infection, although this was not replicated in individuals of recent African descent. Vannberg et al. (2008), investigated the role of the *CD209* -336A/G polymorphism and susceptibility to tuberculosis in sub-Saharan Africans. Significant protection was observed with *CD209* -336G variant allele in individuals from sub-Saharan Africa and, cases with -336GG were significantly less likely to develop tuberculosis-induced lung cavitation. Therefore it has been suggested, that decreased levels of the DC-SIGN receptor may be protective against both clinical tuberculosis and cavitory tuberculosis disease.

8.4 SP110 polymorphisms

Ipr1 gene is attributed to tuberculosis susceptibility gene in mice. Polymorphisms in the human homologue, SP110, have been investigated in various populations and only one study reports an association with TB susceptibility. Eight SP110 polymorphisms in a South African population, including two novel polymorphisms had been investigated. No significant association was found with any of the polymorphisms investigated, including two polymorphisms that were previously found to be associated with TB susceptibility in West African populations (Babb et al., 2007).

8.5 CARD15 polymorphisms

Caspase recruitment domain-containing protein 15 genes (*CARD15*) encodes the nucleotide-binding oligomerization domain 2 proteins (NOD2) and is considered as a susceptibility gene for Crohn's disease (CD). *CARD15* gene was investigated as a candidate gene in Tuberculosis and its product (NOD2) have been recognized as a non-redundant recognition mechanism of *M. tuberculosis*. Moller et al. 2007, genotyped the R702W, G908R and 1007fs variants, in TB cases and controls from the admixed South African Coloured population. No statistically significant differences between cases and controls were observed for these variants. Previously these polymorphisms have been reported to be associated with CD. The CD-associated mutations occur at very low frequencies in this population. The *CARD15* is not a major susceptibility gene for TB in the South African Coloureds.

8.6 BTNL2 polymorphisms

Butyrophilin-like2 gene (*BTNL2*) gene, a MHC class II gene-linked butyrophilin family member, has been recently associated with the inflammatory autoimmune diseases, such as tuberculosis, sarcoidosis, and leprosy. *BTNL2* was investigated as a candidate gene for tuberculosis in the South African Coloured population. Moller et al. (2007) genotyped 18 SNPs in *BTNL2* gene in pulmonary tuberculosis cases and controls. No significant association was detected between the truncating rs2076530 SNP, previously associated with sarcoidosis, and tuberculosis. No other studied SNPs have shown an association with disease and none of the predicted haplotypes showed any association with TB. Comparative analyses of the data from South African, German and American populations revealed that, for a segment of *BTNL2*, the admixed, but not stratified, South African population resembles the African-Americans more than white populations. Six SNPs of *BTNL2* gene in tuberculosis cases and controls in Chinese Han population was investigated by Lian et al. 2010. No significant association was detected between any of the polymorphisms investigated and TB, including rs2076530 SNP that was previously found to be associated with sarcoidosis. Genetic study revealed a significant association between the rs3763313, rs9268494, rs9268492 SNPs in the *BTNL2* gene and tuberculosis. Haplotypes 1–5, and 8 (C/A/G/T/G/A,   C/A/G/T/G/G,   C/A/T/G/C/A,   C/A/T/G/C/G,   and C/G/T/G/C/G, T/A/T/G/C/A) presented a significant association with susceptibility to tuberculosis.

8.7 IL1 B, IL4, IL10, IL12B, IL12RB, IL12RB2, IL18, IFN-γ WNT5A, FZD5 gene polymorphisms

Genes involved in the regulation of inflammatory cytokine, interferon gamma, may influence tuberculosis susceptibility, as interferon gamma is a major macrophage-activating cytokine, during *M. tuberculosis* infection. Cytokine gene polymorphisms and cytokine levels in pulmonary tuberculosis were detected (Selvaraj et al., 2008). Moller et al. (2010), investigated fifty-four polymorphisms in eight candidate genes [Interleukin 4 (*IL4*), interleukin 10 (*IL10*), interleukin 12B (*IL12B*), interleukin 12 receptor beta 1 (*IL12RB1*), interleukin 12 receptor beta 2 (*IL12RB2*), interleukin 18 (*IL18*), wingless-type MMTV integration site family, member 5A (*WNT5A*) and frizzled homolog 5 (*FZD5*)] in tuberculosis cases and healthy controls in South African population. A functional SNP (rs2243250, IL-4 -C590T), has been associated with increased promoter strength, stronger binding of transcription factors and with different levels of IL-4 activity (Luoni et al., 2001; Rosenwasser et al., 1995) but was not associated with TB in study population. The CC genotype of this polymorphism was previously associated with protection against pulmonary TB in south India and Russia (Naslednikova et al., 2009; Vidyarani et al., 2006) but not in Gambia (Bellamy et al., 1998). Two polymorphisms -511 and +3953 in *IL1B* and one in the *IL1RN*, 86 bp VNTR in smear positive TB patients, and control in Gambian individuals (all HIV negative) was investigated. Decreased risk of pulmonary TB was associated with both heterozygosity and homozygosity for the *IL1B* -511-C allele. There was no association between the *IL1B*+3953-T/C polymorphism or the 86 bp *IL1RN* pentallelic repeat and TB in this population. Using an *ex-vivo* whole blood assay, healthy Gambian individuals who are homozygous for the *IL1B* -511-T allele failed to exhibit a significant increase in IL-1β production in response to LPS after IFN-γ priming.

IFN-γ play a central role in the modulation of Tuberculosis disease severity as it is involved in host immune response against *M. tuberculosis* infection. The 12 CA repeat microsatellite allele in the non coding region of the first intron is associated with a high level of *in vitro* cytokine production (Pravica et al., 1999). Recently, it has been reported that, polymorphism at position +874 is associated with risk of tuberculosis in different populations (Rossouw et al., 2003; Lopez-Maderuelo et al., 2003). Ansari et al. (2009) have reported that the ratio of two key cytokines (IFN-γ and IL10) show significant correlation with the severity spectrum of tuberculosis in Pakistani population. In this study frequency of cytokine gene polymorphisms linked to high and low responder phenotypes (IFNγ +874 T/A and IL10 -

1082 G/A) in tuberculosis patients was analyzed. These findings are consistent with the role of IL10 in reducing collateral tissue damage and the protective role of IFNγ in limiting disease in the lung.

A+874T polymorphism on the intron 1 of IFNγ gene, which is associated with the secretory capacity of IFNγ, was reported to be associated with the development of TB among Sicilians, South Africans, Hong Kong Chinese and Spanish, although this association was not found in Malawians54 and in other populations from Houston, West Africa, South India and China. A recent study of 77 TB patients from Japan revealed that the *IFNG + 874 AA* genotype were strongly and independently predictive of a lower likelihood of sputum conversion. Indeed, IL-12, a heterodimeric pro-inflammatory cytokine produced by monocytes, macrophages, DCs and B lymphocytes and SNP in the gene responsible in the expression of this subunit was first described by Hall et al. (2000). Several polymorphisms in promoter, introns and 3'UTR in the IL-12B gene have been reported to be associated with TB in various populations, with inconsistent results. Polymorphisms in the coding sequence of the IL-12 receptor b1 gene have been reported to be associated with TB in Moroccan and Japanese populations, but, again, not in Koreans. Reports indicate that, the *IL-12B* polymorphism is not correlated with susceptibility to tuberculosis in black and white North American populations. Four SNPs, 641 A-G, 684 C-T, 1094 T-C, and 1132 G-C causing three mis-sense variants (Q214R, M365T and G378R) and one synonymous substitution in the extracellular domain of the *IL-12Rβ1* genes have been detected. Investigators have reported that the association of R214-T365-R378 allele (allele 2) is over-expressed in Japanese tuberculosis patients with the homozygosis for R214 - T365 - R378 (the 2/2 allele) being significantly associated with tuberculosis.

8.8 IFNγR1 polymorphisms

Interferon-γ Receptor-1 plays a role in host immune response. Several SNPs in IFNγR1 have been studied in falciparum malaria cases and controls. The frequencies of interferon-γ (IFN-γ) receptor-1 (IFNγR1) promoter polymorphisms (G-611A, T-56C) in tuberculosis patients and controls were not significantly different. Because of these studied SNP affect transcription, the expression of the IFNγR1 gene does not confer susceptibility to disease in patients from Croatia (Bulat-Kardum et al., 2006). A significant association between the protective (CA) n polymorphism (22 repeats, 192 FA1), located in intron five of the IFNγR1 gene and GT promoter haplotype (-611; -56) that showed the strongest expression capacity have been reported. In addition to this cis relationship, the (CA) 22 allele was correlated in trans with an IFN-γ SNP (IFNγ Gþ2109A), which might affect the transcription of the IFNγ gene. These results suggest that a particular combination of IFNγ and IFNγR1 SNP (gene-gene) interaction might provide a better protection against tuberculosis in this population. Several families with Mendelian susceptibility to mycobacterial disease that has mutations in one of two subunits of the *IFN-γ* receptor gene (*IFN-γR1* and *IFN-γR2*) (Ottenhoff et al., 2002) have been discovered.

8.9 NOS2A polymorphisms

Nitric oxide (NO) act as is a free radical and second messenger and has been shown to be important in the development of several diseases, including tuberculosis. NO, produced by NOS2A, plays a major role in the pulmonary host-defense mechanism in response to infections, and is implicated in bacteriostatic as well as bactericidal processes. The cytokines like, TNF-α, IL-1β along with IFN-γ produced by T-cells can induce NO via action of NOS2A. It has been proposed that NO produced by tuberculosis-infected human macrophages and by epithelial cells is anti mycobacterial against *M. tuberculosis* (Liu et al., 2006). A report indicates that the alveolar macrophages from the lungs of patients with tuberculosis express NOS2A in potentially mycobactericidal amounts and this NOS2A can kill mycobacterium *in vitro* (Qidwai & Jamal, 2010). We have review the role of three SNPs (-954G/C, -1173C/T, -1659 A/T), one microsatellite repeat in promoter and one SNP in exon 16 of gene in several case control studies (Qidwai & Jamal, 2010). The promoter polymorphisms (-954G/C, -1173C/T, -1659 A/T) have been shown to increase NO synthesis (Hobbs et al., 2002). This region in the human gene is situated from -0.7 to -2.6 kb upstream of the transcription start and contains important DNA motifs for binding of NF-κB, activator protein 1, signal transducer, and activator of transcription protein 1, and NF-κB repressing factor (Coia et al., 2005). The -954G/C variant is believed to have originated as a consequence of selective pressure of *Plasmodium* in endemic area of Africa. The G allele has been shown to be absent from Caucasian populations (Kun et al., 1998) as well as from the Peruvian population (Martin et al., 1999). In Mexicans, the G allele was not associated with tuberculosis (Flores-Villanueva et al., 2005). Two chromosome 17 genes NOS2A and CCL2 plays a role in susceptibility to tuberculosis in South African population (Moller et al., 2009). Haplotype of two functional (rs9282799 and rs8078340) SNPs in the NOS2A promoter have been significantly associated with tuberculosis. Presence of T allele decreases the DNA-protein complex formation and decreases the duration of DNA-protein interaction, which leads to decrease NO production. The T allele of SNP rs8078340 is over represented in the patients. As NO possess potent antimicrobial effects, having ability to inhibit the growth of many infectious organisms *in vitro*, polymorphism in the promoter alters the level of NOS2A, decreasing the level of NO and thereby increases the susceptibility to tuberculosis.

A case-control association study of TB, patients and controls was performed in African-Americans and Caucasians by Velez et al. (2009). Thirty-nine SNPs were selected from the NOS2A gene, for single SNP, haplotype, and multilocus interaction analyses with other typed candidate genes. In African-Americans, ten NOS2A SNPs were associated with TB. The strongest associations were observed at rs2274894 and rs7215373. The strongest gene–gene interactions were observed between NOS2A rs2248814 and IFNGR1 rs1327474 and NOS2A rs944722 and IFNGR1 rs1327474. Three other SNPs in NOS2A interacted with TLR4 rs5030729 and five other NOS2A SNPs interacted with IFNGR1 rs1327474. No significant associations were observed in Caucasians. These results suggest that NOS2A variants may contribute to TB susceptibility, particularly in individuals of African descent, and may act synergistically with SNPs in TLR4 and IFNGR1.

9. Vitamin D receptor (VDR) polymorphisms

The investigation of the genetic polymorphisms of vitamin D, VDBP, TLR, NOS2A and IFN-γ genes and resistance or susceptibility to *M. tuberculosis* infection was summarized by (Preto, 2009). The vitamin D receptor (VDR) gene is one of the most important candidate genes that play role in susceptibility to tuberculosis. Polymorphisms that affects the activity of the receptor have profound impact. Genetic variants of the natural resistance-associated macrophage protein (*NRAMP1*) and vitamin D receptor (*VDR*) genes are associated with smear-positive pulmonary tuberculosis in Gambian populations (Bellamy et al., 1998a,b;

1999). Vitamin D receptor (VDR) genotypes have been shown to be associated with differential susceptibility or resistance to tuberculosis. The influence of FokI, BsmI, ApaI and TaqI variants of VDR gene on 1, 25(OH)(2) D(3) modulated granzyme A expression of cytotoxic lymphocytes induced by culture filtrate antigen (CFA) of Mycobacterium tuberculosis (Vidyarani et al., 2009). The ApaI aa genotype and bbaaTT extended genotype were associated with a significantly decreased percentage of granzyme A positive cells in normal healthy controls. The study suggest that 1, 25(OH)(2) D(3) suppresses granzyme A probably by down-regulating Th1 cytokine response. Gao et al. (2010), has reviewed published studies on VDR polymorphisms and TB susceptibility and quantitatively summarized associations of the polymorphisms (*FokI*, *TaqI*, *ApaI* and *BsmI*). Among Asians, the *FokI* ff genotype showed a pronounced positive association, a significant inverse association was observed for the *BsmI* bb genotype, and marginal significant associations were found for *TaqI* and *ApaI* polymorphisms. None of the studied polymorphisms have shown a significant association to TB among Africans or South Americans.

9.1 Vitamin D-binding protein

VDBP is a multifunctional, highly expressed, polymorphic serum protein encoded by Gc gene and is the major plasma carrier of vitamin D_3 and its metabolites and ensures that vitamin D is transported to the liver, $25(OH)_2D_3$ to the kidney, and 1, $25(OH)_2D_3$ to target cells and organs. A multi gene cluster at chromosome 4q11-q13 includes albumin, α-fetoprotein and *Gc* gene. Variations in exon 11 of the *Gc* gene at codons 416 and 420 give rise to electrophoretic variants of VDBP, called Gc1 fast (Gc1F), Gc1 slow (Gc1S) and Gc2 differing by amino-acid sequence, as well as by attached polysaccharides. Combinations of the three VDBP or Gc variants result in six common circulating phenotypes: Gc1F/Gc1F, Gc1F/Gc1S, Gc1S/Gc1S, Gc1F/Gc2, Gc1S/Gc2, and Gc2/Gc2 (23). *DBP* polymorphism (Gc phenotype) is related to the VDBP concentration and vitamin D status (Lauridsen et al., 2005). The authors showed a strong correlation between higher, intermediate and lower circulating levels of $25(OH)_2D_3$ and $1,25(OH)_2D_3$ with Gc1-1, Gc1-2 and Gc2-2 phenotypes, respectively, in Danish Caucasian postmenopausal women population. Variations in this property could affect the functioning of the immune system, as *DBP* knockout mice exhibited an impaired immune response to bacterial infections (White & Cook, 2000). A role of *DBP* polymorphism in autoimmune diabetes mellitus and infectious disease in Polynesia and Japan (Hirai et al., 2000) has been suggested. No differences in *DBP* phenotype were seen among patients and the control group. In that study, frequency of Gc2 in tuberculosis patients was slightly but not significantly higher than in the control group and this elevation was at the expense of both Gc1F and Gc1S alleles.

9.2 The Toll-like receptors

The TLRs represent a group of single-pass transmembrane receptors, are expressed on innate immune cells and works as sensors for pathogen-derived molecules, and play a role in host-pathogen interaction (Aderem et al., 2000). TNF-α and NO is induced mostly by macrophages soon after innate recognition of mycobacteria through TLRs (Underhill et al., 1999). The role of TLR in resistance to *M. tuberculosis* was suggested initially by the fact that MyD88-deficient mice are more susceptible to *M. tuberculosis* infection and by the observation that TRL2/TLR1 reduced the viability of intracellular *M. tuberculosis* in human monocytes and macrophages, but not in monocyte-derived DCs (Liu et al., 2006). They have also reported that TLR induces up-regulation of the *VDR*, 1α-vitamin D hydroxylase (enzyme that converts inactive to active vitamin D), and *CYP27B1* gene expression in monocytes and macrophages.

The human TLR2 gene is located on chromosome 4q32 and is composed of 2 non-coding exons and 1coding exon (Haehnel et al., 2002). In TLR2 gene, 89 SNPs have been reported, (26 in the 5'-untranslated region, 17 in the 3'-untranslated region, 29 located in intronic parts of the gene, and 17 modify bases of the third exon of TLR2). Six non-synonymous SNPs of the *TLR2* gene change amino acids in the cytosolic part of this receptor. Out of which, only two have been linked to reducing NF-κB activation and increasing risk of infection. The first SNP changes of C to T replacing arginine (Arg; R) with tryptophan (Trp, W) at position 677, abolishing the binding with MyD88 with TLR2. This specific polymorphism located within the *bb* loop of *TLR2* (Arg677Trp) abolishes activation of NF-κB in response to *M. tuberculosis*, resulting in decreased IL-12 serum level production by 677W carriers. The second *TLR2* SNP changes G to A, which substitutes an arginine for glutamine at position 753. The *TLR2* 753Q seems to be associated with an increased risk of developing tuberculosis for carriers the AA and AG genotypes (Ogus et al., 2004). Thuong et al. (2007) described a strong association of SNP T597C *TLR2* with susceptibility to military tuberculosis patients from Vietnam. Further association was described among Koreans regarding the microsatellite polymorphisms in intron II or *TLR2* (Yim et al., 2006). In addition, *TLR1* polymorphism in a non-synonymous region (I602S) could be associated with TLR1/2 heterodimer binding sites to mycobacterial lipopeptide, since individuals with 602II genotype produced substantially more IL-6 than those with the 602SS variant. Currently, the polymorphism in *TLR2* might be an important risk factor for disease progression. The G to A (Arg753Gln) polymorphism at position 2258 in exon 3 and the guanine-thymine (GT) microsatellite repeat polymorphism (100 bp upstream of the translational start site) in intron 2, have been associated with susceptibility to clinical tuberculosis (TB) disease in Turkish and Korean patients, respectively (Ogus et al., 2004; Yim et al., 2006). TLR2 promoter region, namely, -16934 A>T and -196 to -174 insertion (Ins) >deletion (Del), polymorphisms have been associated with asthma and gastric cancer, respectively (Eder et al., 2004; Tahara et al., 2007).

Patients with pulmonary TB and healthy controls, were examined for TLR2 polymorphisms over locus -100 (microsatellite guanine-thymine repeats), -16934 (T>A), -15607 (A>G), -196 to -174 (insertion>deletion), and 1350 (T>C) (Chen et al., 2010). An association exists between the haplotype [A-G-(insertion)-T] and susceptibility to pulmonary tuberculosis. Patients with systemic symptoms of tuberculosis had a lower -196 to -174 deletion/deletion genotype frequency than those without systemic symptoms. TB patients with the deletion/deletion genotype had higher blood NK cell counts than those carrying the insertion allele whereas patients with pleuritis had a higher 1350 CC genotype frequency than those without pleuritis. Patients of tuberculosis with the 1350 CC genotype had higher blood NK cell counts than those carrying the T allele. TB patients carrying homozygous short alleles for GT repeats had higher blood NK cell counts than those carrying one or no short allele. Thus, an association between the specific TLR2 haplotype and susceptibility to pulmonary TB have been reported. In patients with pulmonary TB, both the -196 to -174 Del/ Del and 1350 CC genotypes were associated with an increased blood absolute NK cell counts.

9.3 TLR4 polymorphism

Toll-like receptor (TLR) 4 has been described to play a main role in the innate immunity against TB. The association between two particular SNPs in human TLR4 (Asp299Gly and Thr399Ile) and active TB has been studied in non-HIV Africans with contradictory results. However, studies focusing on the effect of these TLR4 SNPs in active TB within a Caucasian HIV population are lacking. The association between TLR4 Asp299Gly and Thr399Ile SNPs and active TB, in Caucasian Mediterranean HIV-infected individuals were analyzed by Ildefonso et al. (2010). Asp299Gly were independently associated with active TB and inversely with latent TB prophylaxis. An independent association between TLR4 Asp299Gly SNP and active TB in Caucasian Mediterranean HIV-infected patients was detected.

9.4 Toll-like receptor 8 polymorphisms

Davila et al. (2008) studied TB association and expression of 18 genes involved in the Toll-like receptor (TLR) pathways. The polymorphisms in pulmonary TB patients and controls from Indonesia was genotyped. The four polymorphisms in the TLR8 gene on chromosome X showed evidence of association with TB susceptibility in males, including a non-synonymous polymorphism rs3764880 (Met1Val).They have also genotyped these four TLR8 polymorphisms in an independent collection of pulmonary TB patients and controls from Russia and again found evidence of association in males (for rs3764880). A marked increase in TLR8 protein expression was also observed directly in differentiated macrophages upon infection with M. bovis, bacille Calmette-Gue´rin (BCG). A role for the TLR8 gene in susceptibility to pulmonary TB across different populations have been reported. Polymorphisms (1805 G/T in TLR1, 2258 A/G in TLR2, -857 C/T and -863 A/C in TNF-α and -819 C/T in IL-10) was genotyped in tuberculosis patients and controls by Mai Juan et al. 2010. Multivariate logistic regression analysis revealed that the TT genotype of -857 C/T in TNF-α gene was significantly associated with lower risk of PTB, in comparison with other genotypes. The genetic variant of -863 A/C in TNF-α gene was associated with susceptibility to PTB and clinical severity of disease. The results of the study suggest that the variants in TNF-α gene were associated with susceptibility to PTB and clinical severity of disease, while no significant association have been reported for TLRs and IL-10 genes polymorphisms and tuberculosis.

9.5 PTPN22 gene polymorphism

The PTPN22 gene encodes the lymphoid tyrosine phosphatase that has an important regulatory effect on T- and B-cell activation in immune response. Lamsyah et al. (2009) reported an association of PTPN22 gene functional variants with development of pulmonary tuberculosis in Moroccan population. The two missense polymorphisms of the PTPN22 gene (R620W and R263Q) and susceptibility to TB in the Moroccan population was investigated. A statistically significant difference exists in the distribution of the PTPN22 1885T allele between pulmonary TB patients and healthy controls. In case of PTPN22 R263Q (G788A) SNP, there is an increase of 788A allele frequencies in TB patients compared with those in healthy individuals. These results suggest that PTPN22 gene variants may affect susceptibility to TB in the Moroccan population.

9.6 Human V-ATPase polymorphism

Capparelli et al. (2009) tested for polymorphisms in the intron 15 and the 5'-untranslated region of the gene coding for the a3 isoform of the human ATPase gene in pulmonary tuberculosis patients and controls. Alleles (two at each site) segregated in the form of four haplotype pairs. The double heterozygous patients were protected against tuberculosis and the double homozygous patients were susceptible to the disease.

9.7 MIF, FCGR2A, and FCGR3A gene polymorphisms

The polymorphisms of macrophage migration inhibitory factor (MIF), Fcg receptors CD16A (FCGR3A) and CD32A (FCGR2A) genes and susceptibility to pulmonary tuberculosis (PTB) in the Moroccan population, was analyzed (Sadki et al., 2010). The genotyping for MIF-173 (G/C) (rs755622), FCGR2A-131 H/R (rs1801274), and FCGR3A-158V/F (rs396991) have been done. A statistically significant increase of the MIF -173CC homozygote genotype and MIF -173*C allele frequencies in PTB patients compared with healthy controls was detected. In contrast, no association was observed between FCGR2A-131H/R and FCGR3A-158V/F polymorphisms and tuberculosis disease. The finding suggests that MIF -173*C variant may play an important role in the development of active tuberculosis.

9.8 CCR2, MCP-1, SDF-1a & DC-SIGN gene polymorphisms

Investigation showed that chemokine, chemokine receptor and DC-SIGN gene polymorphisms were associated with susceptibility/resistance to HIV and HIV-TB in south India (Alagarasu et al., 2009). CCR2 V64I (G/A), monocyte chemoattractant protein-1 (MCP-1) -2518 A/G, stromal cell derived factor-1alpha; (SDF-1alpha) 3'UTR G/A and DC-SIGN gene polymorphisms were studied in HIV-1 infected patients without TB, with pulmonary TB (PTB) and extrapulmonary TB, PTB patients without HIV and healthy controls. No significant difference was detected in the genotype frequencies of CCR2 V64I, MCP-1 -2518 and DC-SIGN polymorphisms between the study groups. A significantly increased frequency of GG genotype of SDF-1alpha polymorphism was observed among positive for HIV and PTB patients compared to healthy controls. The GG genotype of SDF-1alpha 3'UTR polymorphism may be associated with susceptibility to PTB in HIV-1 infected patients. Raghavan et al. (2009) have detected the HLA-DR2 subtypes and the possible HLA-A/-B/-DRB1 haplotype combinations that are associated with susceptibility or resistance to HIV and HIV with pulmonary tuberculosis (HIV+PTB+). Overrepresentation of HLA-DRB1*1501 in HIV+PTB- patients and DRB1*1502 in HIV+PTB+ patients as compared to healthy controls was detected. An increased frequency of HLA-A2-DRB1*1501 haplotype in HIV+PTB- patients and HLA-A2-DRB1*1502 among HIV+PTB+ patients compared to healthy controls have been identified. The study suggests that HLA-A2-DRB1*1501 haplotype may be associated with HIV infection while HLA-A2-DRB1*1502 haplotype might be associated with susceptibility to PTB in HIV patients. HLA-B40-DRB1*1501 and HLA-B40-DRB1*04 haplotypes may be associated with susceptibility to HIV infection and to PTB in HIV patients (Raghvan et al., 2009).

9.9 TIRAP polymorphisms and susceptibility to childhood TB

The adaptor protein TIRAP mediates downstream signaling of TLR2 and TLR 4. TIRAP gene polymorphisms have been associated with susceptibility and resistance to tuberculosis

(TB) in adults in South Africa. Dissanayeke et al. (2009), identified 13 SNPs, and found significant differences in frequency of the variants between the two ethnic groups. The frequency of individual polymorphisms or combinations did not vary between TB cases and controls in either cohort. The 558C→T polymorphism previously associated with TB meningitis (TBM) in a Vietnamese population was found to be associated with TBM in the mixed ancestry group. The study suggests that, polymorphisms in TIRAP do not appear to be involved in childhood TB susceptibility in South Africa.

10. Mannose-binding lectin (MBL) polymorphisms

Mannose-binding lectin (MBL) is considered an important component of innate immunity. Four functional MBL2 alterations in codons 52, 54, 57 and in the promoter at position c.1-290 are correlated with significantly lowered MBL serum levels. These variants have been associated with susceptibility to a variety of infectious agents as well as with various immunologic disorders. The gene encoding MBL is located on chromosome 10 and is designated as MBL2. MBL elicits complement activation by binding to mannose- and N-acetylglucosamine sugar groups on various microorganisms. Variations in the serum MBL levels are mainly due to the presence of three common point mutations in exon1 of MBL2 gene at the codons 52 (rs5030737), 54 (rs1800451) and 57 (rs1800450). MBL deficiency is an example of evolutionary selection, as MBL deficiency reduces the capacity of mycobacteria to invade macrophages, thus provide resistance to TB (Garred et al., 1994). Variations at codons 52, 54 and 57 lead to low or near absent serum MBL. A study from South African suggested that hetrozygotes for MBL54 have protection against tuberculosis meningitis (Hoal-Van Helden et al., 1999). TB patients as compared to controls have an increased genotype frequencies for mutant homozygotes at codons 52, 54 and 57in South Indians but no such association have been reported in China, Poland, Turkey, Malawi, Tanzania and Gambia.

10.1 Complement receptor polymorphisms

The complement receptor-1(CR1) present on the surface of the macrophages is associated with phagocytosis of various microorganisms, including *M. tuberculosis*. Homozygotes in one of five CR1polymorphisms (Q1022H) are associated with increased TB risk in Malawi.

10.2 Purinergic P2X7 receptor

Purinergic P2X7 receptors are cationic channels present on the cells in the blood and immune systems. A polymorphism with a 1513 A-C (rs3751143) that replaces the glutamic acid at residue 496 by alanine, was not associated with pulmonary TB in Gambia (Li et al., 2002). No link of 1513 SNP with pulmonary TB was found in Southeast Asian refugees from Australia but a strong association existed between the C polymorphism and extrapulmonary TB (Fernando et al., 2006).

10.3 Association analysis of susceptibility region on chromosome 5q31 for tuberculosis

In the Asian population the chromosome 5q23.2–31.3 has been identified as a region with linkage to tuberculosis (Ridruechai et al., 2010). A putative tuberculosis susceptibility locus was investigated, in a family-based association test between the dense SNP markers within chromosome 5q31 and tuberculosis in Thai trio families. Seventy-five SNPs located within candidate genes covering SLC22A4, SLC22A5, IRF1, IL5, RAD50, IL13, IL4, KIF3A and SEPT8 were genotyped. Association analysis revealed the most significant association with tuberculosis in haplotypes comprising SNPs rs274559, rs274554, and rs274553 of SLC22A5 gene, which remained significant after multiple testing corrections. The two haplotypes within the SLC22A4 and KIF3A region were associated with tuberculosis. Haplotypes of SLC22A5 were significantly associated with the expression levels of RAD50 and IL13. The variants carried by the haplotypes of SLC22A4, SLC22A5, and KIF3A region potentially contribute to tuberculosis susceptibility among the Thai population.

10.4 Genome-wide analysis of genetic susceptibility to tuberculosis

Bellamy et al. (1998b), performed genome-wide analysis of genetic susceptibility to tuberculosis in Africans. A two-stage genome-wide linkage study to search for regions of the human genome containing tuberculosis-susceptibility genes was carried out. Sibpair families that contain two full siblings, affected by clinical tuberculosis were used. 299 highly informative genetic markers, spanning the entire human genome, were typed in 92 sibpairs ffrom Gambia and South Africa in the first round. To identify whether any of these regions contained a potential tuberculosis-susceptibility gene, 22 markers from these regions were genotyped in a second set of 81 sibpairs from the same countries. Markers on chromosomes 15q and Xq showed suggestive evidence of linkage to tuberculosis. These results indicate that genome-wide linkage analysis can contribute to the mapping and identification of major genes for multifactorial infectious diseases of humans. Thye et al. (2009) have identified a genetic variant, which increases susceptibility to tuberculosis (TB) in African populations using genome-wide association (GWA) study. The studies involve analysing hundreds of thousands of genetic markers across the human genomes in search of variants found in patients but not in healthy controls.

Control of the TB epidemic requires more than developing new drugs. The diagnostic and therapeutic facilities of health care centers in developing countries must be improved, and the socioeconomic status and general welfare of patients (including nutritional and HIV status) should be addressed to help eradicate TB. The development of tuberculosis or other mycobacterial diseases is the result of a complex interaction between the host and pathogen influenced by environmental factors. Numerous host genes are likely to be involved in this process. A variety of study methods, have contributed to substantial progress in advancing our understanding of genetic susceptibility to tuberculosis.

11. References

Aderem, A. & Ulevitch, R.J. (2000) Toll-like receptors in the induction of the innate immune response. Nature, 406, 782-787.

Alagarasu, K., Selvaraj, P., Swaminathan, S., Narendran, G. & Narayanan, P. R. (2009). 5' regulatory and 3' untranslated region polymorphisms of vitamin D receptor gene in south Indian HIV and HIV-TB patients. *J. Clin. Immunol.* 29, 196–204.

Aliberti, J., Serhan, C. & Sher, A. (2002). Parasite-induced lipoxin A4 is an endogenous regulator of IL-12 production and immunopathology in *Toxoplasma gondii* infection. *J. Exp. Med*, 196,1253–1262.

Alvarez, C.P., Lasala, F., Carrillo, J., Muñiz, O., Corbi, A.L. & Delgado, R. (2002). C-type lectins DC-SIGN and L-SIGN mediate cellular entry by Ebola virus in cis and in trans. *J. Virol*, 76, 6841–6844.

Ansari, A., Talat, N., Jamil, B., Hasan, Z., Razzaki, T., Dawood, G. & Hussain R. (2009). Cytokine Gene Polymorphisms across Tuberculosis Clinical Spectrum in Pakistani Patients. *PLos One*, 4,1-7.

Ates, O., Musellim, B., Ongen, G. & Topal-Sarikaya, A. (2008). Interleukin-10 and tumor necrosis factor-alpha gene polymorphisms in tuberculosis. *J. Clin. Immunol*, 28, 232-236.

Babb, C., Keet, E.H., Van Helden, P.D. & Hoal, E.G. (2007). SP110 polymorphisms are not associated with pulmonary tuberculosis in a South African population. *Hum. Genet*, 121,521-522.

Bailie, M.B., Standiford, T.J., Laichalk, L.L., Coffey, M.J., Strieter, R. & Peters-Golden, M. (1996). Leukotriene-deficient mice manifest enhanced lethality from Klebsiella pneumoniae in association with decreased alveolar macrophage phagocytic and bactericidal activities. *J. Immunol*, 157, 5221–5224.

Bandeira-Melo, C., Bozza, P.T., Diaz, B.L., Cordeiro, R.S., Jose, P.J., Martins, M.A. & Serhan, C.N. (2000) Cutting edge: lipoxin (LX) A4 and aspirin-triggered 15-epi-LXA4 block allergen-induced eosinophil trafficking. *J. Immunol*. 164, 2267–2271.

Barreiro, L.B., Neyrolles, O., Babb, C.L. & et al. (2006). Promoter variation in the DC-SIGN-encoding gene CD209 is associated with tuberculosis. PLoS Med, 3:e20. *31*.

Bellamy, R., Ruwende, C., Corrah, T., McAdam, K.P., Whittle, H.C. & Hill, A.V. (1998b). Variations in the NRAMP1 gene and susceptibility to tuberculosis in West Africans. *N. Engl. J. Med*, 338, 640-644.

Bellamy, R., Ruwende, C., Corrah, T., McAdam, K.P., Whittle, H.C. & Hill, A.V. (1998a). Assessment of the interleukin 1 gene cluster and other candidate gene polymorphisms in host susceptibility to tuberculosis. *Tuberi. Lung Dis*, 79, 83–89.

Bellamy, R., Ruwende, C., Corrah, T., McAdam, K.P., Thursz, M., Whittle, H.C. & Hill, A.V. (1999). Tuberculosis and chronic hepatitis B virus infection in Africans and variation in the vitamin D receptor gene. J. Infect. Dis, 179, 721-724.

Bergmann, J.S., Yuoh, G., Fish, G. & Woods, G.L. (1999). Clinical evaluation of the enhanced Gen-Probe amplified Mycobacterium tuberculosis direct test for rapid diagnosis of tuberculosis in prison inmates. *J. Clin. Microbiol*, 37, 1419–1425.

Berrington, W.R. & Hawn, T.R. (2007). Mycobacterium tuberculosis, macrophages, and the innate immune response: does common variation matter? *Immunol. Rev*, 219, 167-186.

Boogaard, J., Kibiki, G.S., Kisanga, E.R. & et. al. (2009). New Drugs against Tuberculosis: Problems, Progress, and Evaluation of Agents in Clinical Development. Antimicrobial agents and chemotherapy, pp. 849–862

Bulat-Kardum, L., Etokebe, G.E., Knezevic, J. & et al. (2006). Interferon-g Receptor-1 Gene Promoter Polymorphisms (G-611A; T-56C) and Susceptibility to Tuberculosis. *Scand. J. of Immuno*, 63, 142–150.

Capparelli, R., Palumbo, D., Iannaccone, M. & Iannelli, D. (2009). Human V-ATPase gene can protect or predispose the host to pulmonary tuberculosis. *Genes Immun*, 10, 641-646.

Chen, Y.C., Hsiao, C.C., Chen, C.J. & et al. (2010). Toll-like receptor 2 gene polymorphisms, pulmonary tuberculosis, and natural killer cell counts. *BMC Medical Genetics*, 11:17.

Coia, V., Jüliger, S., Mordmüller, B. & et al. (2005). Analysis of polymorphic sites in the promoter of the nitric oxide synthase 2 gene. *Biochem. Biophys. Res. Commun*, 335, 1123-1131.

Comstock, G.W. (1978). Tuberculosis in twins: a re-analysis of the Prophit survey. *Am. Rev. Respir. Dis*, 117, 621-624.

Cooke, G.S., Campbell, S.J., Bennett, S., Lienhardt, C., McAdam, K.P. & et al. (2008). Mapping of a Novel Susceptibility Locus Suggests a Role for MC3R and CTSZ in Human Tuberculosis. *Am. J. Respir. Crit. Care Med*, 178, 203–207.

Corbett, E.L., Watt, C.J., Walker, N. & et al. (2003). The growing burden of tuberculosis: global trends and interactions with the HIV epidemic. *Arch. Intern. Med*, 163: 1009–1021.

Correa, P.A., Gomez, L.M., Cadena, J. & Anaya, J.M. (2005). Autoimmunity and tuberculosis. Opposite association with TNF polymorphism. *J. Rheumatol*, 32, 219-224.

Davila, S., Hibberd, M.L., Hari Dass, R. & et al. (2008). Genetic Association and Expression Studies Indicate a Role of Toll-Like Receptor 8 in Pulmonary Tuberculosis. *PLoS Genet*, 4(10): e1000218.

Dissanayeke, S.R., Levin, S., Pienaar, S., Wood, K., Eley, B., Beatty, D., Henderson, H., Anderson, S. & Levin, M. (2009). Variation in TIRAP is not associated with susceptibility to childhood TB but may determine susceptibility to TBM in some ethnic groups. *PLoS One*, 4(8): e6698.

Eder, W., Klimecki, W., Yu, L., von Mutius, E., Riedler, J., Braun-Fahrländer, C., Nowak, D. & Martinez FD (2004). ALEX Study Team. Toll-like receptor 2 as a major gene for asthma in children of European farmers. *J. Allergy Clin. Immunol*, 113, 482-488.

Fernando, S.L. & Britton, W.J. (2006). Genetic susceptibility to mycobacterial disease in humans. Immunol. *Cell Biol*, 84, 125-137.

Flores-Villanueva, P.O., Ruiz-Morales, J.A., Song, C.H., et al. (2005). Functional promoter polymorphism in monocytchemo attractant protein-1 is associated with increased susceptibility to pulmonary tuberculosis. *J. Exp. Med*, 202, 1649-1658.

Gao, L., Tao, Y., Zhang, L. & Jin, Q. (2010). Vitamin D receptor genetic polymorphisms and tuberculosis: updated systematic review and meta-analysis. The Int. J. Tuberc. and Lung Dis, 14, 15-23.

Garred, P., Harboe, M., Oettinger, T. & et al. (1994). Dual role of mannan binding protein in infections: another case of heterosis? *Eur. J.Immunogenet*, 21, 125–131.

Gordon, S. (2002). Pattern recognition receptors doubling up for the innate immune response. *Cell*, 111, 927–930.

Guwatudde, D., Zalwango, S., Kamya, M.R., Debanne, S.M., Diaz, M.I. & et al. (2003). Burden of tuberculosis in Kampala, Uganda. Bull. *World Health Organ*, 81, 799–805.

Hachicha, M., Pouliot, M., Petasis, N.A. & Serhan, C.N. (1999). Lipoxin (LX) A4, and aspirin-triggered 15-epi-LXA4 inhibit tumor necrosis factor 1 alpha-initiated neutrophil responses and trafficking: regulators of a cytokine-chemokine axis. *J. Exp. Med*, 189, 1923–1930.

Haehnel, V., Schwarzfischer, L., Fenton, M.J. & Rehli, M. (2002). Transcriptional regulation of the human toll-like receptor 2 gene in monocytes and macrophages. J. Immunol, 168, 5629-5637.

Hanna, S. & James, M. M. (2001). Molecular Diagnosis of Mycobacteria. *Clinical Chem*, 47, 809–814.

Hirai, M., Suzuki, S., Hinokio, Y., Hirai, A., Chiba, M., Akai, H., Suzuki, C. & Toyota, T. (2000). Variations in vitamin D-binding protein (group-specific component protein) are associated with fasting plasma insulin levels in Japanese with normal glucose tolerance. *J. Clin. Endocrinol. Metab*, 85, 1951-1953.

Hoal-Van Helden, E.G., Epstein, J., Victor, T.C. & et al. (1999). Mannose binding protein B allele confers protection against tuberculosis meningitis. *Pediatr. Res*, 45, 459–464.

Hobbs, M.R., Udhayakumar, V., Levesque, M.C., Booth, J., Roberts, J.M. & Tkachuk, A.N. (2002). A new NOS2 promoter polymorphism associated with increased nitric oxide production and protection from severe malaria in Tanzanian and Kenyan children. *Lancet*, 360, 1468-1475.

Ildefonso, P., Manuel, L., Miguel, G., Yolanda, P.M., Maria, E.S. & Sarabia, N.S. (2010). The TLR4 ASP299GLY Polymorphism is a Risk Factor for Active Tuberculosis in Caucasian HIV-Infected Patients. *Cur. HIV Res*, 8, 253-258.

Jamieson, S., Miller, E., Black, G., Peacock, C., Cordell, H. & et al. (2004). Evidence for a cluster of genes on chromosome 17q11-q21 controlling susceptibility to tuberculosis and leprosy in Brazilians. Genes and Immunity, 5, 46–57.

Kwoh, D.Y., Davis, G.R., Whitefield, K.M., Chapelle, H.L., DiMichele, L.J., Gingeras, T.R. (1989). Transcription-based amplification system and detection of amplified human immunodeficiency virus type 1 with a bead-based sandwich hybridization format. *Proc. Natl. Acad. Sci. U S A*, 86,1173–1177.

Krishnamurthy, M.S. (2001). Problems in estimating the burden of pulmonary tuberculosis in India: a review C.N. Paramasivan & P. Venkataraman (2003). Drug resistance in tuberculosis in India pp 377-386

Kun, J.F., Mordmuller, B., Lell, B., Lehman, L.G., Luckner, D. & Kremsner, P.G. (1998). Polymorphism in promoter region of inducible nitric oxide synthase gene and protection against malaria. *Lanc*, 351, 265-266.

Lamsyah, H., Rueda, B., Baassi, L., Elaouad, R., Bottini, N., Sadki, K. & Martin, J. (2009). Association of PTPN22 gene functional variants with development of pulmonary tuberculosis in Moroccan population. *Tissue Antigens*, 74, 228-232.

Lauridsen, A.L., Vestergaard, P., Hermann, A.P., et al. (2005). Plasma concentrations of 25-hydroxy-vitamin D and 1,25-dihydroxy-vitamin D are related to the phenotype of Gc (vitamin D-binding protein): a cross-sectional study on 595 early postmenopausal women. *Calcif. Tissue Int*, 77, 15-22.

Lienhardt, C., Bennett, S., Del Prete, G., et al. (2002). Investigation of Environmental and Host-related Risk Factors for Tuberculosis in Africa. I. Methodological Aspects of a Combined Design. American Journal of Epidemiology, 155, 1066-1073.

Li, C.M., Campbell, S.J., Kumararatne, D.S., et al. (2002). Association of a polymorphism in the P2X7 gene with tuberculosis in a Gambian population. *J. Infect. Dis.* 186, 1458-1462.

Liu, P.T., Stenger, S., Li, H., et al. (2006). Toll-like receptor triggering of a vitamin D-mediated human antimicrobial response. Science, 311, 1770-1773.

Liu, W., Zhang, F., Xin, Z.T., et al. (2006). Sequence variations in the MBL gene and their relationship to pulmonary tuberculosis in the Chinese Han population. *Int. J. Tuberc. Lung Dis.* 10, 1098–1103.

Lopez-Maderuelo, D., Arnalich, F., Serantes, R., Gonzalez, A., Codoceo, R., Madero, R., Vazquez, J.J. & Montiel, C. (2003). Interferon gamma and interleukin-10 gene polymorphisms in pulmonary tuberculosis. Am. J. Respir. Crit. Care Med, 167, 970–975.

Luoni, G., Verra, F., Arca, B., et al. (2001). Antimalarial antibody levels and IL4 polymorphism in the Fulani of West Africa. *Genes Immun*, 2, 411–414.

Mancuso, P., Nana-Sinkam, P., Peters-Golden, M. (2001). Leukotriene B4 augments neutrophil phagocytosis of Klebsiella pneumoniae. *Infect. Immun*, 69, 2011–2016.

Martin, J., Calzada, J.E., Nieto, A. (1999). Inducible nitric oxide synthase (NOS2) gene polymorphism and parasitic diseases. Lanc, 353: 72.

Martin, M.P., Lederman, M.M., Hutcheson, H.B. & et al. (2004). Association of DC-SIGN promoter polymorphism with increased risk for parenteral, but not mucosal, acquisition of human immunodeficiency virus type 1 infection. *J. Virol*, 78,14053–14056.

Miller, E., Jamieson, S., Joberty, C., Fakiola, M., Hudson, D., et al. (2004). Genome wide scans for leprosy and tuberculosis susceptibility genes in Brazilians. *Genes Immun*, 5, 63–67.

Mohan, V.P., Scanga, C.A., Yu, K. et al. (2001). Effects of tumor necrosis factor alpha on host immune response in chronic persistent tuberculosis: possible role for limiting pathology. *Infect. Immun*, 69, 1847-1855.

Moller, M., Nebel, A., Valentonyte, R., van Helden, P.D., Schreiber, S., Hoal, E.G. (2009). Investigation of chromosome 17 candidate genes in susceptibility to TB in a South African population. *Tuberculosis*, 89,189-194.

Moller, M., Nebel, A., Kwiatkowski, R., Van Helden, P.D., Hoal, E.G. & Schreiber, S. (2007). Host susceptibility to tuberculosis: CARD15 polymorphisms in a South African population. *Human and Cellular Probes*, 21, 148-151.

Moller, M., Nebel, A., Van Helden, P.D., Schreiber, S. & Hoal, E.G. (2010). Analysis of eight genes modulating interferon gamma and human genetic susceptibility to tuberculosis: a case-control association study. *BMC Infect. Dis*, 10: 154.

Naslednikova, I.O., Urazova, O.I., Voronkova, O.V., et al. (2009). Allelic polymorphism of cytokine genes during pulmonary tuberculosis. *Bull. Exp. Biol. Med.* 148, 175–180.

Nedwin, G.E., Naylor, S.L., Sakaguchi, A.Y. et al. (1985). Human lymphotoxin and tumor necrosis factor genes: structure, homology and chromosomal localization. Nucleic Acids Res, 13, 6361-6373.

Nicholson, S., Bonecini-Almeida, M.G., Lapa de Silva, J.R., Nathan, C., Xie, Q.W. (1996). Mumford R Inducible nitric oxide synthase in pulmonary alveolar macrophages from patients with tuberculosis. J. Exp. Med, 183, 2293-2302.

Ogus, A.C., Yoldas, B., Ozdemir, T., et al. (2004). The Arg753Gln polymorphism of the human toll-like receptor 2 gene in tuberculosis disease. Eur. Respir. J, 23, 219-223.

Ottenhoff, T.H., Verreck, F.A., Lichtenauer-Kaligis, E.G., Hoeve, M.A., Sanal, O., van Dissel, J.T. (2002). Genetics, cytokines and human infectious disease: lessons from weakly pathogenic mycobacteria and salmonellae. Nat. Genet, 32, 97-105.

Parkinson, J.F. (2006). Lipoxin and synthetic lipoxin analogs: an overview of anti-inflammatory functions and new concepts in immunomodulation. Inflamm. Aller. Drug Tar. 5, 91–106.

Pesut, D.P. (2009). Marinkovic Lung cancer and pulmonary tuberculosis –a comparative population-genetic study. British J. Med. Genetics, 12/2, 45-52.

Pravica, V., Asderakis, A., Perrey, C., Hajeer, A., Sinnott, P.J. & Hutchinson, I.V. (1999). In vitro production of IFN-gamma correlates with CA repeat polymorphism in the human IFN-gamma gene. Eur. J. Immunogenet, 26, 1-3.

Preto, R. (2009). Genetic polymorphisms in vitamin D receptor, vitamin D-binding protein, Toll-like receptor 2, nitric oxide synthase 2, and interferon-γ genes and its association with susceptibility to tuberculosis. Braz. J. Med. Biol. Res, 42, 312-322.

Qidwai, T. & Jamal, F. (2010). Inducible Nitric Oxide Synthase (iNOS) Gene Polymorphism and Disease Prevalence. Scandinavian Journal of Immunology, 72, 375–387.

Raghavan, S., Selvaraj, P., Swaminathan, S., Alagarasu, K., Narendran, G. & Narayanan, P.R. (2009). Haplotype analysis of HLA-A, -B antigens and -DRB1 alleles in south Indian HIV-1-infected patients with and without pulmonary tuberculosis. Int. J. Immunog, 36, 129-133.

Raviglione, M., Snider, D. & Kochi, A. (1995). Global epidemiology of tuberculosis: Morbidity and mortality of a worldwide epidemic. JAMA, 273, 220– 226.

Ridruechai, C., Mahasirimongkol, S., Phromjai, J. & et al. (2010). Association analysis of susceptibility candidate region on chromosome 5q31 for tuberculosis Genes and Immunity, 11, 416-422.

Rosenwasser, LJ, Klemm DJ, Dresback JK, Inamura H, Mascali JJ, Klinnert M. & Borish L. (1995). Promoter polymorphisms in the chromosome 5 gene cluster in asthma and atopy. Clin. Exp. Allergy, 25, 74–78.

Rossouw, M., Nel, H.J., Cooke, G.S., Van Helden, P.D. & Hoal, E.G. (2003). Association between tuberculosis, and a polymorphic NFkappaB binding site in the interferon gamma gene. Lancet, 361,1871-1872.

Sadki, K,, Lamsyah, H., Rueda, B., Akil, E., Sadak, A., Martin, J., El Aouad, R. (2010). Analysis of MIF, FCGR2A and FCGR3A gene polymorphisms with susceptibility to pulmonary tuberculosis in Moroccan population. J. Gent. and Geno, 37, 257-264.

Sakuntabhai, A., Turbpaiboon, C., Casademont, I. & et al. (2005). A variant in the CD209 promoter is associated with severity of dengue disease. Nat. Genet, 37, 507–513.

Schurr, E. (2007). Is susceptibility to tuberculosis acquired or inherited? *J. Intern. Med,* 261,106-111.

Selvaraj, P., Alagarasu, K., Harishankar, M. & et al. (2008). Cytokine gene polymorphisms and cytokine levels in pulmonary tuberculosis. *Cytokine,* 43, 26–33.

Sharma, S., Ghosh, B., Sharma, S.K. (2008). Association of TNF polymorphisms with sarcoidosis, its prognosis and tumour necrosis factor (TNF)-alpha levels in Asian Indians. *Clin. Exp. Immunol,* 151, 251-259.

Sharma, S., Rathored, J., Ghosh, B. & et al. (2010). Genetic polymorphisms in *TNF* genes and tuberculosis in North Indians. BMC Infectious Diseases, 10,165.

Soilleux, E.J., Barten, R., Trowsdale, J. (2000). DC-SIGN; a related gene, DC-SIGNR; and CD23 form a cluster on 19p13. J. Immunol, 165, 2937–2942.

Tahara, T., Arisawa, T., Wang, F. & et al. (2007). Toll-like receptor 2 -196 to 174del polymorphism influences the susceptibility of Japanese people to gastric cancer. Cancer Sci, 98, 1790-1794.

Tailleux, L., Schwartz, O., Herrmann, J.L. & et al. (2003). DC-SIGN is the major Mycobacterium tuberculosis receptor on human dendritic cells. *J Exp Med,* 197, 121–127.

Tassaneetrithep, B., Burgess, T.H., Granelli-Piperno, A., & et al. (2003). DC-SIGN (CD209) mediates dengue virus infection of human dendritic cells. *J. Exp. Med.* 197, 823–829.

Thuong, N.T., Hawn, T.R., Thwaites, G.E. & et al. (2007). A polymorphism in human TLR2 is associated with increased susceptibility to tuberculous meningitis. *Genes Immun.* 8, 422-428.

Thye, T., Nejentsev, S., Intemann, C.D., et al. (2009). MCP-1 promoter variant -362C associated with protection from pulmonary tuberculosis in Ghana, West Africa. *Hum. Mol. Genet,* 18, 381-388.

Underhill, D.M., Ozinsky, A., Smith, K.D. & Aderem, A. (1999). Toll-like receptor-2 mediates mycobacteria-induced proinflammatory signaling in macrophages. Proc. Natl. Acad. Sci. USA, 96, 14459-14463.

Vannberg, F.O., Chapman, S.J., Khor, C.C. & et al. (2008). CD209 genetic polymorphism and tuberculosis disease. *PLoS One,* 3(1):e1388.

Van Kooyk, Y., Appelmelk, B. & Geijtenbeek, T.B. (2003). A fatal attraction: Mycobacterium tuberculosis and HIV-1 target DC-SIGN to escape immune surveillance. *Trends Mol. Med,* 9, 153–159.

Velez, D.R., Hulme, W.F., Myers, J.L., Weinberg, J.B., Levesque, M.C., Stryjewski, M.E., Abbate, E., Estevan, R., Patillo, S.G., Gilbert, J.R. *& et al. (2009).* NOS2A, TLR4, and IFNGR1 interactions influence pulmonary tuberculosis susceptibility in African-Americans. *Hum. Gene,* 126, 643-653.

Vidyarani, M., Selvaraj, P., Raghavan, S., Narayanan, P.R. (2009). Regulatory role of 1, 25-dihydroxyvitamin D3 and vitamin D receptor gene variants on intracellular granzyme A expression in pulmonary tuberculosis. *Exp. Mol. Pathol,* 86, 69–73.

Vidyarani, M., Selvaraj, P., Prabhu, A.S., Jawahar, M.S., Adhilakshmi, A.R., Narayanan, P.R. (2006). Interferon gamma (IFN-γ) & interleukin-4 (IL-4) gene variants & cytokine levels in pulmonary tuberculosis. Indian J. Med. Res, 124, 403–410.

White, P. & Cooke, N. (2000). The multifunctional properties and characteristics of vitamin D-binding protein. *Trends Endocrinol. Metab.* 11, 320-327.

World Health Organization. (2009). Global Tuberculosis Control – Surveillance, Planning, Financing. URL: http://www.who.int. Accessed in 15/11/2009.

W.H.O. Report 2007. Global tuberculosis control. Surveillance, planning and financing. World Health Organization, Geneva, Switzerland.

Yim, J.J., Lee, H.W., Lee, H.S., Kim, Y.W., Han, S.K., Shim, Y.S. & Holland, S.M. (2006). The association between microsatellite polymorphisms in intron II of the human toll-like receptor 2 gene and tuberculosis among Koreans. *Genes Immun,* 7, 150-155.

2

Human Immunodeficiency Virus, Hepatitis B and Hepatitis C Virus Infections Among Injecting and Non-Injecting Drug Users in Inner City Neighborhoods

Lu-Yu Hwang and Carolyn Z. Grimes
Center for Infectious Diseases,
Division of Epidemiology and Center For Infectious Diseases,
School of Public Health,
University of Texas Health Science Center at Houston,
Houston, Texas,
USA

1. Introduction

Substance abuse is a continuing problem in the United States (US), impacting the individual and their social networks, and impacting society, economically and through public health programs. According to the 2004 National Household Survey on Drug Abuse (NHSDA), there were 19.1 million illicit drug users in the US. Drug use is directly and indirectly related to three blood-borne diseases, HIV, HBV and HCV. Direct exposure occurs through needle sharing and sharing other paraphernalia used to prepare and inject drugs [1-5]. The probability of direct exposure to HIV varies in relation to the procurement, preparation, and injection practices of drug users [6-10]. Frequency of injection and duration of injection are major factors for acquisition of HBV or HCV infections [11-13]. IDU is the primary mode of transmission of HCV in the US [14].

Drug use indirectly contributes to HIV exposure by decreasing inhibitions to engage in high-risk sexual activities and/or increased inhibitory effects on achieving sexual satisfaction [8, 15]. The use of cocaine has been shown to affect biological and behavioral processes related to HIV infection [16-19]. Engaging in risky sexual behaviors associated with drug use remains a significant risk factor for the acquisition of HBV, also, by men having sex with men (MSM) or heterosexual transmission. This interrelationship between drug use and high-risk sexual behavior makes it crucial to understanding the drug user population in order to develop appropriate interventions [20].

Houston is the fourth largest city and has the eighth highest AIDS caseload in the US. The number of African American and Hispanic Houstonians diagnosed with AIDS are increasing. The reason for the change in focus of the epidemic in Houston, from MSM to persons of color, may be related to the use of crack cocaine [4, 5]. Smoking crack cocaine, which became widespread in many poor, African American neighborhoods in the mid-1980s, continues to dominate the inner city drug use scene, and crack smokers, in addition to injection drug users, are at elevated risk for HIV infection. HBV and HCV were endemic among injecting drug users, even before HIV was introduced into this population. Common risk factors for these blood-borne viral agents, such as multi-person use of injecting equipment and sexual behaviors, have resulted in a high prevalence of infection of all three viruses among drug users. However, a significant proportion does remain at risk, as our previous studies in Houston have shown [4, 5] and should be targeted for vaccine prevention.

The purpose of this study was to estimate the prevalence of HIV, HBV and HCV infections and associated socio-demographic, drug use and sexual risk factors in a sample of predominantly African American injecting and non-injecting drug users who were recruited for a HBV vaccination study in Houston, Texas.

2. Material and methods

2.1 Study population

A sample of 2,779 injecting and non-injecting drug users was recruited for a community-based HBV vaccine study from February 2004 to October 2007. Participants were recruited from targeted congregation sites such as copping areas, street corners, and crack houses from predominantly two inner city neighborhood communities of Houston, Texas, by using outreach and chain referral recruiting methods. Target neighborhoods were selected based on previous studies [4, 5]. Potential study participants were asked to go to the designated field site in the area where they were recruited. The eligibility criteria for the study were 1) ages 18 and over, 2) local residence, 3) self-report and confirmed urine drug screen, 4) competent and willing to sign an informed consent form for HIV, HBV, and HCV antibody testing. This study had Institutional Review Board (IRB) approval through the University of Texas Health Science Center Committee for the Protection of Human Subjects.

2.1 Data collection

Data collectors received extensive training in obtaining informed consent, keeping participant information confidential, and administering the questionnaire. The interview was conducted confidentially in a private office and was identified only by a unique study identification number. Socio-demographic measures such as age, gender, race/ethnicity, living arrangement, jail history of >24 hours; drug use history including lifetime injection drug use (IDU), times injected drugs in past 7 and 30 days, lifetime and number of times shared needles in past 30 days, duration of IDU, types and frequency of drugs used in past 48 hours, 7 and 30 days, and drug treatment history; sexual behaviors such as number of sexual partners in the past 30 days, sexual orientation, condom use, history of sexually transmitted diseases, and trading sex for money or drugs in the past 30 days; history of blood transfusion and occupational exposure to blood. All interviews were verbally administered and recorded electronically via computer administered personal interview (CAPI, QDS, Bethesda, Maryland).

After the interview was completed, drug use was confirmed via urine drug screen, using OnTrak TesTstik, (Varian Inc,. Palo Alto, CA) to test for the presence of cocaine, opiates, and/or methamphetamines. Participants with a positive drug screen were asked to provide 10 ml of peripheral venous blood. Participants received a gratuity of $10.

2.2 Laboratory methods

Specimens were screened for HIV 1/2 antibodies, hepatitis B surface antigen (HBsAg), and antibodies to HCV (anti-HCV) by Core Combo HIV-HBsAg-HCV (Core Diagnostics, United Kingdom). Verification of HIV occurred by enzyme immunoassay (EIA), anti-HIV, using Abbott PPC Commander system, third generation HIV antibody test (Abbott Laboratories, Chicago, IL) , to HCV (Anti-HCV), hepatitis B surface antigen (anti-HBs) and antibody to hepatitis B core antigen (anti-HBc), by the Abbott AxSYM system, using microparticle enzyme immunoassay (MEIA) (Abbott Laboratories, Chicago, IL).

Case definition for HIV infection was repeatedly reactive specimen by EIA. The detection of HBsAg or anti-HBc, with or without anti-HBs was the definition of HBV infection. HCV infection definition was based on the presence of antibody to HCV. We have 2,779 observations for the HIV analysis, 1,712 for HBV analysis and 1,867 for HCV analysis at the time of manuscript preparation.

2.3 Statistics

Data from the questionnaire was imported into SAS 9.1 (Cary, NC) and laboratory results were entered into a Microsoft Access database. Data analysis was performed using STATA 9.0 (College Station, TX) software. Prevalence of HIV, HBV and HCV infections were estimated for the overall population and stratified by injecting status. Univariate and multivariable logistic analyses were performed. Any variable demonstrating a p-value of 0.2 or less or was biologically plausible was carried forward from univariate to multivariable analyses. Variables in the multivariable analyses that had a p-value of 0.05 or less were retained as the final model. Asian and other race were combined with Hispanic race because of small numbers. Variables with more than 10% missing responses from participants were not considered reliable enough to be examined.

3. Results

3.1 Demographic characteristics of the participants

Out of the 2,779, 85% of participants were African American, 11% White, and 4% Hispanic or other race with the majority (76%) being male. The median age was 43 and ranged from 18 to 76 years. About 3% reported having received a transfusion and the majority (78%) had a history of being in jail > 24 hours. Twelve percent were currently living in a shelter, and 62% had a history of being in a drug treatment program.

Almost 98% of the study participants had smoked crack in the past 7 days, 5% used methamphetamines and 5% were heroin users. About one-third (32%) had a history of injection drug use and 13% had a history of sharing needles. Almost half (43%) reported less than 50% condom use in the past 30 days. Nearly two-thirds (68%) reported a history of STD, with syphilis (42%) and gonorrhea (50%) being the two most prevalent. About one-fifth (19%) of the study population included MSM, more than one-third had traded sex for money/drugs in the past 30 days, and 23% reported having >3 male sexual partners and 40% had >3 female sexual partners in past 30 days.

3.2 Prevalence and risk factors associated with HIV infection

The prevalence of HIV infection in this population was 8.7%. Variables that had a significant association with being HIV infected in the univariate analysis were gender, shelter status, sexual orientation, condom use, MSM, trading sex for money or drugs in the past 30 days, and number of sex partners in the past 30 days (Tables 1 and 2). The drug-related variables explored in this analysis did not demonstrate any significant associations. After adjustment, HIV positive participants were more likely to be African American {OR= 2.8 (95% CI 1.6, 4.9)}, Hispanic and other race {OR= 2.5 (95% CI 1.1, 5.7)}, men having sex with men {OR= 2.5 (95% CI 1.7, 3.5)}, consistent condom users {OR= 2.9 (95% CI 2.0, 4.2)}, and be a male or female that had more than three male partners in the past 30 days {OR= 1.6 (95% CI 1.0, 2.4)} (Table 3). Study participants that lived in a shelter {OR= 0.5 (95% CI 0.3, 0.9)} or a male or female participant that had more than three female partners in the past 30 days {OR= 0.4 (95% CI 0.2, 0.5)} were less likely to be HIV positive (Table 3).

Variables	Total Number (%)	HIV Positive (%)	HBV Positive (%)	HCV Positive (%)
Total	2779 (100%)	8.7%	44.8%	36.1%
Gender				
Male	2111 (76%)	7.8%*	43.7% △	37.5%*
Female	668 (24%)	11.7%	48.8%	30.8%
Age (years)				
≤29	341 (12%)	7.7%	22.5%*	10.3%*
30-39	682 (25%)	10.7%	34.4%	20.7%
40-49	1177 (42%)	9.1%	50.1%	44.2%
>=50	579 (21%)	6.4%	57.5%	54.6%
Race/ethnicity				
Caucasian	302 (11%)	6.0%	37.9%*	53.4%*
Blacks	2354 (85%)	9.0%	46.3%	32.9%
Others	123 (4%)	10.6%	32.9%	55.7%
Currently living in a shelter				
No	2458 (88%)	9.2%*	45.0%	35.6%
Yes	321 (12%)	4.7%	43.3%	39.5%
Ever in drug treatment				
No	1070 (38%)	9.3%	43.3%	30.1%*
Yes	1709 (62%)	8.3%	45.7%	39.7%
Ever received a transfusion				
No	2692 (97%)	8.7%	43.8%*	34.1*
Yes	87 (3%)	8.0%	53.1%	54.0
Ever in Jail >24 hours				
No	613 (22%)	9.5%	41.3%	27.5%*
Yes	2166 (78%)	8.5%	45.6%	38.3%

*P value <0.05

Table 1. Prevalence of HIV, HBV and HCV infections among demographic characteristics in drug users, Houston, Texas.

Variables	Total	HIV positive N(%)	HBV positive N(%)	HCV positive N(%)
Drugs use in past 7 days				
No	16 (1%)	0%	46.2%	23.1%
Yes	2763 (99%)	8.8%	45.0%	36.2%
Marijuana				
No	1289 (46%)	8.5%	45.8%	38.3%
Yes	1490 (54%)	8.9%	43.8%	34.2%
Methamphetamines				
No	2632 (95%)	8.9%	45.1%	35.5%*
Yes	147 (5%)	6.1%	39.0%	47.2%
Cocaine				
No	62 (2%)	11.3%	48.0%	48.2%
Yes	2717 (98%)	8.6%	44.7%	36.0%
Heroin				
No	2636 (95%)	8.8%	43.9%*	34.8%*
Yes	143 (5%)	7.0%	59.8%	61.6%
Ever injected drugs				
No	1829 (66%)	8.6%	36.6%*	17.9%*
Yes	950 (34%)	8.8%	59.6%	70.0%
Duration of Injecting				
≤5 years	2218 (80%)	8.5%	36.0%*	26.5%*
>5 years	561 (20%)	9.4%	63.9%	78.3%
Ever shared needle/work				
No	2407 (87%)	8.7%	43.0%*	30.2%*
Yes	369 (13%)	8.4%	55.1%	72.1%
History of STD				
No	875 (32%)	7.9%	37.0%*	30.1%*
Yes	1904 (68%)	9.1%	48.9%	39.3%
History of Syphilis				
No	1597(58%)	8.5%	41.4%	34.5%*
Yes	1182(42%)	9.1%	51.1%	39.3%
What % of use a condom:				
Never	1095 (41%)	5.7%*	40.9%	35.5%
Sometimes	1137 (43%)	9.2%	40.5%	36.5%
Always	445 (16%)	14.2%	40.3%	33.1%
Sexuality				
Homosexual	112 (4%)	32.1%*	50.0%	32.0%*
Heterosexual	2137 (77%)	7.1%	44.7%	34.7%
Bisexual	530 (19%)	10.2%	44.2%	42.1%
Men had sex with men				
No	2248 (81%)	7.3%*	45.4%	36.1%
Yes	531 (19%)	14.7%	44.7%	36.2%

Variables	Total	HIV positive N(%)	HBV positive N(%)	HCV positive N(%)
Traded sex for money/drugs past 30 days				
No	1832 (66%)	7.3%*	45.1%	36.1%
Yes	947 (34%)	11.4%	44.0%	36.2%
Number of male sex partners in the past 30 days				
0	1732 (63%)	6.0%*	43.9%	37.3%
1-2	401 (14%)	10.2%	45.9%	33.2%
>=3	630 (23%)	15.2%	47.4%	34.4%
Number of female sex partners in the past 30 days				
0	919 (33%)	14.0%*	50.0%*	37.0%
1-2	759 (27%)	6.9%	41.6%	37.7%
>=3	1091 (40%)	5.5%	43.5%	33.9%

*P value <0.05

Table 2. Prevalence of HIV, HBV and HCV Infections by Drug Use and Sexual Behavior Variables in Past 30 Days among Drug Users in DASH Project.

Risk Factors	HIV OR (95% CI)	HBV OR (95% CI)	HCV OR (95% CI)
Race/Ethnicity			
White	1.00		
African American	2.8 (1.6-4.9) *	1.7 (1.2-2.4)*	0.4(0.3-0.6)*
Other	2.5 (1.1-5.7) *	0.9(0.5-1.6)	1.5(0.8-2.8)*
Age (per year)	1.00 (0.98-1.02)	1.05 (1.04-1.06)*	1.10(1.08-1.12)*
Injecting Drug use			
Yes	1.11 (0.8-1.5)	2.7 (2.27-3.5)*	9.4 (7.4-12.1)*
Shelter			
Yes	0.5(0.3-0.9)*	-----	------
History of blood transfusions			
Yes	------	------	1.6 (1.1-2.3)*
Condom use			
Always	2.9 (2.0-4.2) *	------	------
Sometimes	1.5(1.1-2.2)*		
History of syphilis diagnosis			
Yes	------	1.30(1.05-1.61)*	------
Men had sex with men			
Yes	2.5 (1.7-3.5) *	------	------
No. of male sex partners last 30 days			

Risk Factors	HIV	HBV	HCV
	OR (95% CI)	OR (95% CI)	OR (95% CI)
>3	1.6 (1.0-2.4)*	------	------
No. of female sex partners last 30 days			
>3	0.4(0.2-0.5)*	0.6(0.5-0.8)*	------
1-2	0.5(0.4-0.8)*		

*P value <0.05

Table 3. Multivariable Analyses of Risk Factors for HIV, HBV, HCV Infections Among Drug Users, Houston, TX.

To determine if associations differed between females and males and IDUs and non-IDUs, stratification by gender and injecting status were explored. The male study population analysis did not differ from the results from the total study population above (data not shown). Among the 668 female participants, African American race {OR 3.64 (95% CI 1.07-12.36)} and always using condoms in the past 30 days {OR 2.18, (95% CI, 1.10-4.33)} were found to be independently associated with HIV infection. Among non-injectors and injectors, the results from the multivariable analyses were fairly consistent with what was found in the total study population (Table 5).

Stratification also occurred by MSM status (Table 5) to determine if MSM status masked IDU as a risk factor for HIV. IDU status was not a significant risk factor for HIV in either the non-MSM or MSM analyses (Table 5).

3.3 Prevalence and risk factors associated with Hepatitis B virus infection

The prevalence of HBV in this study was 44.8%. Seropositivity for HBsAg (carrier) was 2.0% and for anti-HBc (previous or current infection), 38.5%. Of those with HBV infection, 412 (53.7%) out of 766 were co-infected with HCV. In Table 1 and 2, significant differences were observed between HBV positive and negative participants in variables representing gender, age, race, transfusion history, use of heroin in the past 30 days, number of sex partners in the past 30 days, history of STD, history of injection drug use, and history of sharing needles or works. After adjustment in the multivariable analysis, African American race {OR= 1.7 (95% CI 1.2, 2.4)}, increasing age per year {OR= 1.05 (95% CI 1.04, 1.06)}, history of injection drug use {OR= 2.7 (95% CI 2.3, 3.5)}, and having a history of being diagnosed with syphilis {OR= 1.3 (95% CI 1.05, 1.61)} remained independently associated with HBV infection, while having more than 3 female partners in 30 days, whether male or female, was inversely related to HBV infection {OR= 0.6 (95% CI 0.5, 0.8)} (Table 3).

To determine if non-IDUs shared the same risk characteristics as IDUs for HBV infection, stratification by injection status occurred. After adjusting for confounders in the multivariable analysis, two risk factors for HBV infection remained significant among non-injectors, increasing age and history of STD, while females or males with more than three female partners were less likely to have HBV infection (Table 4). Injectors that had increasing age, of African American race, female and had injected drugs for more than 5 years were all at risk for HBV infection after adjustment (Table 4).

Risk Factors	HBV		HCV	
	NIDU OR (95%CI)	IDU OR (95%CI)	NIDU OR (95%CI)	IDU OR (95%CI)
Gender				
Male	1.0(0.7-1.4)	1.8(1.1-2.9)*	0.9(0.6-1.3)	1.5(0.9-2.5)
Race/Ethnicity				
White				
African American	1.1(0.6-2.1)	1.7(1.1-2.9)*	0.5(0.2-097)*	0.4(0.2-0.7)*
Others	0.4(0.1-1.4)	1.0(0.5-2.2)	1.5(0.5-4.5)	1.3(0.5-3.0)
Age (per year)	1.03(1.01-1.04)*	1.09(1.07-1.12)*	1.09(1.07-1.12)*	1.10(1.07-1.13)*
Transfusion History				
Yes	-----	-----	1.8(1.1-2.93)	-----
History in jail >24 hours				
Yes	-----	-----	2.5 (1.5-4.1)*	-----
Duration of IDU >6 years	-----	2.1(1.4-3.1)*	2.0(1.4-3.0)*	-----
Men sex with men				
Yes	-----		-----	-----
History of STDs				
Yes	1.5(1.1-1.9)*		-----	-----
Number male sex partners >3 partners	-----		-----	-----
Number female sex partners >3 partners	0.6(0.4-0.9)*		-----	-----

*P value <0.05

Table 4. Multivariable Analyses of Risk Factors for HIV Infection Stratified by Injecting Status Among Drug Users, Houston, Texas.

Risk Factors	HIV		HIV	
	NIDU OR (95%CI)	IDU OR (95%CI)	Not MSM OR (95%CI)	MSM OR (95%CI)
Gender				
Male			0.52(0.07-3.84)	-----
Race/Ethnicity				
White	1.00		1.00	1.00
African American	1.9(0.8-4.4)	2.5(1.1-5.5)*	4.93(1.53-15.87)*	2.27(1.04-4.93)*
Others	1.2(0.3-5.0)	3.1(1.2-8.3)*	5.97(1.42-25.07)*	1.71(0.54-5.35)
Age (per year)	1.0(0.98-1.02)	1.0(0.97-1.03)	1.00(0.98-1.02)	1.01(0.98-1.04)
Shelter				
Yes	0.3(0.1-0.9)*		-----	0.39 (0.15-1.00)*
Ever IDU				
Yes	-----		-----	0.61(0.34-1.10)
Men sex with men				
Yes	2.5(1.6-3.9)*	1.8(1.0-3.3)*	-----	-----
History of Chlamydia				
Yes	-----		-----	0.11(0.03-0.38)*
History of genital warts				
Yes	-----		-----	3.28(1.00-10.77)*
Condom				
Never			1.00	1.00
Always	2.1(1.3-3.4)*	5.6(2.8-11.4)*	2.85 (1.81-4.48)*	3.51(1.56-7.88)*
Sometimes		2.7(1.4-5.1)*	1.45(0.95-2.21)*	2.14(1.12-4.09)*
Number male sex partners				
0			1.00	
1-3 partners			4.38(0.58-33.32)	
>3 partners	2.6(1.5-4.5)*		6.92(0.92-52.12)	
Number female sex partners				
0				1.00
1-3 partners				0.26(0.13-0.53)*
>3 partners	0.4(0.3-0.7)*	0.4(0.2-0.7)*		0.16(0.08-0.31)*

IDU stratification adjusted for history in jail for >24 hours, duration of IDU, history of STDs

MSM stratification adjusted for alcohol use, methamphetamine, cocaine use in the past 30 days, crack use in the past 48 hours, duration of IDU, trading for sex/money past 30 days, history of syphilis or genital herpes

*p value<0.05

Table 5. Multivariable Analyses of Risk Factors for HIV Infection Stratified by Injecting Status and MSM Status Among Drug Users, Houston, Texas.

3.4 Prevalence and risk factors associated with Hepatitis C virus infection

The prevalence of HCV infection in this population was 36.1%. Of 668 participants infected with HCV, 61.7% were coinfected with HBV. In Tables 1 and 2, gender, age, race, history of drug treatment, history of transfusion, history of being in jail for >24 hours, sexuality, methamphetamine use, heroin use, history of injecting drugs, history of sharing needles or works, sexuality, history of STD, and history of diagnosis or treatment for syphilis all showed significant differences between HCV positive and negative participants univariately. After adjustment in the multivariable analysis, increasing age {OR= 1.10 (95% CI 1.08, 1.12)}, history of injection drug use {OR= 9.4 (95% CI 7.4, 12.1)}, and having a history of a transfusion {OR= 1.6 (95% CI 1.1, 2.3)}were all still independently associated with HCV infection, while African American race was inversely related to HCV infection {OR= 0.4 (95% CI 0.3, 0.6)} (Table 3).

Because of the striking difference between injectors (70%) and non-injectors (17.9%) in HCV positive study participants, and the overwhelming magnitude of association between injection drug use status and HCV positivity, stratification by injection status was performed to uncover risk characteristics of non-IDUs that may have been masked. In the multivariable analysis, increasing age and having a history of transfusion were found to be independently associated with HCV infection among non-IDUs. African American race was inversely related with HCV infection (Table 4). The significant variables associated with HCV infection among injectors after adjustment were increasing age, having been in jail for more than 24 hours, and injecting drugs for more than 5 years, while African American race remained inversely associated with HCV infection (Table 4).

4. Discussion

This is the first study to evaluate both IDUs and non-IDUs for HIV, HBV and HCV infections in not-in-treatment urban community settings. In this study, prevalence of HIV, HBV, and HCV was 9%, 45% and 36% respectively. The predominant risk characteristics associated with HIV infection in drug users are sexual behaviors, especially MSM, while the predominant risk characteristic associated with HBV and HCV infections is injection drug use. African American race among IDUs is positively associated with HIV and HBV infections and inversely associated with HCV infection. Increasing age is significantly associated with HBV and HCV infections, but not with HIV infection. Duration of injection drug use is also significantly associated with HBV and HCV infections.

Sexual behaviors are the most prevalent risk factors associated with HIV in this study of primarily African American crack cocaine users, which we have found in our previous studies [4, 5]. Any altering substance, such as crack cocaine and methamphetamines, can influence a person to engage in higher frequencies of risky sexual acts, which increases the total number of exposure events, resulting in a higher likelihood of being infected with HIV [17, 21-23]. Crack cocaine is the drug of choice in this study, as 98% of the participants used this drug, with very few using other drugs, such as methamphetamines. Several studies have shown that crack cocaine users engage in more unprotected sexual acts, trade sex for money or drugs and have more sexually transmitted diseases, all factors contributing to greater risk for HIV infection [17, 21, 23-26]. One third of the study participants had a history of injection drug use, but no associations were identified between IDU and HIV infection in males or females in this study, a conflicting finding from other studies [27-31]. Therefore, crack cocaine use and resulting sexual behaviors from its use infer the most likely way HIV is transmitted amongst drug users in this population.

Study participants that had more than 3 male partners were more likely to have HIV than study participants with less male partners in the past 30 days, emphasizing the point of higher frequencies of sexual acts increases exposure. This result remains significant for non-IDU HIV infected study participants and non-MSM female study participants. Non-IDU and IDU HIV infected MSMs show greater likelihood of infection, adding credence to this finding. Two variables to help explain these risky sexual acts, condom use and trading sex for money or drugs, failed to show a significant association in this study, after adjustment for other variables. Men traded sex for money or drugs more often than women in this study, but neither group showed a significant association. However, 40% of the men that traded sex had at least one male sexual partner in their lifetime, clouding the association between HIV infection and trading sex due to the collinearity of "trading sex" and "MSM" variables. Frequency of partners may have also been collinear with trading sex, and they really point to the same issue, whether being male or female, heterosexual or homosexual, the more partners and unprotected acts one has, the increase in likelihood for exposure to HIV. Of note, the measurement tool captured sexual activity in the past 30 days, not lifetime risk, and prevalent data does not necessarily reflect the risk profile of the study participant at the time of HIV acquisition. This is the case with condom use. Study participants were more likely to be HIV infected and always use a condom.

The majority of study participants in this study are African American. It is important to note that studies on African American male sexual behaviors show incongruity between reported sexual identity and actual behavior, greater in African American MSM, but other races as well [32]. Williams et al. [33] conducted qualitative analyses of HIV positive gay identifying and non-gay identifying African Americans, and revealed consequences of alienation, low self-esteem, unsupportive networks, a need to protect their HIV status, and inconsistent condom use after acknowledgement of the importance of condom use due to race and sexual orientation status. The higher prevalence of HIV in African American MSM and their higher level of bisexual activity can put African American women at risk, therefore identifying two high risk groups where sensitive interventions need to be developed and delivered in supportive surroundings. Our study also alludes to the importance of African American MSM and their risk for HIV infection. In the MSM stratification analysis, minority races were significantly more at risk for HIV infection versus Caucasians. Most of our MSM were African American, 69%, followed by Caucasian, 24%, further heightening the urgency to reach this very high risk group. In this group of drug users, having a male partner, whether bisexual or homosexual, is an overwhelming risk factor for HIV infection, and may be interrelated with injection drug use. IDU does not show to be a significant risk factor in this study for HIV infection, however, the correlation between MSM status and IDU status may be masking the true association. It is logical to assume that an MSM-IDU has the greatest risk for HIV infection.

While sexual practices were associated with HIV infection, injecting practices were significant factors associated with HBV or HCV infection in this same population. This study supports previous work that risky injection drug use practices result in the transmission of HBV or HCV [4, 7, 11, 13, 34-36], and the longer one injects, in regards to age and duration, in a high risk population, the more likely the person will be infected [11-13, 37, 38]. However, sharing needles was not associated with HBV or HCV in this study, contrasting a previous study by our principal investigator [4], and others [13]. This most likely reflects the strong correlation between history of injection drug use and sharing paraphernalia occurring in this study.

African American IDUs in this study were less likely to have HCV infection, but were more likely to have HBV infection, a conclusion supported by two other studies that did not stratify by injection drug use [4, 39]. One last finding associated with HCV infection among IDUs is history of being in jail for at least 24 hours or more. Possible explanations that were not explored in this study but were found in other studies are sharing needles in jail, and/or receiving a tattoo in jail, but all consistently found a high prevalence of HCV in the prison/jail systems, heightening the risk for HCV infection [13, 40, 41].

Non-injecting drug users with HBV infection were more likely to have reported a history of STD and be older, but less likely to have more than 3 female sex partners. Non-injectors with HCV infection were associated with transfusion history, increasing age, but less likely to be African American. The median age of the study participants in this study is 43, and documented to be participating in risky drug and sexual behaviors, plus vulnerable to infection, therefore, increasing age is an understandable risk. Sexual behavior in non-injecting drug users may be influenced by stimulant drug activity, especially crack cocaine [17, 21, 23-26], influencing the drug user to participate in risky sexual behaviors, resulting in increased risk for HIV, hepatitis B, and STDs. From our previous studies and others, there was no significant association found between HCV infection and sexual risk behaviors [4, 34]. Transfusion-associated HCV has been documented [42].

HIV, HBV, and HCV infections, drug use behaviors, and social network dynamics vary widely between populations, even at the neighborhood level. This analysis applies directly only to drug users in the urban neighborhoods in Houston, although generalizations about urban drug users may be used to guide further research in other communities. Every attempt to limit recall bias by limiting the reference period for recall of events and reporting bias through using discretion in interviewing and questions deemed appropriate throughout the pilot study was made, but some bias inevitably exists in the data. High-risk activity may have changed with time, either independent of or dependent on, one's HIV or HBV/HCV serostatus, masking true associations that were not covered by the timeframe in question or creating the appearance of spurious associations between HIV or HBV/HCV and current behaviors that had not been expressed at the time of infection.

Characterizing determinants of risk for HIV, HBV, or HCV infection among drug users will improve targeting of health services and prevention education. The greatest association between HIV and drug users in this study was sexual practices, while injecting drug use was the greatest factor associated with HBV and HCV infections. African American drug users are disproportionately affected by these three blood-borne diseases. The vaccine for HBV is being underutilized in high risk drug users, and outreach efforts to understand the barriers to accepting HBV vaccination need to be explored to prevent further HBV transmission. Studies targeting young drug users to prevent initiation into injecting or curb injecting soon after initiation combined with using social networks for counseling about prevention of these three diseases will impact and interrupt transmission cycles.

5. Acknowledgements

We would like to thank the efforts of our field data collection staff, Lawrence Duncan, Madelyn Randle, Janice Robinson, and Edward Johnson, as well as our Field Coordinators, Sandra Timpson, Jay Johnson and Janel Dennison. For supportive data analysis, we would like to thank Shenying Fang and Rui Xia. This study was funded by The National Institute of Drug Abuse (NIDA# 1R01DA017505).

6. References

[1] Shah S.M., Shapshak P., Rivers J. E., Stewart R. V., Weatherby N. L., Xin K. Q. *et al.* Detection of HIV-1 DNA in needles/syringes, paraphernalia, and washes from shooting galleries in Miami: a preliminary laboratory report. *J Acquir Immune Defic Syndr Hum Retrovirol* 1996; 11: 301-6.

[2] Bradshaw C. S., Pierce L. I., Tabrizi S. N., Fairley C. K., Garland S. M. Screening injecting drug users for sexually transmitted infections and blood borne viruses using street outreach and self collected sampling. *Sex Transm Infect* 2005; 81: 53-8.

[3] Mehta S. H., Galai N., Astemborski J., Celentano D. D., Strathdee S. A., Vlahov D. *et al.* HIV incidence among injection drug users in Baltimore, Maryland (1988-2004). *J Acquir Immune Defic Syndr* 2006; 43: 368-72.

[4] Hwang L. Y., Ross M. W., Zack C., Bull L., Rickman K., Holleman M. Prevalence of sexually transmitted infections and associated risk factors among populations of drug abusers. *Clin Infect Dis* 2000; 31: 920-26.

[5] Ross M. W., Hwang L. Y., Leonard L., Teng M., Duncan L. Sexual behaviour, STDs and drug use in a crack house population. *Int J STD AIDS* 1999; 10: 224-30.

[6] Gold R., Skinner M., Ross M. Unprotected anal intercourse in HIV-infected and non-HIV-infected gay men. *J Sex Res* 1994; 31: 59-77.

[7] Koester S., Hoffer L. "Indirect Sharing:" Additional HIV risks associated with drug injection. *AIDS Public Policy J* 1994; 9: 100-05.

[8] McCoy C., Inciardi J. *Sex, Drugs, and Continuing Spread of AIDS.* Los Angeles: Roxbury Publishing Company, 1995.

[9] Kippax S., Campbell D., Van de Ven P., Crawford J., Prestage G., Knox S. *et al.* Cultures of sexual adventurism as markers of HIV seroconversion: A case control study in a cohort of Sydney gay men. *AIDS Care* 1998; 10: 677-88.

[10] Clatts M. C., Heimer R., Abdala N., Goldsamt L. A., Sotheran J. L., Anderson K. T. *et al.* HIV-1 transmission in injection paraphernalia: heating drug solutions may inactivate HIV-1. *J Acquir Immune Defic Syndr* 1999; 22: 194-99.

[11] Gyarmathy V. A., Neaigus A., Miller M., Friedman S. R., Des Jarlais D. C. Risk correlates of prevalent HIV, hepatitis B virus, and hepatitis C virus infections among noninjecting heroin users. *J Acquir Immune Defic Syndr* 2002; 30: 448-56.

[12] Garten R. J., Lai S., Zhang J., Liu W., Chen J., Vlahov D. *et al.* Rapid transmission of hepatitis C virus among young injecting heroin users in Southern China. *Int J Epidemiol* 2004; 33: 182-88.

[13] Samuel M. C., Doherty P. M., Bulterys M., Jenison S. A. Association between heroin use, needle sharing and tattoos received in prison with hepatitis B and C positivity among street-recruited injecting drug users in New Mexico, USA. *Epidemiol Infect* 2001; 127: 475-84.

[14] Daniels D., Grytdal S., Wasley A. Surveillance for acute viral hepatitis-United States, 2007. *MMWR Surveill Summ* 2009; 58: 1-27.

[15] Gordon C.M., Carey M., Carey K.B. Effects of a drinking event on behavioral skills and condom attitudes in men: implications for HIV risk from a controlled experiment. *Health Psychol* 1997; 16: 490-95.

[16] Booth R.E., Watters J. How effective are risk-reduction interventions targeting injecting drug users? *AIDS* 1994; 8: 1515-24.

[17] Edlin B. R., Irwin K. L., Faruque S., McCoy C. B., Word C., Serrano Y. *et al.* Intersecting Epidemics--Crack Cocaine Use and HIV Infection among Inner-City Young Adults. *N Engl J Med* 1994; 331: 1422-27.

[18] Wilson T., DeHovitz J. A. STDs, HIV, and crack cocaine: a review. *AIDS Patient Care STDS* 1997; 11: 62-6.

[19] Petry N. M. Alcohol use in HIV patients: What we don't know may hurt us. *Int J STD AIDS* 1999; 10: 561-70.

[20] Siegal H. A., Falck R. S., Wang J., Carlson R. G. History of sexually transmitted diseases infection, drug-sex behaviors, and the use of condoms among midwestern users of injection drugs and crack cocaine. *Sex Transm Dis* 1996; 23: 277-82.

[21] Jones D. L., Irwin K. L., Inciardi J., Bowser B., Schilling R., Word C. *et al.* The High-Risk Sexual Practices of Crack-Smoking Sex Workers Recruited From the Streets of Three American Cities. *Sex Transm Dis* 1998; 25: 187-93.

[22] Campsmith M. L., Nakashima A. K., Jones J. L. Association between crack cocaine use and high-risk sexual behaviors after HIV diagnosis. *J Acquir Immune Defic Syndr* 2000; 25: 192-98.

[23] Booth R. E., Watters J. K., Chitwood D. D. HIV Risk-Related Sex Behaviors among Injection Drug Users, Crack Smokers, and Injection Drug Users Who Smoke Crack. *Am J Public Health* 1993; 83: 1144-48.

[24. McCoy C. B., Lai S., Metsch L. R., Messiah S. E., Zhao W. Injection Drug Use and Crack Cocaine Smoking: Independent and Dual Risk Behaviors for HIV Infection. *Ann Epidemiol* 2004; 14: 535-42.

[25] Kral A. H., Bluthenthal R. N., Booth R. E., Watters J. K. HIV Seroprevalence among Street-Recruited Injection Drug and Crack Cocaine Users in 16 US Municipalities. *Am J Public Health* 1998; 88: 108-12.

[26] Hudgins R., McCusker J., Stoddard A. Cocaine use and risky injection and sexual behaviors. *Drug Alcohol Depend* 1995; 37: 7-14.

[27] Nguyen T. A., Hoang L. T., Pham V. Q., Detels R. Risk factors for HIV-1 seropositivity in drug users under 30 years old in Haiphong, Vietnam. *Addiction* 2001; 96: 405-13.

[28] Kozlov A. P., Shaboltas A. V., Toussova O. V., Verevochkin S. V., Masse B. R., Perdue T. et al. HIV incidence and factors associated with HIV acquisition among injection drug users in St Petersburg, Russia. *AIDS* 2006; 20: 901-6.

[29] Ruan Y., Qin G., Liu S., Qian H., Zhang L., Zhou F. et al. HIV incidence and factors contributed to retention in a 12-month follow-up study of injection drug users in Sichuan Province, China. *J Acquir Immune Defic Syndr* 2005; 39: 459-63.

[30] Kawichai S., Celentano D. D., Vongchak T., Beyrer C., Suriyanon V., Razak M. H. et al. HIV voluntary counseling and testing and HIV incidence in male injecting drug users in northern Thailand: evidence of an urgent need for HIV prevention. *J Acquir Immune Defic Syndr* 2006; 41: 186-93.

[31] Barrio G., De La Fuente L., Toro C., Brugal T. M., Soriano V., Gonzalez F. et al. Prevalence of HIV infection among young adult injecting and non-injecting heroin users in Spain in the era of harm reduction programmes: gender differences and other related factors. *Epidemiol Infect* 2007; 135: 592-603.

[32] Millett G., Malebranche D., Mason B., Spikes P. Focusing "down low": bisexual black men, HIV risk and heterosexual transmission. *J Natl Med Assoc* 2005; 97(7Suppl): 52S-59S.

[33] Williams J. K., Wyatt G. E., Resell J., Peterson J., Asuan-O'Brien A. Psychosocial issues among gay- and non-gay-identifying HIV-seropositive African American and Latino MSM. *Cultur Divers Ethnic Minor Psychol* 2004; 10: 268-86.

[34] Hammer G. P., Kellogg T. A., McFarland W. C., Wong E., Louie B., Williams I. et al. Low incidence and prevalence of hepatitis C virus infection among sexually active non-intravenous drug-using adults, San Francisco, 1997-2000. *Sex Transm Dis* 2003; 30: 919-24.

[35] Bialek S. R., Bower W. A., Mottram K., Purchase D., Nakano T., Nainan O. et al. Risk factors for hepatitis B in an outbreak of hepatitis B and D among injection drug users. *J Urban Health* 2005; 82: 468-78.

[36] Hagan H., McGough J. P., Thiede H., Weiss N. S., Hopkins S., Alexander E. R. Syringe exchange and risk of infection with hepatitis B and C viruses. *Am J Epidemiol* 1999; 149: 203-13.

[37] Nyamathi A. M., Dixon E. L., Robbins W., Smith C., Wiley D., Leake B. et al. Risk factors for hepatitis C virus infection among homeless adults. *J Gen Intern Med* 2002; 17: 134-43.

[38] Garfein R. S., Vlahov D., Galai N., Doherty M. C., Nelson K. E. Viral infections in short-term injection drug users: the prevalence of the hepatitis C, hepatitis B, human immunodeficiency, and human T-lymphotropic viruses. *Am J Public Health* 1996; 86: 655-61.

[39] Butterfield M. I., Bosworth H. B., Stechuchak K. M., Frothingham R., Bastian L. A., Meador K. G. et al. Racial differences in hepatitis B and hepatitis C and associated risk behaviors in veterans with severe mental illness. *J Natl Med Assoc* 2004; 96: 43-52.

[40] Babudieri S., Longo B., Sarmati L., Starnini G., Dori L., Suligoi B. et al. Correlates of HIV, HBV, and HCV infections in a prison inmate population: results from a multicentre study in Italy. *J Med Virol* 2005; 76: 311-17.

[41] Hennessey K. A., Kim A. A., Griffin V., Collins N. T., Weinbaum C. M., Sabin K. Prevalence of infection with hepatitis B and C viruses and co-infection with HIV in three jails: a case for viral hepatitis prevention in jails in the United States. *J Urban Health* 2009; 86: 93-105.

[42] Armstrong G. L., Wasley A., Simard E. P., McQuillan G. M., Kuhnert W. L., Alter M. J. The prevalence of hepatitis C virus infection in the United States, 1999 through 2002. *Ann Intern Med* 2006; 144: 705-14.

3

Isolator System For Laboratory Infectious Animals

Xin Pan

Animal Biosafety Level 3 Laboratory,
Second Military Medical University, Shanghai,
China

1. Introduction

The international mutual acceptance of safety data in certification and accreditation system have led to high-level bio-safety laboratories becoming an irreplaceable hardware in peacetime for the study of pathogen in emerging and re-emerging infectious disease, and in important international activities for detection and identification high-risk pathogen in antiterrorism security.

In an effort to minimize the risks for scientists exposure to the infectious environment and avoiding infectious incident, high-level bio-safety laboratories are designed and constructed to improve experimental safety by preventing laboratory infectious waste causing harm to people or the environment. The possibility of high-risk pathogens spread to the public environment with flow of people and materials and water and air is strictly controlled by improvement physical protection to reduce human infection rates and incidence of environment contamination to zero. The air flow safety, including interior mechanical ventilations and the suction and exhaust process in large working process equipments, is ensured by installing air conditioning system, air filter system, one working and one on standby extraction blowers, constant or variable air volume damper in pipes, automation and monitoring system, and power supply system (including dual power supply system and online emergency power supply) to maintain suitable directional negative filtering air flow with constant temperature and humidity working conditions for the operators. The materials flow safety, including experimental materials, laboratory animals and laboratory infectious waste, is mastered by installing transfer system (including delivery window and double port transfer exchange system) and sterilization system (double-doored autoclave). The liquid flow safety, including launching and softened water, is controlled by reverse osmosis disinfection system and independent sewage discharge system (including high temperature and high pressure sterilizer and chemical disinfection tank). The people flow safety, including walking around in the laboratory, carrying out experimental procedures, changing protective clothing, and physiological activity such as respiration, is protected by primary barriers (including biological safety cabinet and negative-pressure isolator), secondary barriers (building envelope and facility construction), third barriers (personal protective equipment, PPE), communication systems between the lab and outside, visual monitoring devices and alarm system.

In high-level bio-safety laboratories, animals infected with Risk Group 3 pathogens (as defined by the World Health Organization) must be housed in isolation chambers (World Health Organization, 2004). Animal isolation system is used broadly in laboratory research, pharmaceuticals and medical areas, gene modified animals, and gnotobiotic animals. Isolators were developed for studying the disease of scrub typhus in 1940 during the Second World War (Bantin, 2004). Today, the isolators are much more advanced, especially the commercial rodent isolator systems (Wathes & Johnson, 1991). But for infectious medium-sized animal (sheep, pigs, goats, nonhuman primates, dogs, cats, rabbits and chickens) research, the market normally supplied semi-open negative pressure cabinet. This kind of cabinet can not provide completely physical barrier for safeguarding animal and occupational health and the odors and allergens environment, because the directly face-to-face manipulation exist between animal and operator in the research procedure. The Class III biological safety cabinet (glove box) was mainly used for experiment operation (Kruse et al., 1991), its internal work area was maintained negative pressure during running state, it was able to provide security, even in the physical prevent contamination system failure. The requirements for wind speed and pressure were relatively higher to maintain the glove box internal laminar flow, but were not conducive to animal care, the occupants had to suffer high stress and uncomfortable environment under the high velocity air flow. If the glove box was simply expanded to an isolator, large area filtration equipment was easy to plug, animal welfare was difficult to achieve in insufficient space (limited height) (Huang, 2005). Recently we developed a set of automatic multi-functional isolation system for feeding (Pan et al., 2010) and dissection and micrurgy laboratory animals carrying infectious diseases. The isolation system, including the transfer chain, disinfection chain, negative air pressure isolation system, animal welfare system and the automated system, are designed to meet all biological safety standards.

Isolator was mainly designed to separate the internal controlled environment from external environment, and the operator from the experimental process and products. The primary aim was to prevent the leakage of the contaminated products within the internal environment to the external environment, or the penetration of substances of the external environment into the internal environment, or both simultaneously (Tattershall, 2006). Isolators were used to improve operators and process safety, avoid operator wearing too many protective suits, improve operator comfort and flexibility and personnel availability, improve safety level against operator errors, completely control the contaminated material and minimize the contaminated area (Sawyer et al., 2007).

There are many types of isolators, mainly included positive pressure isolators and negative pressure isolators. Specified-pathogen-free (SPF) laboratory animals housed in positive pressure isolators for the protection of any animals inside the isolator from outside contaminants (Clough et al., 1995). Infectious animal housed in negative pressure isolators to prevent migration of hazardous contaminants to the outside (Wathes & Johnson, 1991).

In general, the commonly used physical separation mainly included rigid and soft barriers (ISO 14644-7:2004). Rigid barriers can be made of many different materials, and the more rigid the material, the more reliable the physical barrier. Construction of these rigid barriers usually makes of plastic enclosures, metal profile enclosures or hot-worked metal enclosures (ISO 10648-1:1997). The isolation chamber is designed to house a living animal, and therefore continuous airflow inside the enclosure is needed to drive out heat and moisture generated by the animal's metabolism and to decrease the concentration of odor, dust, and infectious substances (Hillman et al., 1992). The resulting exhaust gas is subject to a filtering system designed to prevent pathogen contamination of the external environment (Institute of Laboratory Animal Resources Commission on Life Sciences, National Research Council, 1996). The aerodynamic is joined in the physical separation cabinet to allow for one-way flow or turbulence of the airflow inside the isolation chamber, negative pressure relative to the environment. Supply and exhaust air can be passed through high-efficiency particulate air filters (HEPA) to prevent the formation of aerosols that could potentially escape into the environment (Runkle et al., 1969).

Double port transfer exchange (DPTE) system is used in the isolator to allow the transfer of experiment materials from one container to another without exposing the experiment material to the outside environment (Allen et al., 2009). The technology was developed in the early 1960s by a French company for the French nuclear industry to greatly reduce Alpha and Beta exposures and Gamma dose. The acronym DPTE was originally derived from the French phrase 'double porte de transfert etanche', meaning double door sealed transfer or double door transfer port. A newly validated rapid transfer port boasts bi-directional transfer as one of its features, a system also known as an Alpha-Beta transfer port or rapid transfer port (RTP) (Michael et al., 2004). The biological sciences involving dangerously toxic or infectious materials (such as poisons, bacteria or viruses) also need to use DPTE system as the transfer tool to enclose the dangerous materials without escaping into the surroundings.

Laboratory animal models are often susceptible to a number of diseases and parasites found in humans or economic animals (Tauraso et al., 1969). The similarities of genetic, physiological, and behavioral characteristics between research objects and laboratory animal models, and the occurrence of similar pathological changes upon infection, have led to laboratory animal models becoming an irreplaceable experimental materials for the study of pathogen infection, the screening of anti-pathogen drugs, and vaccine evaluation (Pan & Sun, 2004; Conly & Johnston, 2008). Because of the critical role that laboratory animal models play in the study of these pathogens, it is critical to find safe and reliable methods for their physical containment.

2. Isolator system composition and structure

The structure of stainless-steel medium-sized animal breeding isolator and acrylic mice breeding isolator and acrylic anatomy isolator and acrylic micrurgy isolator include top ventilation unit, isolator working zone, lower part of control system and isolator support frame (Fig. 1).

The isolation chamber is supported by type 304 stainless-steel isolation chamber support stand. The ventilation unit is on the top of the isolation chamber. Stainless-steel slideways are mounted on the top of the isolation chamber box. The pipes, air blower, valve, and adjustable illumination lamp are fastened to the reserved mounting holes or mounting plates of the slideways by a fixing screw.

Two extraction blowers share one exhaust port in which an anemometer is installed. Each of the extraction blowers is connected with its own coupling clamp to the outlet ventilation pipe, exhaust ventilation pipe and exhaust electronic control ball valve to form an exhaust channel. The two exhaust channels have a parallel connection. Two sets of sterilizing agent bypass tubes have a series connection with an ipsilateral sterilizing agent bypass electronic control ball valve, and a parallel connection with the same side of the exhaust ventilation pipe on two ends of the exhaust electronic control ball valve. All of the valves are automatically controlled by the programmable logic controller (PLC).

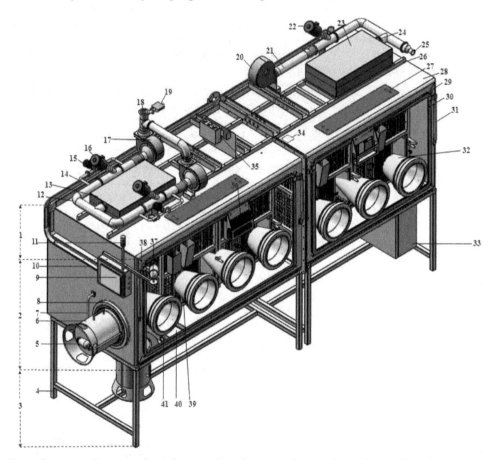

Fig. 1. Structure diagram of stainless-steel medium-sized animal breeding isolator. 1. top ventilation unit; 2. isolation chamber working zone; 3. lower part of the control system; 4. isolation chamber support stand; 5. transfer bin container HEPA filter; 6. DPTE 270 transfer bin container; 7. water inlet pipe; 8. DPTE 270 α door; 9. control touch panel; 10. cable duct; 11. alarm indicator light tower; 12. exhaust ventilation pipe; 13. Two in series HEPA exhaust filters; 14. sterilization bypass pipe; 15. sterilization bypass electric control ball valve; 16. exhaust electronic control ball valve; 17. extraction blower; 18. exhaust export; 19. anemometer; 20. inlet air blower; 21. inlet ventilation pipe; 22. inlet air electronic control ball valve; 23. inlet HEPA filter; 24. coupling clamp for inlet ventilation pipe; 25. sterilization reagent import; 26. top installation slideway; 27. adjustable illumination lamp; 28. stainless-steel box; 29. television-installed box; 30. front door; 31. damping-brace for the front door; 32. glove and sleeve system; 33. control cabinet; 34. temperature humidity sensor; 35. micro-differential pressure sensor; 36. flat television; 37. rotatable camera; 38. installed camera base; 39. animal cage; 40. disinfection pool; 41. drain valve.

The airflow direction through the isolation chamber via the air inlet and outlet is shown in Figure 1. Room air is drawn into the interior of the isolation chamber through the inlet pre-filter, inlet air blower, inlet ventilation pipe, inlet air electronic control ball valve, and inlet HEPA filter in the animal breeding mode. The air from the isolation chamber is drawn out of the exhaust export through two exhaust HEPA filters arranged in series, exhaust ventilation pipe and exhaust electronic control ball valve via an extraction blower. The HEPA filters are arranged in series to ensure that if one fails, the other can still ensure exhaust security and prevent pathogens from being discharged into the atmosphere.

The isolation chamber interior pressure is controlled by automated instrumentation that is connected to the supply and exhaust ventilation system. The automatic pressure regulation system is capable of maintaining the relative pressure inside the isolation chamber via the exhaust ventilation system, which can account for transient volume changes such as glove entry or withdrawal.

The isolation chamber working zone is composed of chamber, doors, glove-sleeve system and DPTE system. The welded box of medium-sized animal breeding isolator is manufactured using dumb-gloss stainless-steel 316L with a thickness of 3 mm. The adhesion acrylic isolator is manufactured with 10mm polymethylmethacrylate (PMMA).

The stainless-steel isolation chamber front door includes damping braces on each front side with dual-pistons mechanism for holding the front door securely open to let the animal cages in, operation panels with stainless-steel 316L framework and the door hinges connected to the stainless steel box. The operation panel is made of transparent PMMA. The transparent front door allows for visualization of the contents of the isolation chamber. Silicone seals around the PMMA panel ensure that the system is air tight. The front door is manually fastened onto the box framework with a hammer bolt. One gas-tight water service valve with a serrated hose is mounted on one side interior. A spray gun is connected to the serrated hose for cleaning the isolator. Animal cages can be placed on the stainless steel cage slideways in the isolator. The slideways are attached to the isolator bottom in a manner that allows cage movement in a direction along the axis perpendicular to the axis of the isolator front door. The type of animal cages can be changed, but each time just only one kind of animal species cages can be inside. In a breeding isolator all the cages share the same air space so the same microbiologically or genetically must be assure.

One door is used as a sidewall in the acrylic isolator. It allows the internal equipments and frames entry. The door can be fixed on the PMMA panel by compressing the gasket and pressure ring around the edge of the door until all the screws are tightened.

There are circular polyethylene (PE)-machined glove ports on the operation panels. The glove-sleeve port inner diameter is 300 mm and the center-to-center spacing of each port is 450 mm. The glove port assembly includes a glove port ring, glove port gasket, pressure ring and glove port inner-securing ring. The glove port ring and glove port inner-securing ring are jointed with a thread connection. The glove port ring edges are fixed on the PMMA panel by compressing the glove port gasket and pressure ring on each side of the PMMA panel by tightening a fixing screw.

The changeable sleeve and glove combination is mounted on the glove port through a sleeve fixing ring that secures the elastic Hypalon sleeve onto the glove port inner-securing ring. A glove port bung connects the glove and sleeve. Neoprene glove shapes are ambidextrous.

The transfer system for the isolation chamber is composed of DPTE systems. The DPTE system with an alpha transfer door is built into one wall of the isolation chamber using a transfer port assembly kit. The transfer port assembly kit includes the DPTE transfer port external flange, DPTE transfer port external flange sealing ring and DPTE transfer port internal flange. The DPTE transfer port external flange is fixed onto the inside isolation chamber wall by compressing the DPTE transfer port external flange sealing ring on the outside of the isolation chamber wall with a tightening fixing screw.

The transfer container is autoclavable and contains a beta door that can be manually docked to the port. The depth of the transfer container can be changed according to the research projects, its volume is enough to transfer the animal or material into the isolator. The transfer container can be autoclaved without compromising its containment and can be opened with a specialized tool to remove the sterilized waste. It also can be opened with the specialized tool in the negative pressure exhaust hood, the samples (such as animal blood samples) can be moved out for further analysis (e.g. centrifugation), while the transfer container is closed and put into a sterilizable plastic bag for autoclaving. This system works very well for rapidly and safely transferring experimental materials and animals and waste.

A videotape system mounted on the control touch panel stainless-steel box on the side of the medium-sized animal breeding isolator includes a rotatable camera and camera-installation base. The camera installation base is fastened to the control touch panel stainless-steel box by fixing screws. The position of the rotation camera can be adjusted by using the telescopic locking nut and rotating locking nut. This system enables recording of both the scientist's experimental procedures and the status of animals living in the isolation chamber. The video is displayed on the personal computer (PC) screen and saved automatically in the central control room through the control interface connected to the videotape system.

To ensure the comfort and welfare of animals in the isolation chamber, chambers are equipped with an automatic light control system and a television entertainment system. The automatic light control system includes adjustable illumination lamps and a lampshade. The adjustable illumination lamps are composed of three cold light lamps and their conditioners. The illumination system can be used to meet the needs of the animal's physiology, as well as experimental requirements.

The television entertainment system consists of a flat television and the transparent television installation box fastened to the front door by fixing screws. The animal can watch the appropriate television program to reduce depression associated with the space constraints faced by the animals and to ensure the ethical treatment of the animals.

The videotape system and lamps and television do not mount on the acrylic isolators. The videotape system and lamps in the laboratory can provide related services for transparent acrylic isolators.

The composition of the isolation control system includes an alarm indicator light tower, liquid crystal display (LCD) touch screen and control cabinet. The liquid crystal display touch screen is fastened on the outside of the isolation chamber by a fixing screw.

The PLC is built into the control cabinet. The control cabinet, which has a fan and a filter cover, is mounted onto the stainless steel shelf of isolator support stand through fasteners and fixing screw.

3. Intelligent control of isolator system

Simatic Manager Step 7 software installed in the PLC central processing unit (CPU), and through the LCD touch screen enables users to automatically control a variety of options. The animal breeding mode program, leakage test program, sterilization program, auto/manual control mode, maintenance mode, and custom procedure can all be automatically controlled by the PLC CPU and associated touch screen (Pan et al., 2010).

The management system for isolator touch screen is developed by Simatic Wincc flexible software. The operation and any system failures can be recorded and printed. The data interchange between PLC and touch screen is made possible through an industrial trunk Profibus decentralized periphery (DP).

The temperature, humidity, illumination, atmospheric pressure and air flow velocity are measured by appropriate sensors, and the values are imported to the PLC through control lines. Normal value ranges for each parameter can be programmed into the PLC, and if the parameter values deviate from the set upper and lower limits, the PLC automatically adjusts the interior environment of the isolator to match the programmed values. For example, the levels of humidity, illumination and ventilation can all be controlled by the PLC to adjust values back to pre-determined normal levels. If the PLC is unable to bring the parameter back into a normal range, the digital output module in the PLC lights an alarm bulb and sounds a buzzer, as all alarms are indicated with both a warning light and sound.

The control system controls alarms for a variety of isolation chamber problems including major equipment error alarms (such as the air blower or HEPA), major parameter alarms when values are out of the desirable ranges (such as temperature, humidity, illumination, atmospheric pressure, air exchange rate and air flow velocity), an alarm when switching to the uninterruptible power supply (UPS) / emergency power supply (EPS) and alarms for experimental failure or error (such as negative pressure breeding mode procedures or pressure test procedures).

To control pressure, a micro-differential pressure sensor is mounted on the side of the first exhaust filter. The analog module in the PLC compares the values of program settings with the values collected from the micro-differential pressure sensor, and automatically conducts proportional-integral-differential (PID) regulation. The adjusted output values are used to control blower velocity through the output module of the PLC, regulating the isolation chamber internal pressure. If a plug or leak occurs, the micro-differential pressure sensor transmits the detected signal to the PLC. If the detected values are beyond the scope of the pre-loaded high and low pressure settings, the exhaust electronic control ball valve and inlet air electronic control ball valve automatically shut down to maintain the isolation chamber as a fully-contained environment and to prevent the escape of pathogens into the outside environment. At the same time an alarm indicator light tower would start to sound an Alarm, and the touch-screen would display information on the alarm. The alarm information would then be transmitted to the lab server through the industrial Ethernet module in the PLC. The alarm message displayed is recorded onto the lab server for analysis at a later date.

The blower rotation rate and frequency are automatically controlled by the PLC system to ensure that the airflow velocity, air exchange rate, and atmospheric pressure match the set values. If one exhaust blower fails, the PLC system responds by switching to another backup exhaust blower to ensure ventilation safety and the internal negative pressure state of the isolation chamber.

The cold light lamp regulator is controlled by the PLC digital output module to automatically adjust the illumination time according to animal behavior. The illumination time and intensity can be set from the touch screen by the operator and automatically executed. The lamps also can be switched on or off manually to meet different lighting requirements during an experimental operation.

Temperature and humidity sensors are equipped within the isolator. The isolator internal temperature is maintained within $18\sim29°C$, and relative humidity is kept within $40\sim70\%$. The isolator internal temperature and humidity electrical signals are collected by the PLC analog module, visualized as the project value (actual values of temperature and humidity), and automatically displayed and recorded on the touch screen. The values also recorded on the lab server.

4. Installation isolator system in high-level biosafety laboratory

The design of isolator system in high-level biosafety laboratory must consider about types and groups of laboratory animals, shape and actual area of the experiment field in order to the effective utilization of the independent negative-pressure ventilation system of the robust isolator offering maximizing population density and the welfare of animals. The isolator support frames and box bodies can be assembled after laboratory partitions and self-leveling floors and cable ducts on the sidewall all being in the right place. Once the large-scale isolators have been installation, the movements are quite difficult.

The vent thread hose mounted on the exhaust export of the isolator is connected to laboratory heating, ventilation and air conditioning (HVAC) exhaust main pipe via constant volume venturi valve and dynamoelectric airtight valve. The airflow velocity through each open glove port can be regulated using the external venturi valve. The air from the type 304 stainless-steel main pipe is drawn out of the exhaust export through the exhaust in-place scan testable HEPA filter combination unit via the laboratory extraction blower. This connection can reduce the exhaust exports of the building and comply with environmental protection requirements.

The isolator locating leaks may be detected by placing a dish of ammonia and using compressed air to pressurize with a positive pressure of up to 1000 Pa. Suspected areas will turn blue for the leaked ammonia reacts with bromine on the covered yellow bromide developing cloth. Leaks are commonly in soft and hard junction. The gel has to be removed and the sealing ring has to be cleaned or replaced and resealed with gel.

5. Detection the technology performance parameters of isolator system

The technology performance parameters of isolator system are established according with related China national standards and European standards and international standards (Table 1).

TSI8386A-M-GB multi-parameter ventilation meter is used to detect airflow differential pressure, vertical section airflow velocity and air velocity into open glove port. BCJ-1 airborne particle counter is used to measure air cleanliness. TES-1350A sound level meter is used to monitor noise. Testo540 luxmeter illumination tester is used to measure illumination. MARK- Ⅱ micro manometer was used to test alarm function. TSI8386A-M-GB and HM34C humidty / temperature meter are used to checkout pressure integrity. Test procedures are carried out according to the protocol as GB50591-2010, GB19489-2008 and ISO10648-2:1994 described.

Apply power and clean compressed air to the isolator before testing. The main power on the control cabinet is first turned on. Turn on the lock-controlled switch. The experimental personnel exit the lab to start and run the high-level biosafety laboratory HVAC in central control room. Personal protective clothing should be worn when entering the running normally lab to perform testing work. Detecting equipments are transferred into isolation chamber by DPTE container. The starting and stopping control and the setup of operating parameters of isolator can be controlled by staff to adopt computer technology to remote control in central control room, or to implement on-the-spot control with control touch panel of the isolator. The current operating parameters are displayed on the touch screen interface and can be adjusted by the operator following the interface prompts.

The room lamps are turned off in order to measure the independent illumination system of the stainless-steel isolator. The illumination of acrylic isolator without independent lamp is detected by using the lab illumination system.

The accuracy temperature control of air-conditioning system with all fresh air in the lab is 0.5°C. The HVAC has to be turned off when using pressure change method to test the isolator leak tightness. The leak rate test data are obtained by detecting in relatively stable room temperature. The glove-sleeve systems need to be changed by blind plates. Each overexpansion glove-sleeve in 1000Pa can create tiny deformation to change volume during the pressure changing and the air volume changes can result in significant pressure attenuation during the multi-glove-sleeve system detection stage. Flexible film windows of micrurgy isolator also have to be changed by blind plates.

The glove-sleeve system must be in place during operation and a breach in glove integrity can be serious consequence. The multi-glove-sleeve system cannot complete extension into the isolator in -250 Pa. The guideline for ABSL-4 building enclosure integrity test on GB19489-2008 is selected for measurement the isolator with the multi-glove-sleeve system or flexible film windows or both in place. The natural attenuation of pressure is less than 250 Pa in 20 min when the isolator internal air pressure down to -500Pa. This test is also a good

Testing Items	Parameters	Reference
Temperature, °C	18～29	Architectural and technical code for
Diurnal temperature, °C ⩽	4	laboratory animal facility. GB50447-
Relative humidity, %	40～70	2008
Vertical section airflow velocity, m/s ⩽	0. 2	
Air changes per hour, ACH	8～50	Laboratory animal- requirements of
Airflow differential pressure, Pa	20～150	environment and housing facilities.
Air cleanliness, class	100～10000	GB14925-2001
Settling microbe, cfu/(Φ90mm • 0. 5h)	0	
Light / dark rhythms, h	12/12 or 10/14	
Animal illumination, lux	5～200	
Working illumination, lux ≥	150	
Noise, dB ⩽	68	Architectural and technical code for biosafety laboratories. GB50346- 2004
Air velocity into open glove port, m/s ≥	0. 7	Biotechnology-Performance criteria for microbiological safety cabinets. EN 12469:2000
-1000 Pa hourly leak rate (rateacceptance test), h^{-1} <	2. 5×10^{-3}	Containment enclosures - Part 2: Classification according to leak tightness and associated checking methods. ISO10648-2:1994
-500 Pa pressure attenuation in 20 min (glove- sleeve in place), Pa ≤	250	Laboratories-General equirements for biosafety. GB19489-2008

Table 1. The technology performance parameters of isolator.

way to perform to be sure the leak rate is in the tolerable range before starting the experiment. This kind of periodic testing should be established and recorded for comparison preventative maintenance requirements.

The test results of isolator system have been compiled together in table 2 and they all meet technology criterion. The isolator internal dust concentration test indicate that the result for particle size ≥0.5 μm is ≤3.5 particles/L, for particle size ≥5.0 μm is 0 particles/L. It is supposed that the air cleanliness in isolator internal is Class 100. The temperature of the isolator internal is 0.1-0.5°C below room temperature. The relative humidity of the isolator internal is determined by the lab atmosphere.

Isolator -1000 Pa pressure decay test results show in figure 2. During the acceptance test, inlet air blower, inlet air electronic control ball valve, sterilizing agent by-pass electronic control ball valve, exhaust electronic control ball valve and extraction blower are all closed. Part of the inlet ventilation pipes, an inlet HEPA filter, two exhaust HEPA filters arranged in series, part of exhaust ventilation pipes and part of sterilizing agent bypass tubes are all in the range of pressure integrity testing. If leakage present in the installed HEPA filters, the negative or positive pressure tests will be failure. Anyway the isolators pass through the

Type of isolator	Vertical section airflow velocity (m/s)	-1000Pa hourly leak rate(h⁻¹)	-500Pa pressure attenuation in 20min (Pa)	Air velocity into open glove port (m/s)	Airflow differential pressure ΔP(pa)	Interior dust concentration (Particles/L)				Noise [dB(A)]	Illumination (average values) (lux)	
						Maximum average values of measuring points		Statistical mean values in isolator working zone			Animal illumination	Working illumination
						≥0.5µm	≥5.0µm	≥0.5µm	≥5.0 µm			
medium-sized animal breeding isolator	0.03	1.54x10⁻³	76.1	0.72	-55.9	0	0	0	0	60.8	17	162
mice breeding isolator	0.06	1.59x10⁻³	31.4	0.72	-65.8	0	0	0	0	67.3	/	282
anatomy isolator	0.04	1.03x10⁻³	132.6	0.71	-62.5	0.24	0	0.15	0	64.7	/	349
micrurgy isolator	0.02	0.96x10⁻³	101.4	0.70	-51.6	0.47	0	1.10	0	67.1	/	367

Table 2. Measuring results of isolators.

leakage rates tests in both positive and negative states. During normal operation, the directional air flow from the isolation chamber to the exhaust export and into the attached thread chimney should pass through two exhaust HEPA filters arranged in series. Airborne contaminants in the isolator are removed by the two HEPA filters, so the vent thread hose and the part of the exhaust ventilation pipes installed behind the electronic control ball valves need not do the leak rate test with the isolator. Even the leakage present among the hoses, the laboratory is in the negative pressure atmospheric conditions, the emitted particles can be mechanical captured by the lab filters. The exhaust in-place scan testable

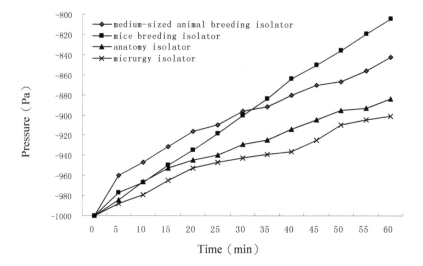

Fig. 2. Negative 1000Pa pressure decay test of isolator.

HEPA filter combination housing assembly is another important downstream exhaust filter devices of isolators and the lab before the air flow can disperse to the environment. The airborne contaminants can be detected by the leakage detection device of the unit if the leaks occur in-service. The actual test results of the exhaust filter units downstream are zero particles/L.

The maximum airflow rate of the isolator is 180 m³/h and the maximum air exchange rates is 36 ACH. The airflow rates of the laboratory are 740 ~ 3900 m³/h and are excessively greater than the airflow rate of the isolator. The isolators are turned on or off one by one via remote control by the dedicated computer in the central control room, and the lab pressure changes being observed actually have no significant effect.

Testing of the alarm system of isolator is essential to ensure proper function. The value of negative pressure is reduced by manually exposing the glove port when the isolation chamber running normally. Buzzer alarm of the isolator alarms as loss of pressure when the negative pressure absolute value of the isolator internal is less than 20Pa. The resistance of exhaust HEPA filter is increased artificially covering the isolator filter with plastic membrane. Buzzer alarms as filter blocking.

6. Operation method of isolator system

The isolation chamber should be monitored for 48 hours to ensure that it is running normally in a Class 10000 high-level bio-safety laboratory. This includes supplying filtered air to the isolator and ensuring that the exhaust air is cleaned by the double in-line HEPA filters and passed through the exhaust air system into the open air. Fresh air exchanges should be conducted at a rate of about 36 air changes per hour. Following 48 hours of monitoring, the inside temperature is 22~23 °C, the relative humidity is 60%, the working negative pressure in the isolation chamber is adjusted to -50 Pa with respect to the laboratory. Healthy animals should be passed through the quarantine system and transferred into the isolation chamber via the DPTE system.

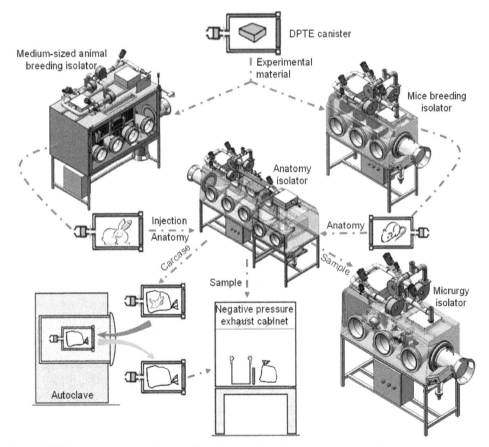

Fig. 3. DPTE systems are used to realize the transfer of experiment materials among different types of isolators and associated instruments.

The experiment in isolator systems can be carried out according to the protocol showing in figure 3.

The feeds and aseptic water can be kept enough in the isolator to minimize disturbances to breeding animals. The glove-sleeve systems allow direct complete animal feeding operations without compromising the health status or contamination of the animals within the isolator. Rapid pressure changes when operating under transient volume changes such as glove entry or withdrawal are adjusted via a variable frequency drive inlet air blower and extraction blower.

Non-human primates breeding need special approval by government, so New Zealand white rabbits are the first residents in the medium-sized animal breeding isolators. The animal excrement and other waste materials are cleaned out by DPTE container and sent to sterilize by autoclave every week. The rabbits selected for immunity with inactive pathogen are moved to the anatomy isolator with large space in an independence room by DPTE system to perform the operation of injection. The animal is sent back to the breeding isolator in the breeding room by transfer container after injection.

The ventilation performance of mice breeding isolator in mice breeding room allows using ordinary transparent mice cages and water bottles, and an extended cage-changing period up to one month (6 mice per cage, ~15g/mice). The changed cages without mice are transferred to autoclave by DPTE system.

The operation of animal anatomy can be performed in the anatomy isolator. Blood of immunity rabbit can be transferred to negative pressure exhaust cabinet by transfer canister. The β-door of the canister can be opened with a specialized tool, and the blood samples can then be removed to the biological safety cabinet for further stages of analysis (e.g., centrifugation), while the transfer canister is closed and sent into autoclave. The Leica CM1100 cryostat in the anatomy isolator can be used to rapid freezing and manual sectioning of animal tissue specimens. The frozen section slides of mice infected by attenuated strain of pathogen are packaged and transferred to micrurgy isolator for immunostaining assays and observing under a fluorescence microscope in the micrurgy isolator. It is determined by the fluorescence microscopy that the attenuated strain of pathogen in mice tissues is specific binding with its strain-specific rabbit antiserum. The image data are sent out from the lab local area network. The dead animal and experimental waste materials in the isolator are collected respectively into plastic bags for autoclaving by DPTE canister.

The animal experiment should be performed according to bio-safety operation standard procedures. If the gloves are removed during the operation, a low pressure audible/visual alarm system is activated, and a minimum velocity value of 0.7 m/s in the center of the glove port is maintained. If a glove is damaged by a needle, the blowers are capable of maintaining the isolation chamber pressure at -50 Pa but the alarm system would not be activated because the micro-differential pressure sensor is not sensitive enough for a leak of this size. Proper procedure dictates that the small hole be labeled by the operator and a new glove exchanged. All of the feeds, experimental material, waste, feces and other materials can be transferred into or out of the isolation chamber by the DPTE system. There are several breeding isolation chambers in one room, and the autoclave does not connect with any of them. Instead, DPTE beta canisters are filled with items and are then sterilized in the autoclave. After sterilization, the sterile items are removed after opening the beta door with specialized tools. The sterile items are then sent to a centralized disposal center for medical waste. Following the completion of studies with single animals, each animal is treated as dictated by bio-safety operation standards and general animal welfare. The cadavers are autoclaved in beta canisters and sent to animal carcass disposal sites.

7. Isolator system decontamination

The isolator systems need biodecontamination after finishing the breeding program and experiment. The choice of sterilant depends on what kind of devices in the isolator. If only the cages are in the isolator, or there is nothing in the isolator, the stainless-steel or acrylic isolation chamber can be connected to the peracetic acid sterilizer to sterilize the interior of the isolation chamber. During the sterilization process, inlet air blower, inlet air electronic control ball valve, exhaust electronic control ball valve and extraction blower are all closed. Raven Labs offered *Bacillus atrophaeus* spore strips can be used for sterility testing by Soproper in isolator sterilization environments. Amount (A) of Soproper in the evaporation reservoir of peracetic acid sterilizer can be calculated with the formula: A (mL) = T×70mL/h+150mL, where T = sterilization time (h). The sterilizing agent by-pass electronic control ball valve is opened. The sterilizing agent in the peracetic acid sterilizer evaporation tank is heated and its vapors are pushed by compressed air into the volume to be sterilized by a sterile connecting hose, a sterilization reagent import, a coupling clamp for the inlet ventilation pipe and an inlet HEPA filter. The sterilizing vapors escape from the interior of the isolator through two in series HEPA filters, a sterilizing agent by-pass tube, a sterilizing agent by-pass electronic control ball valve and an extraction blower to the exhaust export. The sterilization time using Soproper vapor is 12h for the interior chamber with 400cm(L)×120cm (W)×120cm(H) dimensions sterilization. *B. atrophaeus* spore strips placed in 13 critical locations of the isolator internal surface (such as DPTE α door, stainless-steel cages, glove-sleeve systems, the end of HEPA filter) were all destroyed.

Minncare dry fog system is also a good disinfection device for breeding isolator. This system can be transferred into the isolator with 30% hydrogen peroxide in the reservoir. The nozzle allows for rapid vapor dispersion and ensures that the entire isolator space is exposed to dry fog when compressed air source connected with the dry fog system. The isolator is maintained under positive 750 Pa for 5 min, and then the isolator internal pressure allows natural attenuation to zero. All *Bacillus atrophaeus* spore strips placed in the isolator were inactive. Anyway the system always sprays out some large droplets at the beginning, then stride forward to 7.5 μm normal droplets. So it is still not be used for decontaminating equipments.

Hydrogen peroxide vapor technology used by BioQuell Z system has been developed to be the effective system available for rapid and secure biodecontamination of equipment and facilities. The anatomy isolator and micrurgy isolator and their internal equipments can be decontaminated simultaneity with the laboratory terminal disinfection. There are conditioning, gassing, dwell and aeration four phases as described by the Z manufacturers. The gassing time (T) can be calculated with the experience formula: T= V×5 (g/m³) /20 (g/min), where V = room volume (m³). Apex Laboratories offered *Geobacillus stearothermophilus* spore stainless steel discs can be used for sterility testing by 30% hydrogen peroxide in isolator and its located room sterilization environments. The anatomy isolator and micrurgy isolator are in the independent 63 m³ room respectively. The isolator negative pressure sets as -20 Pa. The lab ventilation is off, four desktop fans are on. The room temperature is 16°C, relative humidity is 40%~70%. Connected the Z well, and check area to be bio-decontaminated no people or animal. All doors and windows are shut and secured, and seal the door with tape. The gassing time sets as 15 min, dwell time sets as 25 min. The injection rate of hydrogen peroxide during dwell phase is 5g/min as to maintain the concentration necessary for decontamination. At the end of aeration, the concentration of hydrogen peroxide within the room is reduced down to zero, and the Z can be stopped. The total time is 8h for the isolator and its interior equipment and the room sterilization. *G. stearothermophilus* spore discs placed in 13 critical locations of the isolator internal surface (such as DPTE α door, stainless-steel frame of equipment, glove-sleeve systems, the bottom and surface of equipment, the end of HEPA filter) were all inactive. The black paint on the microscopy are disappear after 20 times of this kind of disinfection, but the other paints still keep well, and the optical system of microscope is also not affected.

8. Conclusions

The isolator systems achieve multiple technical improvements: (1) By using variable frequency drive blowers as the inlet air and extraction blowers, adjustments for rapid pressure changes (e.g., insertion of gloves) can occur automatically without breaching the inert atmosphere. The extraction blowers contain an integrated backup system with one blower running at full strength and another on standby to act as a backup. Negative or positive pressure states are kept stable and at a safe level through the automatic control system. The pressure is adjusted depending on different requirements for different animals and/or experimental conditions. (2) The control cabinet installation is comprised mainly of the programmable logic controller, electric element (which includes the voltage transformer, secure alternating current contactor, circuit breaker, electric cable, indicating lamp and button), network port (for data output) and industrial Ethernet interface (which allows for the remote data control of multiple isolation chambers by the WINCC 6.0 program system). Automatic control and monitoring of the isolation chamber and sterilization system are achieved by the exchange of data between the touch screen and control cabinet through the industrial bus Profibus DP to meet different laboratory animal research project parameter requirements such as pressure, humidity, temperature, illumination and disinfection. A human operator can set the isolation chamber environment parameters according to the requirements of the infectious animals or for cleaning animals, allowing for the acquisition of adequate and authentic data. (3) Animal welfare is ensured by installing adjustable illumination lamps, a rotatable camera, a flat television, a micro-differential pressure sensor and temperature humidity sensor to maintain comfortable living conditions for the animal.

9. Acknowledgements

This work was supported by the Natuional Natural Science Foundation of China (30972633).

10. References

World Health Organization, (2004). Laboratory biosafety manual, 3rd ed. World Health Organization, Geneva.

Bantin GC. (2004). A comparison between the application of flexible film isolators and individual ventilated cages. Shanghai Laboratory Animal Science. 24(1):3-6.

Wathes CM, Johnson HE. (1991). Physical protection against airborne pathogens and pollutants by a novel animal isolator in a level 3 containment laboratory. Epidemiol Infect. 107(1):157-170.

Kruse RH, Puckett WH, Richardson JH. (1991). Biological safety cabinetry. Clin Microbiol Rev. 4(2):207-241.

Huang R. (2005). Isolator of using negative prcssure for big animals. CN Patent Publication number 1625942A.

Pan X, Long M, Liang H, Chen X, Li H, Li GB, Zhao ZY. (2010). Development of a multifunction isolator system for the care of medium-sized laboratory animals harboring infectious diseases. J Med Devices. 4(4): 041004.

Tattershall SF. 2006. Enclosure for handling hazardous material. US Patent No.: US7077486 B2.

Sawyer J, Bennett A, Haines V, Elton E, Crago K, Speight S. (2007). The effect of microbiological containment systems on dexterity. J Occup Environ Hyg, 4(3):166-173.

Clough G, Wallace J, Gamble MR, Merryweather ER, Bailey E. (1995). A positive, individually ventilated caging system: a local barrier system to protect both animals and personnel. Lab Anim. 29(2):139-151.

Wathes CM, Johnson HE. (1991). Physical protection against airborne pathogens and pollutants by a novel animal isolator in a level 3 containment laboratory. Epidemiol Infect. 1991;107(1):157-70.

ISO 14664-7:2004，Cleanrooms and associated controlled environments —Part 7: Separative devices (clean air hoods,gloveboxes, isolators and minienvironments). International Organization for Standardization, Geneva.

ISO 10648-1:1997, Containment enclosures — Part 1: Design principles. International Organization for Standardization, Geneva.

Hillman P, Gebremedhin K, Warner R. (1992). Ventilation system to minimize airborne bacteria, dust, humidity, and ammonia in calf nurseries. J Dairy Sci. 75(5):1305-1312

Institute of laboratory animal resources commission on life sciences, National research council. (1996). Guide for the care and use of laboratory animals. Washington,D.C: National Academy Press.

Runkle RS, Allendale NJ, Marsh RC, Albuquerque NM. (1969). Unit for providing environmental control of animals. US Patent No.: 3630174.

Allen JR, Burgess M, Aiken SC. (2009). Container lid gasket protective strip for double door transfer system. US Patent Pub.No.: US2009/0212054 A1.

Michael A, Szatmary FT, Worth TX. (2004). Rapid transfer port. US Patent No.: US6779567 B1.

Tauraso NM, Norris GF, Sorg TJ, Cook RO, Myers ML, Trimmer R. (1969). Negative-pressure isolator for work with hazardous infectious agents in monkeys. Appl Microbiol. 18(2):294-297.

Pan X, Sun Y. (2004). Expression of SARS-CoV spike protein functional receptor ACE2 in human cornea and conjunctiva tissues. High Technology Letters. 10 (supplement): 273-277.

Conly J, Johnston B. (2008). The infectious diseases consequences of monkey business. Can J Infect Dis Med Microbiol. 19(1):12-14.

Pan X, Qi JC, Long M, Liang H, Chen X, Li H, Li GB, Zheng H. (2010). New technique: Development of a large-scale isolation chamber system for the safe and humane care of medium-sized laboratory animals harboring infectious diseases. J Zhejiang Univ Sci B. 11 (10): 771-778.

GB50447-2008, Architectural and technical code for laboratory animal facility. National Standard. China.

GB14925-2001, Laboratory animal- requirements of environment and housing facilities. National Standard. China.

GB50346-2004, Architectural and technical code for biosafety laboratories. National Standard. China.

EN 12469:2000, Biotechnology-Performance criteria for microbiological safety cabinets. European Standard. European Committee for Standardization.

ISO10648-2:1994, Containment enclosures - Part 2: Classification according to leak tightness and associated checking methods. International Organization for Standardization, Geneva.

GB19489-2008, Laboratories-General equirements for biosafety. National Standard. China.

GB50591-2010, Code for construction and acceptance of cleanroom. National Standard. China.

Development of Therapeutic Interventions for Emerging Diseases

Nigel J. Silman

Research & Development, Health Protection Agency Porton,
Porton Down, Salisbury,
UK

1. Introduction

New infectious diseases emerge with a high regularity; it has recently been estimated that a novel infectious disease agent either emerges or re-emerges approximately every 8 months. This latter statistic is supported by the observation that there have been over 335 emerging infectious disease (EID) events between 1940 and 2004 (Jones *et al.*, 2008). Of course, not all of these EID events represent a threat to human health, indeed many of these are infections of animals, although approximately 60% are also zoonotic infections (which by definition can be transmitted between animals and humans); another additional proportion also have the potential to cross the species barrier. Since 1970 there have been approximately 30 new species of pathogen emerge which cause human infection. Table 1 lists these pathogens (taken from World Health Organisation, 1999).

Year	Pathogen	Year	Pathogen
1972	Small Round Structured Viruses	1989	Hepatitis C virus
1973	Rotavirus	1990	Human herpesvirus-7
1975	Astrovirus	1990	Hepatitis E virus
1975	Parvovirus B-19	1991	Hepatitis F virus
1976	*Crytosporidium parvum*	1992	*Vibrio cholerae* 0139:H7
1977	Ebola virus	1992	*Bartonella henselae*
1977	*Legionella pneumophila*	1993	Sin Nombre virus
1977	Hantaan virus	1993	Hepatitis G virus
1977	*Cambylobacter jejuni*	1994	Sabia virus
1980	HTLV-1	1994	Human herpesvirus-8
1981	Toxigenic *Staphylococcus aureus*	1995	Hendra virus
1982	HTLV-II	1996	Prion (BSE/vCJD)
1982	*Borrelia burgdorferii*	1997	Influenza A virus (H5N1)
1983	*E.coli* 0157:H7	1997	Transfusion-transmitted virus
1983	HIV	1997	Enterovirus 71
1983	*Helicobacter pylori*	1998	Nipah virus
1988	Human herpesvirus-6	1999	Influenza A virus (Hong Kong 'flu)
1989	*Ehrlichia* spp.	1999	West Nile virus

Table 1. Emerging Infectious Disease Pathogens, 1972-1999.

An emerging infectious disease may be defined as one that has appeared in a population for the first time, or that may have existed previously but is rapidly increasing in incidence or geographic range (World Health Organisation [WHO]). This definition is quite generic and many consider EID's as those which are either genuinely novel infectious disease pathogens (examples include the SARS coronavirus which emerged in 2003) or those where there has been a paradigm shift in their genotype or phenotype such that it poses a new threat to health (examples include the appearance of multi-drug resistant *Mycobacterium tuberculosis* and other bacterial pathogens). These latter pathogens are frequently referred to as re-emerging infectious diseases, to discriminate them from completely novel disease agents. Because of the apparent rise in the incidence of EIDs during the 1980's and 90's (HIV/AIDS, vCJD *etc.*), factors involved in the process of emergence were analysed by a number of workers. One such study (Taylor *et al.*, 2001), concluded that although over half of EIDs were zoonotic in origin, the route of transmission had no effect on the likelihood of emergence, rather it was the taxonomy of the organism that was the root cause. They concluded that viruses and bacteria were of much higher likelihood of emergence, whereas parasites such as Helminths, were very unlikely to ever emerge.

Despite the advances in medical science, infectious diseases still constitute a threat to human survival, health and well-being and have done since human life began. Immediately following the discovery of penicillin, there was a mood of optimism that felt that the conquest of infectious diseases was a war that had been won; rather it seems it was merely the first skirmish in a very long-lasting battle. In the first decade of the 21st century, we know that infectious diseases represent a major global threat, accounting for some 41% of the global disease burden and in the UK alone, infectious diseases now account for approximately 70,000 deaths per annum and 40% of the population in the country consult a medical practitioner each year because of infection (Donaldson, 2001). It is clear, therefore, that infectious diseases remain a major global threat and that the burden of disease with an infectious aetiology is very high. There are a large number of interventions that can be applied to the control of infectious disease and for health protection. Interventions include simple public health control measures (hand-washing, quarantine, supply of clean water *etc.*), diagnostic tests, therapeutic treatments and vaccines. These different aspects will be discussed in greater depth in the following sections.

2. Vaccination

Vaccination is the process by which the adaptive immune system is stimulated to produce a deliberate response. Typically, vaccines comprise an antigenic component (or components) which are administered by a variety of routes and mimic the infection against which protection is sought. Modern vaccination was probably first described by Edward Jenner (there are reports that a similar approach had been used some years earlier) in 1796; indeed it was Jenner who coined the phrase vaccination. The term is derived from the Latin word *vacca* meaning "cow", so derived since the first "vaccination" used material from cowpox viral lesions on a milk-maids hands as protection against Smallpox infection (reviewed in Lombard *et al.*, 2007). Strictly, vaccination may be considered to be the process of introducing a foreign antigen into the body for the purpose of protection against infectious disease, whereas, immunisation is the process by which a vaccine induces an immune response against a foreign antigen – a subtle difference in meaning, although in practice the two terms are often used interchangeably. From these early beginnings, there are 26 currently licensed vaccines widely available and administered as components of vaccination programmes. These 26 vaccines are shown in Table 2 below.

Vaccine	Vaccine
Anthrax	Pertussis
Cervical cancer (papilloma virus)	Pneumococcal infection
Chicken pox virus	Poliomyelitis
Cholera	Rabies
Diphtheria	Rotavirus
Group A & C Meningococcal infections	Rubella
Hib infection	Shingles
Hepatitis A	Smallpox
Hepatitis B	Tetanus
Japanese encephalitis	Tuberculosis
Influenza	Typhoid Fever
Measles	Varicella
Mumps	Yellow Fever

Table 2. Licensed Vaccines Currently Available for Use.

The table above illustrates that there are available vaccines for many of the "common" infectious diseases, yet despite this availability, there still exists a considerable disease burden for many of the diseases shown in Table 2. One might reasonably question why this is so, and the answer is multi-fold. Firstly the aspect of vaccine efficacy needs to be considered; the availability of a licensed vaccine does not, of course, indicate that use will result in 100% protection of the recipient. Due to the very different immune profiles observed within the human population, there will be a response curve which at one end results in next to no (or at least very low) levels of protection, whereas at the other end of the scale, recipients will show good protection. Taken on a population level, this means that there will always be a proportion of the population which are unprotected and thus the disease is still able to circulate. The above reasoning also assumes that take-up (and indeed availability) of any vaccine is 100% within a population; it is not due both to the cost involved in vaccinating entire populations and the choice which some make not to receive vaccination when offered. This latter point is very well illustrated by the recent issues surrounding the MMR (Measles, Mumps & Rubella) tri-valent vaccine within the UK. Adverse scientific publications (for an update on the current scientific evidence and lack of any link between these events see DeStefano & Williams, 2004), indicating a link between receipt of the vaccine and autism in children has meant that many parents decided not to allow their children to receive the vaccine and the UK now has a considerable measles outbreak due to much higher levels of susceptibility within the population (see ECDC measles Surveillance Report, 2011). It is of note, though, that the risk of real adverse events with the MMR vaccine are very low; the risk of brain damage due to receipt of the vaccine is calculated to be approximately 1/100,000 (this is due to the measles component of the vaccine), whereas the risk of brain damage if a child catches measles is approximately 1/1000, a figure which is considerably higher.

2.1 Types of vaccine

There are basically three ways of making vaccines against infectious diseases, all rely on a level of knowledge about the pathogenesis of the disease and ideally about the virulence factors which the pathogen employs. That vaccination is an effective method to protect the health of a population is well known and documented; the figure below illustrates the reduction in numbers of ill and in numbers of deaths for a fictitious respiratory disease, spreading with a population of approximately 60 million people (Fig. 1). A large number of assumptions have been made in running this very simple Susceptible, Infected, Recovered (SIR) model, one of which was that a new vaccine had to be developed and that the time taken to both produce a crude, whole-cell vaccine, plus manufacture enough to be used widely, resulted in an approximately 50% reduction in the overall numbers of fatalities (C. Norris & N J Silman, Unpublished). Of course, modelling the same disease, but making the assumption that a vaccine already exists can reduce the impact of the disease even more than that shown in Fig.1.

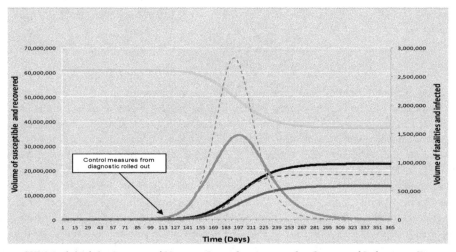

Fig. 1. SIR Model of the Impact of Vaccine Introduction on the Course of Infectious Disease. Key: ____ Susceptible population; _ _ _ Infected population; ___ Infected population after vaccine introduced; _ _ _ Fatalities if vaccine not used; _____ Fatalities when vaccine used; ___ Numbers Recovered

This figure is shown merely to illustrate the point that development of a new vaccine in the event of an emerging disease can have a very profound effect on the outcome of the disease (this point was well made during the recent H1N1 influenza pandemic). The illustration also includes an element of diagnostic roll-out, where we made the assumption that in the early stages of a newly emerged pathogen, simple public health control measures would be invoked to control person to person transmission and that these measures would be supported by a diagnostic test.

The three different approaches to vaccine development will be discussed in greater detail in the sections which follow, and their potential for use in producing vaccines against rapidly emerging pathogens will be discussed further.

2.1.1 Whole-cell vaccines

The simplest vaccines comprise growing up the pathogen and inactivating a crude, unfractionated preparation. This is an approach which has been used for a considerable length of time and vaccines made using this relatively simple rationale are still widely used. Examples taken from table 2 include Anthrax, Japanese encephalitis, influenza, yellow fever and typhoid fever; the reader will note that both bacterial and viral vaccines are made using the same approach and both types can show good efficacy in use. There are, of course, a number of examples where such an approach is not successful; examples here include vaccines that were produced against Cholera, Plague, meningitis and Smallpox. These vaccines failed because of a paucity of understanding of the mechanisms of virulence (*e.g.* the major virulence factor for Cholera is a toxin and thus a crude whole-cell preparation would not contain this secreted component). However, it is still considered that this method of rapidly producing a vaccine could be used in the event of a newly emerging infectious disease that had a high mortality rate and was highly transmissible within the population. Although there are examples of vaccines for both bacteria and viruses produced by this method, it is generally considered that the approach is probably more suited to production of viral vaccines due to their lower complexity. Probably the most commonly used vaccine of this type which is still produced and updated year on year is the split virion influenza vaccine that is produced seasonally. This vaccine comprises an unpurified preparation of virus typically grown in egg-culture (although there are notable examples of cell-culture grown influenza virus vaccines which are licensed for use or in clinical trial) and inactivated. The rationale is that the major antigenic components of the influenza virus are the haemagglutinin and neuraminidase, both of which are surface proteins against which considerable immune responses are mounted. Interestingly, despite the longevity of use of this vaccine and the considerable number of clinical trials and research work that has been conducted, the correlates of protection for influenza are still unknown (Montomoli *et al.*, 2011).

Looking at the list of recently emerged pathogens shown in Table 1, it is interesting to note that this approach has been used to develop vaccine candidates for a number of the pathogens. The most notable example is HIV/AIDS, for which there is still no effective vaccine and that an inactivated viral preparation did not exhibit high protective efficacy. Thus, for this method of vaccine development to be of value for an emergent pathogen a number of criteria need to be fulfilled, some of which will not be obvious when the disease first emerges. Firstly, the disease needs to have a high mortality rate, such that use of a vaccine is absolutely required. Secondly, it must be highly transmissible, since an infection with a low rate of transmission (R_0) can be controlled by other public health measures, a good example of such a pathogen was the SARS coronavirus, which was transmissible but had a relatively low R_0 and thus was adequately controlled by quarantine. Thirdly, natural infection should induce a protective immunity, otherwise an inactivated preparation is unlikely to induce immunity if the natural infection is incapable of so doing. This last consideration is very unlikely to be understood at the point when the pathogen emerges and will only be fully understood after a considerable length of time, most probably once an epidemic or pandemic situation has passed. The speed that a vaccine must be deployed is illustrated in Fig.2, which shows the effect on the numbers of infectious people within a population as the reproduction rate of the infectious disease pathogen is varied.

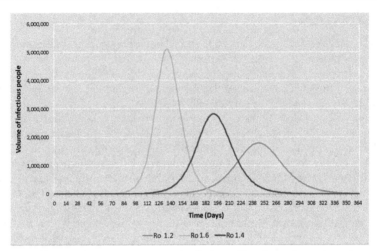

Fig. 2. Effect of Varying R_0 on the Number of Infectious People within a Population.

This figure illustrates a modest range of R_0 values between 1.2 and 1.6, the point to note is that even with small variations in the R_0 value, large differences in the numbers of infected people are observed and the time that maximum numbers of people are infected varies between approximately 130 and 240 days. This should be compared with the reproduction rate of typical influenza viruses which may be up to $R_0 = 3$ (that is, 3 uninfected people are infected by each infectious member of the population). The lower values used in this illustration were seen with the SARS coronavirus and perhaps illustrate why a vaccine was not developed against this pathogen during the epidemic phase.

2.1.2 Attenuated vaccines

Another approach to the rational design of vaccines for existing or emerging pathogens is the attenuation of virulent strains. Here, a strain is used which is not able to produce fulminant infection as a result of its' attenuation. In contrast to the inactivated vaccines described in section 2.1.1, these vaccines comprise live micro-organisms. Historically, attenuated strains were first obtained by serendipity often following prolonged sub-culture or passage (for example see Barrett *et al.*, 1990). Good examples of this occurrence are the Yellow fever 17D strain which was naturally attenuated by repeated passage and has been used as a vaccine against this disease since the 1950's. Interestingly, the mechanism of attenuation is still not known, although the vaccine has a long history of safe use, except in those members of the population with an egg allergy (the virus is propagated in egg culture). Another well-known example of an attenuated vaccine strain is the Polio virus vaccine, of which there are two vaccines in use. The first, the Salk vaccine is an inactivated viral preparation whilst the second, called the Sabin strain is an attenuated Polio virus (see Pearce, 2004). The Sabin vaccine was trialled between 1957 and 1962, when it was licensed for widespread use. The vaccine is taken orally and was attenuated by repeated passage in the brains of mice. By the seventh passage the virus was found to be no longer capable of infecting mice via the neurological route. A further 2 to 3 passages through rats confirmed the attenuation and the strain was considered safe for human inoculation. The development of polio vaccines in the 1950's was a response to the large burden of disease caused by this virus and delivery of the Salk and Sabin vaccines constitutes the first mass-immunisation programmes. At the current date, Polio is still yet to be eradicated, despite efforts which began in 1988 between the WHO, UNICEF and the Rotary Foundation, however the hope is that this virus will soon be committed to history.

As the above example illustrates, the process of attenuation is not one which can be undertaken rapidly. There is no rational way of determining whether a strain may be attenuated by simple repeated passage or not and therefore the utility of such an approach is of limited value in responding to emergence of new infectious diseases. There are, of course, alternative ways of attenuating pathogenic strains of microorganism. For example, in the time between isolation of the Sabin strain and the present day, the mutations which are responsible for this strains lack of neuro-infectivity have been mapped to the internal ribosome entry site (IRES) of the virus in the currently used strain, a derivative of the original Sabin isolate. Extensive characterisation of the series of viruses that have been used as live-attenuated Polio vaccines has indicated that there are fifty-seven nucleotide substitutions which distinguish the attenuated Sabin 1 strain from its virulent parent (the Mahoney serotype), with a two further nucleotide substitutions between the Sabin 2 and parent strain, and ten more substitutions are involved in further attenuating the Sabin 3 strain (Kew *et al.*, 2005).

An alternative to repeated passage is the rational deletion of one or more genes from the genome of the organism. This approach requires in-depth knowledge of the virulence or pathogenicity factors which the infectious micro-organism uses to achieve infection in the human host. There are a number of examples where this approach has been successfully used. In view of the subject within this chapter to look at prospects for emerging infectious diseases, the live attenuated influenza vaccine (LAIV) will be used as a discussion example to illustrate this approach. There is currently only one licensed influenza vaccine based upon this LAIV technology, although, like other influenza vaccines, the virus backbone is used to construct vaccines against currently circulating strains by recombination with the genomic segments encoding the haemagglutinin and neuraminidase genes from the currently circulating strains. The LAIV is licensed in the USA by FDA and sold under the trade name of FluMist™. The backbone strain used for this vaccine is a cold-adapted strain which is attenuated since it is not able to complete the cycle of replication at normal human body temperatures. The relatively small genome of the influenza virus has been completely sequenced from this strain and many nucleotide substitutions have been made to ensure that the strain cannot revert and also to improve its growth properties in cell, rather than egg culture as this is a more scalable technology for rapid vaccine manufacture than is egg culture.

A similar approach may be envisioned for viral groups such as the Flaviviruses. This is an important group of viruses, whose members have been responsible for several infectious disease outbreaks during the last two decades. Their members include Yellow fever virus, West Nile virus and Dengue virus and they are viruses with segmented RNA genomes. One of the key factors in the emergence of new pathogens is the presence of an RNA genome as this allows rapid recombination, mutation and hence evolution and adaptation. This group is therefore of great importance when horizon scanning for the next emergent viral disease and only one flavivirus already has a licensed vaccine (Yellow fever). There are vaccines against Dengue virus in clinical trial, since this is a disease with a worldwide distribution and serious complications can be observed if re-infection with a different serotype occurs (Dengue haemorrhagic fever). West Nile virus is a classic example of an emergent viral infection; it arose in the West Nile delta in North Africa and was transported by cervid birds into North America where, as it is a mosquito vector-transmitted disease, it has caused seasonal outbreaks in every subsequent year (see Campbell *et al.*, 2002). Chikungunya virus has similarly spread across the Indian Ocean and has also been imported into Europe where it caused a limited outbreak in Italy during 2009 (Beltrame *et al.*, 2007). It is likely that infection with one flavivirus induces an immunity against some other viruses within the group, based on the observation that antibodies against many of these viruses cross-react with flaviviral antigens in ELISA assays and thus make clinical infection with a particular virus impossible to diagnose by serology alone. By comparing different flaviviruses with the Yellow fever 17D vaccine, it should be possible to produce vaccines against this range of viruses by using the same approach to attenuate different viruses. What is unknown, once again, are the correlates of immunity for not only Yellow fever infection but for any of the other flavivirus infections. Care will also be needed to avoid any complications by priming the immune system as are seen in Dengue virus infection. As a method of rapidly producing a vaccine strain, attenuation by repeated passage is not useful due to the extensive length of time that it may take to produce an attenuated virus and the additional time required to demonstrate irreversible attenuation.

2.1.3 Sub-unit vaccines

Probably the most rapid way to make a vaccine against a newly emerging pathogen is to use a recombinant technology approach and identify a single immunogenic antigen, clone out and express the gene encoding that particular antigen. A common theme that we have observed whilst discussing vaccinology, is that rational vaccine design has an absolute requirement for good understanding of both the factors which affect pathogen virulence as well as those which contribute to immunity in the host. Although this has been discussed previously, it bears repeating that in the event of a newly emerging pathogen, these data will not be available and that the second best approach is to fall back to an inactivated whole pathogen preparation. Assuming, however, that we are aiming to develop a vaccine against a pathogen which is similar to one about which we have considerable knowledge, then a rational sub-unit approach is likely to be used. Once again the caveat is that a single sub-unit(s) may not induce complete protective immunity, as there may well be multiple components involved in protection following natural infection. There are numerous examples where single sub-unit vaccine candidates fail to provide complete or even any protection, a good illustration of this observation is the lack of complete protection afforded by single sub-unit vaccines in HIV infection (inactivated virus also fails to induce protection though).

Yersinia pestis, the bacterial causative agent of plague, is a re-emergent infection as it has caused recent outbreaks in geographical areas that have previously not experienced infections caused by this organism. Fig. 3 below illustrates that although there are a large number of surface antigens, against which an immune response is induced (as determined by the presence of human antibody response), only two are associated with protective immunity, these are the F1 and V antigens and both are virulence factors encoded by transferrable plasmids. A vaccine containing the F1 and V-antigens is being developed, although because of the low prevalence of disease, it is unlikely to be widely used. As an exemplar of the approach that can be taken with emerging and re-emerging diseases, it illustrates perfectly the requirement for a thorough understanding of the pathogenesis of the organisms as well as understanding the host immune response.

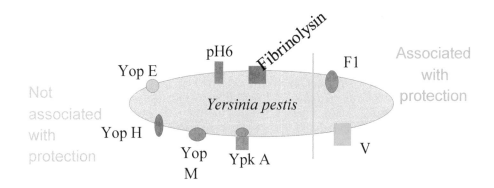

Fig. 3. Identification of Protective Antigens in *Yersinia pestis*.

3. Therapeutic interventions

There are a great number of therapeutic interventions that can be applied to the control of infectious diseases. The key type of interventions are discussed in greater detail below, and as a general trend, we have observed a move towards more targeted approaches to design of therapeutic compounds. During the last 30 years, the period under discussion when considering emerging infectious diseases, there has been a marked change in the scientific approaches to discovery of therapeutic molecules. There were a great many researchers using natural product libraries during the 1970's and 80's to discover compounds with activity against a wide range of biological activities; of relevance to infectious diseases are those which exhibited antimicrobial activity. A consequence of these high-throughput screening programmes was that several new classes of antibiotic were discovered during this time, but subsequently there have been very few new discoveries and there is now a real shortage of new antimicrobial compound groups to counteract the rise of antimicrobial resistance. Future research to meet clinical unmet needs, must incorporate the rational design and discovery of new ways of combating antimicrobial resistance, be it new antibiotics or other therapeutic approaches.

3.1 Antimicrobial compounds

The majority of currently licensed antibiotics were discovered between 40 and 60 years ago and modern drugs are mostly derivatives of existing classes of drug. Despite the increased need to treat expanding populations against micro-organisms exhibiting increasing levels of resistance, there has been a reduction in the effort by the major pharmaceutical companies to discover new antibiotics (Marinelli, 2009). There have been a number of high, but unrealised expectations driven by high-throughput screening, combinatorial chemistry and microbial genome sequencing that have failed to deliver the new compounds required. It is interesting to note that during the "Golden Age" of antibiotic discovery (1940-1960) approximately 12,000 compounds were screened and resulted in 160 licensed products (0.01%). This statistic played a major part in the evolution of antibiotics where research effort was directed towards the improvement of existing chemotypes (increased potency, stability and pharmokinetics, reduced side-effects) rather than discovery of novel compound classes. Those that did continue to invest research funds into discovery rather than improvement were rewarded by the discovery of some new chemotypes such as thienamycin, daptomycin and echinocandins. One of the main confounders to the discovery of new compounds was the high rate of re-isolation of existing compounds, requiring a different approach to screening assays from the traditionally used inhibition of bacterial growth that has been used since Alexander Fleming discovered Penicillin in 1928. This need has led to the introduction of functional, cell-free assays, but this has not resulted in the desired increase in discovery of novel compounds. Moreover, the availability of whole genome sequence data for a wide range of pathogenic bacteria and viruses similarly has not resulted in discovery of novel chemotypes, despite high investment by the pharmaceutical companies.

There are, however, several prospects for the discovery of new classes of chemotype. The first of these is to harness the wealth of structural data that are now available, but this approach requires an in-depth knowledge of the biology of the target micro-organism. There are a number of documented examples of this approach being coupled with virtual high-throughput screening (VHTS) against virtual compound libraries. One example is that described by Reddy et al. (2006) for the rational discovery of small molecule inhibitors of prion protein, a key emergent disease. Here a virtual compound library was screened for molecules that would theoretically bind and inhibit prion protein from entering cells. A similar approach has been taken to the design of inhibitors of the Anthrax toxin cell-binding component (protective antigen; PA) which combines with two further toxin components to exert the toxic effects, which typically result in death of the animal or human host. The protein crystallography data were used for the PA molecule and the cell-receptor binding site was identified from published research (Bradley et al., 2001). This crystal structure was screened using VHTS and small-molecule inhibitors of this binding reaction were identified and then synthesised and screened in vitro using functional assays for one of the two Anthrax toxins (lethal toxin, a combination of PA and lethal factor). Many of the molecules screened using this approach were subsequently found to have significant activity in the in vitro assays; approximately 3% of the compounds screened were found to possess activity, compared with the 0.01% that are typically obtained by high-throughput screening of compound libraries (B. Chen, personal communication). This approach clearly holds much promise for the rational design of novel chemotypes of antimicrobial compound and the approach works irrespective of whether the pathogen is a virus or bacteria. This is therefore, an attractive approach for the development of targeted inhibitors of a range of processes involved in the pathogenesis of disease. The main caveat, though, is that a thorough understanding of the virulence factors and pathogenesis of the disease are needed, along with suitable structural data to enable this approach to be used to combat emerging diseases. Clearly, when a pathogen first emerges, it is completely uncharacterised and such a directed approach is not possible.

Other approaches to the discovery of new chemotypes are the screening of compound libraries derived from different sources. This approach somewhat mimics the approach used during the "Golden Age", in that compound libraries are screened using high-throughput methods and inhibition of microbial growth at this stage is a precursor to further characterisation. The libraries from which most antibiotics were derived are soil organisms, but there are also untapped resources in the oceans, where there is a large number and range of micro-organisms and from plant extracts where a number of compounds have already been shown to possess antibacterial and/or antiviral activity. Examples are the extracts from the garlic and clove plants (Arora & Kaur, 1999). A range of spice plants were screened for activity and only these two extracts exhibited antimicrobial activity, however, they were active against a range of Gram positive and Gram negative bacteria and yeasts.

As an adjunct to antimicrobial compounds, we should also consider those compounds which modify activity of existing drugs. Such examples include ß-lactamase inhibitors such as clavulanic acid (used as a proprietary preparation in conjunction with amoxicillin and other ß-lactam antibiotics) and efflux inhibitors which maintain an elevated drug concentration within cells and hence improve antimicrobial efficacy.

3.2 Therapeutic antibodies

An alternative therapeutic approach to emerging infectious diseases is the use of antibodies to treat disease. This is a concept which has existed for a considerable time, however, only relatively recently have therapeutic antibodies really been used against infectious diseases. As of 2006, there were 20 therapeutic antibodies approved as therapeutics by the FDA (Das, 2006), but they offer considerable potential for the rapid treatment of emerging infectious diseases. One may question why this should be; the answer is straightforward, since protection from infection by pathogenic micro-organisms may be either active, and induced by immunization using prophylactic vaccines (see section 2.1), or passive. One of the issues discussed in section 2 was that prophylactic vaccines take a considerable time to make and formulate and these can be too slow for a pathogen with a high rate of reproduction (R_0) in a susceptible population. Passive immunity, where specific antibodies are administered, is a viable alternative here and also for the treatment of diseases where antimicrobial therapy may exacerbate the disease symptoms and also result in higher transmissibility (*e.g.* ulcerative colitis caused by *Clostridium difficile* infection and toxin). Many advances have been seen over the past decade which has allowed improved antibody engineering technologies along with improvements in safety and efficacy. These developments, along with a greater understanding of the immunomodulatory properties of antibodies, have paved the way for the next generation of new and improved antibody-based drugs for the treatment of human diseases. One major factor that makes this an attractive technology is that antibody "factories" can be rapidly turned around to produce a stock of antibodies for therapeutic use. This approach was recently described by Rogers *et al.* (2008) where they developed a panel of neutralising antibodies against the SARS coronavirus, a recently emerged pathogen, using a novel DNA display method. They describe their approach which involved panning the library using whole SARS virus rather than just the spike protein (which had been used by others, being a primary virulence factor for cell binding and entry). Other therapeutic antibody approaches in development include those to treat toxigenic effects following bacterial infection (*Clostridium difficile,* verotoxigenic *E.coli,* Anthrax toxin).

The use of therapeutic antibodies certainly holds much promise for the treatment of infectious diseases and is particularly attractive due to the rapidity that recombinant antibodies may be selected, produced and manufactured at scale.

3.3 Other therapeutics

There are a considerable number of other therapeutic approaches in development or at the research stage, far too many to comprehensively review here. Instead, we will concentrate on some of the key areas where there are noteworthy developments.

3.3.1 Therapeutic vaccines

Firstly, we will consider therapeutic vaccines. In section 2 previously, we have considered the use of vaccines for induction of prophylactic immunity. There is an alternative use of some vaccines, however, and this is for prophylaxis following exposure to an infectious disease micro-organism. A good example is the AIDS virus, HIV, which emerged in 1983 and for which, despite many attempts, there is no prophylactic vaccine. The Norwegian biotech company, Bionor Pharma recently released results from a study of its therapeutic HIV vaccine, Vacc-4x. There are recent data showing that the vaccine lowered patients' viral loads and negated the need for antiretroviral therapy (Fierce Vaccines, 2011).

3.3.2 Phage therapy

Phage therapy entails the use of bacteriophage viruses that infect bacteria for the treatment of bacterial infections. Phages are ubiquitously found in bacterial populations and control the growth of bacteria in many environments, including in the intestine, the oceans, and the soil. Phage therapy was in used in the 1920s and 1930s in the USA, Western & Eastern Europe, however, success rates of this therapy have never been firmly established, because only a limited number of clinical trials testing the efficacy of phage therapy have ever been conducted. These studies were performed mainly in the former Soviet Union. The development of antibacterial-resistant bacteria has once again sparked renewed interest in phage therapy with several companies, universities and foundations across the world now focusing on phage therapeutics. One of the main difficulties is that of delivery of the phage to the site of infection, making them potentially more suitable for treatment of respiratory or skin diseases than for deep-seated infections. There is also the safety concern about giving live viruses to human subjects.

3.3.3 Bacteriocins

Bacteriocins are peptides that can potentially be more readily engineered than small combinatorial chemistry generated molecules and are potential alternatives to conventional antibacterial compounds. Different classes of bacteriocins have different potential as therapeutic agents. Small-molecule bacteriocins (*e.g.* microcins and lantibiotics) are similar to the classic broad-spectrum antibiotics whereas colicin-like bacteriocins possess a much narrower activity spectrum, and require pathogen identification (and susceptibility testing) prior to therapy. Limitations of large-molecule antibacterials include reduced transport across membranes and within the human body. For this reason, they are usually used topically or gastrointestinally.

3.3.4 Chelation

A novel approach relies on the removal of essential nutrients for bacterial growth within the host by chelation. These compounds are not suitable for use alone, but may have utility in combination with conventional antibacterial compounds. A similar approach forms the basis of a treatment for lymphoblastic leukaemia, where bacterially-derived L-asparaginase is used as a therapeutic to remove L-asparagine, an essential amino acid for leukaemia cells to grow and divide, from the circulating blood stream and hence effectively "starving" the cancer cells.

3.3.5 Probiotics

Probiotics consist of live cultures of bacteria, which may become established as competing commensal organisms and thus inhibit or interfere with colonization by microbial pathogens. This approach has been used to reduce nasal carriage with Methicillin-resistant *Staphylococcus aureus* (MRSA) by replacement therapy using a skin commensal *Corynebacterium* sp. (Uehara *et al.* 2000).

4. Diagnostic tests

Diagnostic testing is not a therapeutic intervention, of course, but like other public health control measures, this chapter would be incomplete without mention of its use. In the early stages of an outbreak caused by any infectious disease pathogen, the public health control measures are inevitably supported by diagnostic testing. When a new disease emerges, the only factor that can be used for diagnosis is the clinical presentation. This is frequently compounded by the observation that many diseases present at the early stage with non-specific symptoms that are common with many less severe diseases. For example, the early symptoms of the SARS virus are very similar to many other respiratory infections caused by a range of viral pathogens, most of which do not require any intervention. Thus the power and value of a good diagnostic is in the differentiation of a pathogen causing severe infection from seasonally circulating infections of much lower consequence. Recently the Health Protection Agency undertook a study to model the value of rapid diagnostics development in the control of an outbreak caused by an emerging infectious disease (C. Noris & N. J. Silman, unpublished). The conclusion was that the diagnostic was of value only early in an outbreak when differential diagnosis was used to drive a policy of "containment" of the disease, that is, preventing onward transmission by preventing non-infected persons coming into contact with those who were infectious. Of course, quarantine cannot be enforced, but it was an effective tool used in controlling the spread of the H1N1 "swine" influenza pandemic during 2009. At the stage of the outbreak where containment is no longer possible, *i.e.* there are sufficiently high numbers of cases, then laboratory diagnosis ceases to have any real value in the CONTROL of the pandemic. That is not to say that it is of no value at all though.

5. Public health control measures

Although this chapter is focussing on the different therapeutic interventions that may be used to tackle the problems of emerging infectious diseases, it would be incomplete without mention of non-therapeutic means of controlling spread of infectious disease. In the initial stages of responding to an emergent infectious disease, the only tools available to limit spread of the disease and prevent nosocomial infection of clinical staff are non-therapeutic public health interventions. Perhaps the earliest described successful approach was in 1854 when John Snow removed the handle from a water pump in Broad Street, Soho, London. Before the discovery of pathogenic micro-organisms, Snow, a physician, was sceptical about the "miasma" theories that surrounded what we know to be infectious disease outbreaks. Miasma theory suggested that the cause of disease was a form of pollution or bad air. Snow carefully pieced together the evidence surrounding the distribution of the Cholera cases in the Soho area of London and concluded that the water pump in Broad Street was the common denominator; he removed the pump handle to prevent people from drawing and hence consuming water contaminated by *Vibrio cholerae* and very effectively curtailed the outbreak.

The same general, non-therapeutic approach may be taken with newly emerging diseases. For example, many of the diseases that have emerged in the last 30 years have an insect vector involved in the dissemination of the infectious disease pathogen (Jones *et al.*, 2008). The most effective intervention for vector-borne diseases is the eradication or reduction in the numbers of the insect vector using pesticides, rather than prophylaxis (not generally available) or therapeutics (Rose, 2001). Another recent example is the reduction in the numbers of cases of hospital acquired infection (HCAI). A contribution to this reduction is the reminder that good hand hygiene is vital and re-education of medical and nursing staff in the UK on good hand-washing practice, as well as the introduction of hand sanitizer gels (Grayson *et al.*, 2009). Thus these important interventions, although mostly quite simple can have very pronounced outcomes in the control of infectious diseases.

6. Conclusion

There are a number of therapeutic interventions that can be used to combat emerging infectious diseases. When a new pathogen emerges and subsequently causes a widespread outbreak, the interventions that can be applied differ during the course of the outbreak. At the early stage, recognition of the disease is heavily reliant upon clinical case definition, as was used in differentiating the new variant H1N1 influenza virus in 2009, prior to the development of a molecular diagnostic assay. We have seen that the development of a diagnostic assay is used in support of clinical case definition. The most effective interventions are therapeutic or prophylactic ones, however, since they are able to either treat those infected or protect onward spread by inducing herd immunity within a population. The downside of a therapeutic approach against a newly emerging disease is the length of time that is required to develop an effective vaccine or therapeutic against any specific pathogen. Here we require more generic, broad-spectrum interventions such as antimicrobials. What is evident is that more investment in R&D to discover new therapeutic molecules that can be used against newly emerging pathogens. Currently we are relatively well-served by the availability of broad-spectrum antibiotics, but increasingly widespread multi-drug resistance is a major problem and new chemotypes are urgently required. Perhaps the greatest hope is available by using recombinant antibody technology, where using the high-throughput genome sequencing approaches now available, we can rapidly sequence newly emerged pathogens, clone out and express surface antigens for rapid development of therapeutic antibody preparations. Many countries have invested heavily in infrastructure to build rapid vaccine facilities that can be turned around quickly in the event of the emergence of a new highly infectious pathogen and these sorts of adaptable facilities are of potentially great value in combating emerging infectious diseases.

7. References

Arora, D, S, & Kaur, J. (1999). Antimicrobial activity of spices. *Int. J. Antimicrob. Agents.* 12, pp. 257-262.

Barrett, A, D, T, Monath, T, P, Cropp, C, B, Adkins, J, A, Ledger, T, N, Gould, E, A, Schlesinger, J, J, Kinney, R, M, & Trent, D, W. (1990). Attenuation of wild-type yellow fever virus by passage in HeLa cells. *J. gen. Virol.* 71, pp. 2301-2306.

Beltrame, A, Angheben, A, Bisoffi, Z, Monteiro, G, Marocco, S, Calleri, G, Lipani, F, Gobbi, F, Canta, F, Castelli, F, Gulletta, M, Bigoni, S, Del Punta, V, Iacovazzi, T, Romi, R, Nicoletti, L, Grazia Ciufolini, M, Rorato, G, Negri, C, & Viale, P. (2007). Imported Chikungunya Infection, Italy. *Emerg. Inf. Dis.* 13, pp. 1264-1266.

Bradley, K, A, Mogridge, J, Mourez, M, Collier, R, J, & Young, J, A, T. (2001). Identification of the cellular receptor for anthrax toxin. *Nature* 414, pp. 225-229.

Campbell, G, L, Marfin, A, A, Lanciotti, R, L, & Duane J Gubler, D, J. (2002). West Nile Virus. *Lancet Inf. Dis.* 2, pp. 519-529.

Das, R, C. (2006). Antibody Therapeutics: Product Development, Market Trends, and Strategic Issues, Revised Edition. *Drug and Market Development Publishing.* Available from: http://www.researchandmarkets.com/reports/354677

DeStefano, F, & Thompson, W, W. (2004). MMR vaccine and autism: an update of the scientific evidence. *Ex. Rev. Vaccines* 3, pp. 19-22.

Donaldson, L. (2001). Getting Ahead of the Curve: A strategy for combating infectious diseases. *A Report by the Chief Medical Officer, Dept. of Health.* Available from: http://www.dh.gov.uk/en/Publicationsandstatistics/Publications/PublicationsP olicyAndGuidance/DH_4007697

ECDC Measles Surveillance Report. (2011). Eurpoean Monthly Measles Monitoring (EMMO). Available from: http://ecdc.europa.eu/en/publications/Publications/2011_June_measles_montly. pdf

Fierce Vaccines. (2011). Results From Phase IIB Placebo Controlled Study of Bionor Pharma's Vacc-4x Show Excellent Safety Profile. Available from: http://www.fiercebiotech.com/press-releases/results-phase-iib-placebo-controlled-study-bionor-pharmas-vacc-4x-show-exce

Grayson, M, L, Melvani, S, Druce, J, Barr, I, G, Ballard, S, A, Johnson, P, D, R, Mastorakos, T, & Birch, C. (2009). Efficacy of Soap and Water and Alcohol-Based Hand-Rub Preparations against Live H1N1 Influenza Virus on the Hands of Human Volunteers. *Clin. Inf. Dis.* 48, pp. 285-291.

Jones, K E, , Patel, N G, Levy, M A, Storeygard, A, Balk, D, Gittleman, J L, & Daszak, P. (2008). Global trends in emerging infectious diseases. *Nature,* 451, pp. 990-994, doi:10.1038/nature06536.

Kew, O, Sutter R, de Gourville, E, Dowdle, W, & Pallansch, M (2005). Vaccine-derived polioviruses and the endgame strategy for global polio eradication. *Annu Rev Microbiol.* 59, pp. 587–635. PMID 16153180

Lombard, M, Pastoret, P P, & Moulin A M. (2007). A brief history of vaccines and vaccination. *Rev Sci Tech*. 26, pp. 29-48. PMID: 17633292

Marinelli, F. (2009). Antibiotics and *Streptomyces:* the future of antibiotic discovery. *Microbiology Today* February 2009. Available from: http://www.sgm.ac.uk/pubs/micro_today/pdf/020903.pdf

Montomoli, E, Capecchi, B, & Hoschler, K. (2011). Correlates of protection against influenza. In *Influenza Vaccines for the Future*. Eds: Rappuoli, R & Del Giudice, G. pp. 199-222. Springer. Retrieved from http://www.springerlink.com/content/p2l4v614p282h828/

Pearce, J (2004). Salk and Sabin: poliomyelitis immunisation. *J Neurol Neurosurg Psychiatry* 75, pp. 1552. PMID 15489385

Reddy, T, R, K, Mutter, R, Heal, W, Guo, K, Gillet, V,J, Pratt, S & Chen, B. (2006). Library Design, Synthesis, and Screening: Pyridine Dicarbonitriles as Potential Prion Disease Therapeutics. *J. Med. Chem.* 49, pp. 607-615.

Rogers, J, Schoepp, R, J, Schröder, O, Clements, T, L, Holland, T, F, Li, J, Q, Lewis, L, M, Dirmeier, R, P, Frey, G, J, Tan, X, Wong, K, Woddnutt, G, Keller, M, Reed, D, S, Kimmel, B, E, & Tozer, E, C. (2008) rapid discovery and optimization of therapeutic antibodies against emerging infectious diseases. *Prot. Eng. Des. Sel.* 21, pp. 495-505.

Rose, R, I. (2001). Pesticides and public health: integrated methods of mosquito management. *Emerg. Inf. Dis.* 7, pp. 7-23.

Taylor, L H, Latham, S M, & Woolhouse, M E J. (2001). Risk factors for human disease emergence. *Phil. Trans. R. Soc. Lond.*, 356, pp. 983-989.

Uehara, Y, Nakama, H, Agematsu, K, Uchida, M, Kawakami, Y, Abdul Fattah, A, S, M, & Maruchi, N. (2000). Bacterial interference among nasal inhabitants: eradication of *Staphylococcus aureus* from nasal cavities by artificial implantation of *Corynebacterium* sp. *J. Hosp. Inf.* 44, pp. 127-133.

World Health Organisation. (1999). Emerging issues in water and infectious diseases. *A Report by the World Health Organisation*. Available from: http://www.who.int/water_sanitation_health/emerging/emergingissues/en/

5

Oxidative Stress in Human Health and Disease

Isaac K. Quaye
University of Botswana School of Medicine,
Faculty of Medicine and Health Sciences, Gaborone,
Botswana

1. Introduction

Oxidative stress arises when the antioxidant capacity of cells to scavenge the excess production of reactive oxygen species(ROS) falls short. It may also be due to changes in the redox status of the cell. In health, pro-oxidants engage in useful signaling pathways that are important for growth and cellular health. Overstimulation of signaling pathways leads to sustained pro-oxidant production in the form of ROS that disrupt cellular structures and impair function leading to disease. Normally, antioxidants counteract the activity of pro-oxidants to retain cellular homeostasis and therefore a state of health.

In this review the cellular sources of reactive oxygen species (ROS) will be discussed in addition to its effect on macromolecular structures, cellular function and health. The ROS referred to in the text are:superoxide, hydrogen peroxide, hydroxyl radicals; reactive nitrogen species (RNS) nitric oxide and peroxynitrite.

The primary source of ROS is molecular oxygen (O_2). In aerobic cells during electron transport about 10% of reducing equivalents from NADH leaks to produce superoxide (O_2^- ·) and hydrogen peroxide (H_2O_2). These diffuse out of mitochondria and form the starting materials for subsequent generation of ROS through a serial one electron acceptor process. RNS (NO) also fuel ROS generation through a similar interaction with cytochrome c oxidase to give rise to O_2^-·/H_2O_2 or react with O_2^- ·to generate peroxynitrite (ONOO-).

The oxidative stress effect on health is discussed from the point of view of infectious/communicable diseases, non-infectious/non communicable diseases, genetic diseases and oxidant stress factors (mutation/hemolysis).

The respective infectious/communicable and non communicable diseases that are discussed are malaria, HIV/AIDS, and diabetes, obesity, sickle cell disease and ageing. Except for ageing, the biology of the diseases is briefly outlined and host immunological responses to the disease state that augments ROS generation and its effects are discussed.

The review ends with a brief on oxidative stress and ageing and a summary of how oxidative stress is at the core of the physiological processes that maintain a healthy body and longevity.

2. ROS activity in normal cell function

The designation 'reactive oxygen species' refers to the unpaired electrons on an oxygen atom, molecule or ion that confers reactivity to the species (1, 2). By this definition oxygen molecule is the weakest radical as the ground state has two unpaired electrons (1) although it is unreactive. Multicellular organisms maintain a network of signals to ensure growth, defense and repair. These signals begin outside of the cell, with ligand receptor interaction, followed by conformational changes in the receptor that enables it to be activated through phosphorylation by kinases and inhibition of phosphatases (3, 4). The signal is then carried by second messengers for transduction into the cell nucleus (5, 6). Transcription factors constitute the terminal signal receivers to initiate gene expression critical for normal cell function. ROS act as second messengers in signal transduction in normal housekeeping cell functions (7, 8). ROS signaling can also be through regulation of ion channels, in particular potassium and calcium ion channels to modulate nerve conduction and apoptosis (9).

In normal cell function ROS is generated constitutively by non-phagocytic cells and in response to injury, trauma or infection by phagocytic cells (10, 11). A common functional attribute of the two sources of ROS is that moderate amounts is largely associated with signaling activity while increasing amounts is important in cellular defense and or repair (12). Moderate amounts of ROS are generated through electron transport, vascular smooth muscle cell (VSMC) and endothelial cell (EC) activities (13). Other cellular sources of ROS that may be limited by the changes in cellular metabolic activity include lipoxygenases, cyclooxygenase, cytochrome P450 enzyme activities and lipid peroxidation (7).

2.1 ROS generation in non phagocytic conditions

Non phagocytic generation of superoxide occurs constitutively and intracellularly in fibrobrast , smooth muscle cells (14), renal mesanglial cells (15), hematopoietic stem cells, neurons, hepatocytes, vascular endothelium and for the cellular organelles mitochondria, peroxisomes and the cytochrome P450 system. When generated, ROS participate in the maintenance of baseline signal transduction needed for normal cell function in the absence of activation (16-18). The non phagocytic oxidases (NOX) are transmembrane proteins that transport electrons across cell membranes to reduce oxygen to superoxide. To date six human isoforms have been isolated (Nox 1, 3, 4, 5, and Duox 1 and 2) (19, 20). They utilize a system that is dependent on NADPH, although, NADH can also be used as substrate (21). As a result they are referred to as NAD(P)H oxidases (12, 22). A large component of the non-phagocytic ROS is from mitochondria during electron transport under normal physiological conditions (23). The primary ROS is superoxide generated from reduction of oxygen. It has a short half-life and so its availability is limited, making it a poor signaling molecule (24). In low pH environments as in phagosomes however, the reactivity of superoxide is enhanced by conversion to hydrogen peroxide (25). Unlike superoxide, hydrogen peroxide which is generated from superoxide dismutation (26), is stable and can selectively diffuse through membrane pores to stimulate distant targets, including downstream kinases (27, 28). It also activates the antioxidant function of p53 which potentiates the activity of glutathione peroxidase to convert it to water (29). A summary of ROS generation in the mitochondria in normal physiology and some effects attributed to ROS is presented in Figure 1.

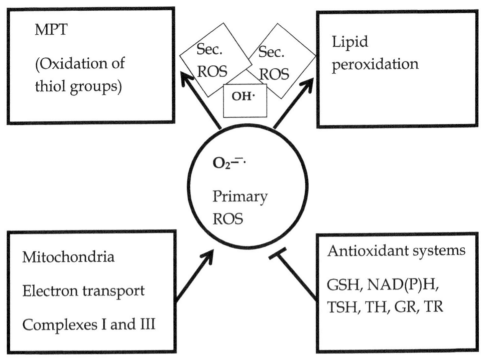

Fig. 1. Mitochondrial ROS generation sites by partial reduction of oxygen through a series of one electron acceptance and a role in oxidative stress effects.

2.2 ROS generation in the electron transport chain

At the end of the electron transport chain, molecular oxygen receives 4 electrons and is reduced to water providing energy for ATP synthesis. When oxygen is incompletely oxidized through the sequential acceptance of one electron, it gives rise to oxygen radicals that are more reactive than the molecule. These are in order of one electron acceptance, O_2^-; H_2O_2 and OH (30, 31). Acquisition of an electron by molecular oxygen generates $O_2^-\cdot$ as the primary ROS. The sites in the electron transport chain known to significantly contribute to ROS are complex I and III. Complex I ROS production is mediated by NADH coenzyme Q reductase while in complex III ROS production is through the binding of NO to ubiquinol cytochrome c oxidase to produce $O_2^-\cdot$ and H_2O_2 (31-33). Mitochondrial nitric oxide synthase produces NO, the primary RNS which reacts with $O_2^-\cdot$ to give peroxynitrite. Therefore NO production is central to the generation of $O_2^-\cdot$ and H_2O_2 in the electron transport chain (34, 35). Mitochondria also functions as an oxygen sensor under hypoxia to produce hydrogen peroxide which stabilizes hypoxia inducible factor (HIF) to modulate its effect on hypoxia (36-38). HIF is degraded by the hydroxylation of prolyl residues and requires iron as an obligatory cofactor, so when ROS oxidizes iron, it is unavailable for hydroxylation thereby retaining cellular response to hypoxia (38). In normal cellular metabolism, low to moderate ROS/RNS are generated as part of the signaling pathways, cellular response to growth and in innate and adaptive immune response against danger signals (39).

2.3 ROS generation in VSMC and EC

ROS generation in non-phagocytic cells other than mitochondria, is through the activity of non-phagocytic NAD(P)H oxidase (Nox) following ligand binding to the cognate receptor (cytokines, growth factor and G-protein coupled receptor agonists, e.g. angiotensin II) (40, 41). Of particular note is the binding of vascular endothelial growth factor (VEGF), platelet derived growth factor and epidermal growth factor (EGF) to their cognate receptors that lead to receptor dimerization, auto-phosphorylation and signaling to activate redox sensitive transcription factors (eg. NF-κB) responsible for the expression of target genes (40).

2.4 Functional significance of ROS/RNS generation

ROS generated by non-phagocytic cells channel signals to induce cell migration, proliferation and vessel wall formation (42). This activity is particularly important for angiogenesis and in ischemia/reperfusion response (27). In order to sustain signal transduction, ROS generated from ligand receptor interactions can oxidize cysteine residues in phosphatases to inhibit their function and sustain signal transduction to the nucleus (43, 44). Within the endothelial cell (EC), hydrogen peroxide or angiotensin II (Ang II) stimulation of ROS production activates eNOS to produce NO which facilitates cell migration and proliferation (2, 45, 46).

2.5 ROS and danger sensing

The cells of the innate immune system sense danger by recognizing highly conserved pathogen associated molecular patterns (PAMP) present on all the major pathogens; bacteria, parasites, viruses and yeast, or danger associated molecular patterns (DAMP) through germ line encoded pattern recognition receptors (PRR) (47-50). While PAMP enables ROS generation in response to an infection, DAMP enables cellular response to danger (damage, stress) in the absence of an infection (51-53). These molecules that signal cell damage or stress include ATP, nucleotides and uric acid (54). Through ligand receptor interactions and phagocytosis, ROS signaling molecules (hydrogen peroxide and superoxide) are generated intracellularly to promote signaling cascades on one hand and/or activate inflammasome (55). The inflammasome is a descriptive term for cytosolic pattern recognition receptors belonging to members of the caspase-1 activating platform, nucleotide oligomerization domain (NOD) like receptor family (NLR) or AIM2 DNA binding proteins (56, 57). The proteins activate the expression of pro-inflammatory cytokines (IL-1β and IL-18) necessary to amplify ROS generation against pathogen elimination or containment through pyroptosis (57, 58). ROS can be generated extracellularly when a ligand binds to a receptor. This source of phagocytic ROS is through NADPH oxidase, largely in neutrophils engaged in phagocytosis, when activated by PAMP. Activated neutrophils undergo a burst of ROS production to eliminate the offending organism (59).

3. ROS in oxidative stress

Oxidative stress arises when the activity of oxidant species (ROS) overwhelms the cells capacity to counteract with antioxidants (60-65). In oxidative stress, excess ROS (O_2^-, H_2O_2, OH·) are involved in three main activities:

a. Causing damage to cellular macromolecules (DNA, proteins and membrane lipids) due to their chemical reactivity,

b. Causing changes in membrane potential, which in the inner mitochondrial membrane directly causes mitochondrial permeability transition (MTP) and

c. Acting as a sink for cellular antioxidants.

Whereas superoxide and hydrogen peroxide target Fe-S clusters and cysteine residues respectively, hydroxyl radical appears to be indiscriminate on targets, including oxidation of thiol groups in membrane proteins, making it the most damaging oxygen species (66-68).

a. ROS effect on macromolecules

DNA damage

The type of DNA damage attributed to ROS species may fall into several forms: single and double strand breaks; (69), sister chromatid exchange, DNA-DNA and DNA protein cross links and base modifications (71). Single strand breaks may be due to oxidation of phosphodiester bonds by direct abstraction of hydrogen by OH· from the deoxyribose-phosphodiester backbone giving rise to abnormal 3′ and 5′ ends which are not recognized by DNA polymerases (72). The bases may undergo hydroxylation or part of the ring may open up particularly for pyrimidine bases (73). Hydroxyl radicals also interact with DNA bases to form adducts. For instance reaction with guanine generates 8-oxo-7,8-dihydro-2′-deoxyguanosine (8-oxodG) adducts (74). Peroxynitrites generated from the reaction between NO and superoxide also react with guanine to form adducts (8-nitodG) (66, 71, 75, 76). The formation of DNA adducts can lead to loss of the bases giving rise to apurinic or apyrimidinic (AP) sites (77, 78). These adducts also contribute to accelerated telomere shortening, which regulates senescence. They can also lead to G→T transversion and microsatellite instability, a recipe for cell transformation (79). ROS attacks DNA to form hydroperoxides and peroxides (80-82). Lipid peroxidation by ROS is mediated through the Fenton reaction ($Fe^{2+} + H_2O_2 = Fe^{3+} + OH·$) to produce lipid hydroperoxides (LOOH) and 4-hydroxynonenal (4-HNE) (1, 67, 83). These reactive metabolites impair membrane function and lead to changes in Ca^{2+} flux (84). They also serve as signaling molecules for activating or inhibiting apoptosis through the activity of serine/threonine kinase Akt in the PI3K/Akt pathway (85). Lipid peroxides are the major end products for stress induced oxidative damage that mediate apoptosis (86).

Protein damage

Oxidative ROS damage of proteins can lead to disruption of several vital cellular activities such as replication, transcription, and protein synthesis (78, 87, 88). The breakdown of amino acids occurs largely through the reactivity of hydroxyl radicals. Hydroxyl radical is generated by Fenton Chemistry through superoxide in the Haber-Weiss reaction ($O_2^- + H_2O_2 \rightarrow O_2 + ·OH + OH^-$) (88). It attacks amino acids abstracting hydrogen atom from the alpha carbon to generate the alkyl radical as the primary radical (89). This then undergoes a series of reactions to generate alkyl peroxide and alkoxyl radicals. These radicals not only disrupt the protein backbone but also engage in peptide bond cleavages to disrupt protein function (90). ROS can also oxidize almost all amino acid side chains, in particular sulphur containing amino acids, cysteine and methionine (1, 91). Other well-known targets are glutamyl and prolyl side chains to induce peptide bond cleavage. RNS also contribute to amino acid oxidation (nitration of tyrosine residues, nitrosation of cysteine sulfhydryl groups and oxidation of methionine) through the activity of peroxynitrite generated from a reaction between NO and superoxide (87). Oxidized amino acids have a higher tendency to cross link which affects folding and function. A major physiological impact of protein oxidation is accelerated ageing (92-94). This is attributed to increased degradation of oxidized proteins, limiting function (83, 87, 91, 95).

b. ROS and changes in mitochondrial membrane potential

Oxidation of mitochondrial membrane sulfhydryl groups is associated with membrane permeability transitional states (65). Mitochondrial membrane permeability transition (MPT) occurs when the inner membrane becomes non selectively permeable leading to accumulation of Ca^{2+}, loss of matrix components, impairment in mitochondrial function, excessive fluid accumulation and outer membrane burst (64, 96, 97). This leads to loss of cytochrome c and a drive towards apoptosis (96, 97). Currently, it has been shown that changes in mitochondrial redox status due to oxidation of NAD(P)H by ROS serves as the starting point for MPT (64, 98). NAD(P)H is critical for maintaining mitochondrial redox status through reduction of oxidized glutathione (GSSH) and thioredoxin (TSSH) necessary for reducing thiol groups in the inner membrane (27, 99, 100). Oxidized thiol groups in membrane proteins, cross link and aggregate to form the non selective permeability pores that disrupt mitochondrial function (101).

4. ROS in infectious diseases

4.1 Oxidative stress in malaria

Malaria is caused by parasites belonging to the genus *Plasmodium*. In humans four major species are responsible for the disease: *P. falciparum*, *P. vivax*, *P. ovale*, and *P. malariae* (102). Recently, *P. knowlesi* has been shown to be a major cause of malaria in parts of South East Asia (Borneo) (103, 104).The parasites are obligate and belong to the Phylum Apicomplexa (105). *P. falciparum* accounts for most severe malaria globally (106). The major vector for parasite transmission is the female anopheline mosquito (107). During a blood meal, sporozoites are inoculated under the skin and travel through the blood stream, liver sinusoids to settle in a hepatocyte after traversing several (108-111). This journey usually takes approximately 1 hour (112). Each sporozoite in a parasitophorous vacuole in the liver divides to generate between 10,000 to 30,000 merozoites (110). In *P. ovale*, *P. malariae*, and *P. vivax* some sporozoites turn to hypnozoites which can remain dormant for months or several years and then get reactivated (113, 114). Merozoite maturation occurs within two weeks in a process called tissue shizogony. The merozoites invade RBCs and develop into ring forms, trophozoites and blood schizonts which repeat the cycle of RBC invasion leading to significant hemolysis. The cycle repeats every 48 hours for *P. falciparum*, *P. ovale*, and *P vivax* called tertian malaria and every 72 hours for *P. malariae* called quartan malaria. Each RBC can harbor up to 20 trophozoites. Following a cycle of blood schizogony some merozoites develop into gametocytes which are the sexual forms. These are taken up in a next meal to undergo sexual reproduction and eventually generate sporozoites ready for inoculation(115) .

4.2 Generation of ROS in plasmodium infection

When Plasmodium species infects an individual, the clinical presentation may be described as uncomplicated (asymptomatic or mild) or complicated (severe). In uncomplicated malaria host exposure to the parasite is significant enough to generate protective immunity such that the parasite burden is limited (116). This is usually seen in endemic areas (116, 117). In contrast, in low endemicity and low parasite exposure, because of lack or low host immune response, infection can lead to severe disease. It has been shown that whether an infection is uncomplicated or severe, there is a higher generation of ROS that is host and parasite derived (118). Host derived ROS generation arises from interaction of parasite ligands with host receptors during sporozoite invasion leading to phagocytosis and activation of NADPH dependent oxidases for ROS release (119). In addition polymorphonuclear neutrophil attraction to the site of infection and activation is associated with significant release of ROS as a defense mechanism for parasite clearance (120-122). This mechanism also occurs during blood schizogony to inhibit merozoite invasion of RBCs. During the period of blood schizogony, significant quantities of heme are released into circulation that overwhelms the scavenging activity of hemopexin, so that free heme is available to induce further neutrophil migration and catalyze its activation (123). Free heme also binds to and oxidizes lipoproteins in membranes increasing RBC breakdown (124, 125). Malaria parasites release a large quantity of ROS in the infected RBC in the process of converting heme to hemozoin for heme detoxification (126). It has been shown that hemozoin (Pf, Hz) mediates peroxidation of unsaturated fatty acids and contributes to the production of 4-hydroxynonenal (HNE) which reacts with proteins to form adducts disrupting their function (127). The impact of disrupted protein function is down regulation of receptors required for gene expression and cell division. This is suggested to be a factor in decreased erythropoiesis and malaria induced anemia. An additional source of ROS recently identified is from infected rbc membrane microparticles which enable activation of macrophages and increase ROS generation.

4.3 Oxidative stress in HIV infection

The classical pathway of HIV infection is through binding of the envelope glycoprotein to CD4+ cells mediated by the coreceptors CXCR4 and CCR5 chemokine receptors (128) .HIV-1 isolates that replicate primarily in activated CD4 T-lymphocytes in vitro are said to be T-tropic whereas isolates replicating in primary macrophages are M-tropic (129). Dual tropism is shown by isolates with the ability to infect both cells efficiently. CXCR4 and CCR5 act as coreceptors for T-tropic and M-tropic isolates respectively (129-131). CCR5 target cells appear to be important in the early phase of transmission switching to CXCR4 as the disease progresses (129, 132). For the most part however both receptors are expressed on known target cells (CD4+ T cells, monocyte/macrophages, dendritic cells, Langerhans cells and rectal and vagina mucosa) (133). Recently it has been shown that HIV-1 can be transmitted into cells directly by a tunneling mechanism independent of receptor functions (134). HIV-1 has been divided into nine subtypes called clade A-D, F-H, J and K based on variation in the viral envelope. Clade B is predominant in Europe, the Americas and Australia, while the rest are found in Africa and Asia (135).

A common comorbidity in HIV infection is dementia, which is a combination of behavioral, cognitive, and motor dysfunction following HIV infection (134, 136). It is estimated that in adults below the age of 40, HIV accounts for the most cause of dementia (137, 138). Data accumulated to date shows that oxidative stress is an underlying cause of HIV associated dementia (HAD) (139). Brain polyunsaturated fatty acids readily undergo peroxidation by free radicals to generate the 4-HNE which breaks bonds in cysteine, histidine and lysine residues to disrupt protein function (140). 4-HNE also disrupts mitochondrial function to generate ROS aggravating oxidative stress in the process (141). Lipid peroxidation and protein oxidation also contribute to the generation of carbonyl groups, which characterize HIV dementia (142, 143). Some of the proteins that are affected due to lipid peroxidation include ATPases and glucose transporters. HIV regulatory protein Tat and structural protein gp120 are known to exert neurotoxicity by increasing ROS generation and lipid peroxidation (140). HIV gp41 is documented to induce iNOS expression and NO generation to react with superoxide forming peroxynitrite. Peroxynitrites cause nitration of tyrosine residues to disrupt protein function while its decomposition gives rise to hydroxyl radicals, a highly potent lipid peroxidizing agent (138). Over production of NO has been suggested to also increase HIV-1 replication. HIV-1 infection not only causes an increase in ROS generation but also leads to depletion of protective antioxidants in particular, glutathione (138, 144). Thus HIV disease is characterized by chronic oxidative stress which drives disease pathogenesis.

5. ROS in non communicable diseases

5.1 ROS in type 2 diabetes

Diabetes is a metabolic disease caused by derangement in carbohydrate and lipid metabolism due to defects in insulin secretion, action or both (145). Two major forms are defined, type 1 and 2. Type 1 is due to an absolute deficiency in insulin secretion attributed to autoimmune destruction of the β cells of the Islet and genetic factors (145, 146). Type 2 is a combination of insulin resistance and inadequate compensatory insulin secretory response. It is now confirmed that diabetes is an inflammatory disease with elevated plasma concentrations of IL-6, CRP, orosomucoid and sialic acid (146-148).

5.2 ROS in pancreatic β cell damage

In type 1 diabetes β cell damage partly initiates from cellular response to the danger signal, dsRNA which leads to overexpression of Toll like receptors (TLR3, 4). The TLR then activates redox sensitive transcriptions factors including NF-kB (149).The major source of ROS in pancreatic β cells is from mitochondria and activity of non phagocytic NADPH oxidase (98, 150, 151). When ROS generation is high, the β cell which is known to have lower levels of antioxidants (catalase, glutathione peroxidase and superoxide dismutase) compared to other cell types is damaged leading to decreased insulin secretion. It is also reported that autoimmune activities fuel an inflammatory phenotype to damage β cells. In insulin sensitive tissues glucose is transported intracellularly by specific membrane transporters (GLUT). Once inside the cell glucose is phosphorylated by glucokinase and goes through the glycolytic pathway (152, 153). Increased glycolytic activity feeds into higher ATP production, closure of K+ channels and increased intracellular Ca^{2+} which can stimulate ROS generation by mitochondria (153). The increased Ca^{2+} flux can also promote NADPH oxidase activity to produce more ROS (154). As previously noted, low levels of ROS generated by glucose metabolism, is important for glucose stimulated insulin secretion while higher levels damage β cells of the Islets and induce insulin resistance through activation of redox sensitive intracellular signaling pathways (6). Changes in glucose and lipid metabolism contribute to ROS generation through the formation of diacylglycerol (DAG), advanced glycation end products (AGE), increased polyol formation and increased hexosamine pathway flux (155, 156). The polyol pathway involves the conversion of glucose to sorbitol when hyperglycemia persists. Metabolism of sorbitol generates fructose in a dehydrogenation reaction so that the NADH/NAD+ ratio increase favoring DAG synthesis. DAG potently stimulates protein kinase C, for activating non phagocytic NADPH oxidases (157). In addition increase in mitochondrial NADH/NAD ratio increases the proton gradient and probability of electron donation to molecular oxygen to generate superoxide (156). The β cell is insulin independent for glucose uptake so under elevated plasma glucose, the cells fail to down regulate glucose entry by insulin resistance. Free available reducing sugars (eg.glucose), can react with free amino groups to form a Schiffs base which rearranges into an Amadori glycation product (158-160). When accumulated in proteins, these AGEs modify protein function and or contribute to generation of ROS thereby damaging the cell (151). Another mechanism is the hexosamine pathway flux which functions under normal metabolism but is increased under hyperglycemia. In this process glucose metabolism in glycolysis is channeled into glucosamine phosphate from fructose 6-phosphate. The end product of the pathway is UDP-N-acetylglucosamine, which acts as a substrate for glycosylation of intracellular proteins, including transcription factors (161). Therefore, the expression of several genes including insulin is affected.

5.3 ROS and insulin resistance

In general insulin resistance leads to a sustained inflammatory state (162). Overt insulin resistance occurs from an initial impairment in insulin mediated glucose up take (IGT) (146, 163, 164). If this state is sustained, the impaired insulin response becomes blunted to constitute resistance (146, 164-166). In the end the blunted response leads to overt type 2 diabetes as glucose uptake is severely compromised leading to derangement in lipid metabolism (167, 168). Target tissues (muscle and adipose tissues) may fail to respond to insulin because of the diminished secretion or decreased sensitivity. Hyperglycemia, raised serum free fatty acids (FFA) and increased inflammatory phenotype indicated by high TNFα, CRP, IL-6 and IL-1β ((165, 167, 169) predominate in insulin resistance. High FFAs repress translocation of GLUT4 transporters to the plasma membrane and resistance to insulin mediated glucose uptake in muscle and adipose tissues, particularly (167). High FFA gives rise to elevated fatty acid metabolites; DAG, ceramides and fatty acyl CoA which activate protein kinase C resulting in activation of serine/threonine cascades (170). In skeletal muscle and adipose tissue the insulin receptor is phosphorylated at tyrosine sites upon binding by insulin (171, 172). The receptor in turn causes phosphorylation of substrates: insulin receptor substrate 1 and 2 (IRS1 and IRS2), which activates PI3-kinase, Akt/protein kinase B to recruit GLUT4 to the plasma membrane for glucose uptake ((167, 173). Elevated lipid metabolites scuttle this mechanism, and instead cause phosphorylation of serine sites on insulin receptor substrates, which inhibit their activation of phosphatidyl-inositol 3-kinase (PI3-kinase) and induce failure of transport of GLUT4 to the cell membrane (150, 171, 174). Also these metabolites decrease downstream signaling activities whereby insulin receptor substrates are activated for insulin secretion and response. ROS can also mediate these responses by inhibiting insulin receptor substrates 1 and 2 (IRS-1, and IRS-2) tyrosine auto-phosphorylation, while increasing phosphorylation of serine sites (173-175). Inhibition of tyrosine phosphorylation limits gene expression, cell growth and differentiation of the Islets.

5.4 ROS in obesity

Obesity is defined as a body mass index greater than or equal to 30 kg/m^2 (176). It is established to be a state of chronic low grade inflammatory disease (meta-inflammation) grouped together with insulin resistance, type 2 diabetes, cardiovascular disease and fatty liver disease as the metabolic syndrome (167). Excess calories stored in adipose tissue, causes it to expand, accompanied by infiltration of macrophages (176-179). The macrophages drive production of pro-inflammatory cytokines (TNFα, IL-6. iNOS, TGF-β, MCP-1) through toll like receptor 4 (TLR4) and so present the inflammatory phenotype (176, 180). In addition, increasing adiposity is associated with changes in the expression of adipokines (leptin, adiponectin, IL-6, resistin and TNF-α) which regulate energy intake and insulin sensitivity (176). With the exception of adiponectin, the expression of all the adipokines is increased with increasing fat mass (166, 178, 181). Adiponectin promotes insulin sensitivity by reducing fat and glucose storage. In Obese individuals, insulin resistance is characterized by upregulation of TNF-α by resident macrophages, a mechanism that is similar to that seen in type 2 diabetes (177). The location of the increased fat mass is known to affect the degree of inflammation. While visceral adipocity exacerbates, lower body fat mass has limited effect (177, 182). Enhanced DAG synthesis also affects downstream signaling pathways required to synthesize protein for Islet cell differentiation. As result islet cell differentiation is limited; this in turn affects insulin secretion and regulation of metabolic pathways (173).

5.5 ROS in sickle cell disease

Sickle cell disease arises from a mutation in the beta globin gene with substitution of glutamate for lysine at the 6th codon of β-globin to give hemoglobin S (HbS) variant (183-185). A homozygous HbSS is referred to as sickle cell anemia, while a heterozygous globin mutant with HbS constitutes sickle cell disease (186). The abnormal Hb has defining characteristics: it undergoes polymerization under low oxygen tension, precipitates when polymerized leading to generation of ROS which oxidizes the rbc membrane and makes it fragile and brittle (187). In sickle cell disease, the vascular endothelium becomes dysfunctional and shows increased inflammatory state, adhesiveness, and activation, concomitant with decreased NO bioavailability (188, 189). The disease makes subjects amenable to ischemic stroke, ischemia reperfusion injury, chronic renal disease, pulmonary hypertension, priapism, fetal wastage and growth retardation (190).

The propensity towards sickling is greatly enhanced if the transit time of rbc in the capillaries is increased. In the inflammatory state such delays become common place leading to severer hemolytic episodes and 'crisis'. Sickle cell anemia has high hemolytic episodes. The average life span of a normal rbc of 120 reduces to 14 days in sickle cell disease (190). The enhanced hemolysis contributes significantly to instigate a proinflammatory phenotype as free heme and hemoglobin are strong oxidants (191). Heme can donate electrons or Fe to membrane lipids through the fenton reaction to generate ROS that contributes to membrane damage and sustained hemolysis(188). Under sustained hemolytic conditions, the cellular mechanisms for scavenging hemoglobin and heme are overwhelmed (haptoglobin and hemopexin respectively) so that free heme and Hb are present intravascularly to initiate inflammation (192, 193). Extravascular hemolysis arising from ineffective scavenging of rbcs worn out or damaged, and ineffective erythropoiesis also contribute to heme and Hb leak into circulation. So in essence, sickle cell anemia is a typical systemic proinflammatory disease with sustained ROS production. Typical sources of ROS include activated NADPH oxidases from activated monocytes and endothelium, increased Xanthine oxidase expression and diminished NO availability (194, 195, 196). Activated endothelium increase expression of adhesion molecules for binding leukocytes and rbcs which contribute to hemostasis, rbc lysis and increased inflammatory phenotype (194).

5.6 ROS and endothelial dysfunction

The endothelium is the organ situated at the interface between the wall of the blood vessel and blood stream, functioning as a sensor for modulating vasomotor function, hemostasis and inflammation (197). Endothelial dysfunction refers to impairment of these functions associated with vascular remodeling and vascular growth, but more commonly to impairment of endothelium dependent vasodilation due to depletion of NO in the vessel wall (198). The factors released by the endothelium may lead to vasodilation or constriction. Some of these factors are NO, prostacycling, C-type natriuretic peptide, and endothelium derived hyper polarizing factors which act as vasodilators. ROS along with Ang II, endothelin 1 (ET-1) and thromboxane A_2, act as vasoconstrictors and up regulate adhesion molecules, intercellular adhesion molecule (ICAM-I), vascular cell adhesion molecule (VCAM-I) and E-selectin (197). The major sources of ROS in the endothelium are mitochondria, lipoxygenases, cyclooxygenases, cytoP450s, xanthine oxidases and NADPH oxidases (2, 14, 198, 199).

5.7 NO depletion and endothelium

In endothelial dysfunction NO synthesis is reduced. This affects vasodilation, inflammation and hemostasis. NO synthesis is by eNOS using L-arginine as substrate in the endothelium. Suggested mechanism for reduced NO synthesis is substrate unavailability, reduced eNOS synthase activity and quenching of NO when synthesized (200-204). ROS constitutes a major quencher of NO bioavailability. Reaction of NO with superoxide generates peroxynitrite which in turn reacts with proteins, lipids, and eNOS cofactor tetrahydrobiopterin (BH_4). By oxidizing BH_4 to generate BH_2, eNOS synthase activity is uncoupled, so that instead of producing NO, more ROS is generated from increased reductase activity of eNOS (199, 205). ROS up regulates the expression of adhesion molecules, ICAM-1, VCAM-1 and chemoattractant molecules (MCP-1) for neutrophil and macrophage attraction and activation (206, 207). eNOS synthase may also be competitively inhibited by asymmetric dimethylarginine (ADMA). It has been shown that increased ADMA concentration correlates with high blood pressure (BP) as renal plasma flow is impaired while flow resistance is increased leading to high BP (208, 209). As protein degradation increases in the cell, ADMA concentration also rises and is excreted in the kidneys or degraded to citrulline by the enzyme dimethylarginine dimethylaminohydrolase (DDAH) (208, 210, 211). As DDAH concentration increases in the cell, ADMA levels correspondingly decrease, associated with increased eNOS activation and reduced BP (211). Recently, the degree of endothelial dysfunction has been shown to inversely correlate with amount of endothelial progenitor cells in circulation. Endothelial progenitor cells have the capacity to develop into endothelial cells and are used to repair endothelial lesions (212, 213).

5.8 ROS in ageing

The free radical theory of ageing postulates that accumulated cellular damage by ROS over a period of time is associated with shortened life span (214). This includes effect on telomere shortening, dementia, accumulation of glycation end products and changes in signaling pathways that affect cellular function. A rise in the intracellular ROS generation as outlined previously damages cells, macromolecules and affects signaling pathways (1, 39, 214). These cumulatively drive cellular ageing.

6. Summary

Cumulative evidence shows that ROS is like a 'double edged sword' that on one side enables normal physiological cellular functions to be sustained and provides defense against invading organisms. However when in excess shown as oxidative stress, it plays a destructive role leading to cellular damage, senescence or death. These life attributes make ROS an essential investigative target in the biochemistry and physiology of health and pathological mechanisms of disease.

7. References

[1] Valko M, Leibfritz D, Moncol J, Cronin MT, Mazur M, Telser J. Free radicals and antioxidants in normal physiological functions and human disease. Int J Biochem Cell Biol 2007;39:44-84.

[2] Taniyama Y, Griendling KK. Reactive oxygen species in the vasculature: molecular and cellular mechanisms. Hypertension 2003;42:1075-81.

[3] Ha H, Lee HB. Reactive oxygen species amplify glucose signalling in renal cells cultured under high glucose and in diabetic kidney. Nephrology (Carlton) 2005;10 Suppl:S7-10.

[4] Lee SR, Kwon KS, Kim SR, Rhee SG. Reversible inactivation of protein-tyrosine phosphatase 1B in A431 cells stimulated with epidermal growth factor. J Biol Chem 1998;273:15366-72.

[5] Reth M. Hydrogen peroxide as second messenger in lymphocyte activation. Nat Immunol 2002;3:1129-34.

[6] Bogeski I, Kappl R, Kummerow C, Gulaboski R, Hoth M, Niemeyer BA. Redox regulation of calcium ion channels: Chemical and physiological aspects. Cell Calcium 2011.

[7] Reth M, Wienands J. Initiation and processing of signals from the B cell antigen receptor. Annu Rev Immunol 1997;15:453-79.

[8] Mahadev K, Wu X, Zilbering A, Zhu L, Lawrence JT, Goldstein BJ. Hydrogen peroxide generated during cellular insulin stimulation is integral to activation of the distal insulin signaling cascade in 3T3-L1 adipocytes. J Biol Chem 2001;276:48662-9.

[9] Reth M, Dick TP. Voltage control for B cell activation. Nat Immunol 2010;11:191-2.

[10] Lau AT, Wang Y, Chiu JF. Reactive oxygen species: current knowledge and applications in cancer research and therapeutic. J Cell Biochem 2008;104:657-67.

[11] Endemann DH, Schiffrin EL. Nitric oxide, oxidative excess, and vascular complications of diabetes mellitus. Curr Hypertens Rep 2004;6:85-9.

[12] Bedard K, Krause KH. The NOX family of ROS-generating NADPH oxidases: physiology and pathophysiology. Physiol Rev 2007;87:245-313.

[13] Spooner R, Yilmaz O. The role of reactive-oxygen-species in microbial persistence and inflammation. Int J Mol Sci 2011;12:334-52.

[14] Griendling KK, FitzGerald GA. Oxidative stress and cardiovascular injury: Part I: basic mechanisms and in vivo monitoring of ROS. Circulation 2003;108:1912-6.

[15] Shiose A, Kuroda J, Tsuruya K, Hirai M, Hirakata H, Naito S, Hattori M, Sakaki Y, Sumimoto H. A novel superoxide-producing NAD(P)H oxidase in kidney. J Biol Chem 2001;276:1417-23.

[16] Starkov AA. The role of mitochondria in reactive oxygen species metabolism and signaling. Ann N Y Acad Sci 2008;1147:37-52.

[17] Balaban RS, Nemoto S, Finkel T. Mitochondria, oxidants, and aging. Cell 2005;120:483-95.

[18] Nabeebaccus A, Zhang M, Shah AM. NADPH oxidases and cardiac remodelling. Heart Fail Rev 2011;16:5-12.

[19] Guichard C, Pedruzzi E, Fay M, Ben Mkaddem S, Coant N, Daniel F, Ogier-Denis E. The Nox/Duox family of ROS-generating NADPH oxidases. Med Sci (Paris) 2006;22:953-9.

[20] Cai H, Griendling KK, Harrison DG. The vascular NAD(P)H oxidases as therapeutic targets in cardiovascular diseases. Trends Pharmacol Sci 2003;24:471-8.

[21] Kim JA, Neupane GP, Lee ES, Jeong BS, Park BC, Thapa P. NADPH oxidase inhibitors: a patent review. Expert Opin Ther Pat 2011;21:1147-58.

[22] Krause KH, Bedard K. NOX enzymes in immuno-inflammatory pathologies. Semin Immunopathol 2008;30:193-4.

[23] Bedard K, Lardy B, Krause KH. NOX family NADPH oxidases: not just in mammals. Biochimie 2007;89:1107-12.

[24] Reeves EP, Nagl M, Godovac-Zimmermann J, Segal AW. Reassessment of the microbicidal activity of reactive oxygen species and hypochlorous acid with reference to the phagocytic vacuole of the neutrophil granulocyte. J Med Microbiol 2003;52:643-51.

[25] Klebanoff SJ. Myeloperoxidase: friend and foe. J Leukoc Biol 2005;77:598-625.

[26] Geiszt M, Witta J, Baffi J, Lekstrom K, Leto TL. Dual oxidases represent novel hydrogen peroxide sources supporting mucosal surface host defense. FASEB J 2003;17:1502-4.

[27] Hoek JB, Rydstrom J. Physiological roles of nicotinamide nucleotide transhydrogenase. Biochem J 1988;254:1-10.

[28] Li JM, Shah AM. Mechanism of endothelial cell NADPH oxidase activation by angiotensin II. Role of the p47phox subunit. J Biol Chem 2003;278:12094-100.

[29] Fujita T, Maruyama M, Araya J, Sassa K, Kawagishi Y, Hayashi R, Matsui S, Kashii T, Yamashita N, Sugiyama E, Kobayashi M. Hydrogen peroxide induces upregulation of Fas in human airway epithelial cells via the activation of PARP-p53 pathway. Am J Respir Cell Mol Biol 2002;27:542-52.

[30] Genova ML, Bianchi C, Lenaz G. Structural organization of the mitochondrial respiratory chain. Ital J Biochem 2003;52:58-61.

[31] Genova ML, Pich MM, Biondi A, Bernacchia A, Falasca A, Bovina C, Formiggini G, Parenti Castelli G, Lenaz G. Mitochondrial production of oxygen radical species and the role of Coenzyme Q as an antioxidant. Exp Biol Med (Maywood) 2003;228:506-13.

[32] Bianchi C, Fato R, Genova ML, Parenti Castelli G, Lenaz G. Structural and functional organization of Complex I in the mitochondrial respiratory chain. Biofactors 2003;18:3-9.

[33] Nohl H, Jordan W. The mitochondrial site of superoxide formation. Biochem Biophys Res Commun 1986;138:533-9.

[34] Packer MA, Porteous CM, Murphy MP. Superoxide production by mitochondria in the presence of nitric oxide forms peroxynitrite. Biochem Mol Biol Int 1996;40:527-34.

[35] Szabo C, Ischiropoulos H, Radi R. Peroxynitrite: biochemistry, pathophysiology and development of therapeutics. Nat Rev Drug Discov 2007;6:662-80.

[36] Muller FU, Neumann J, Schmitz W. Transcriptional regulation by cAMP in the heart. Mol Cell Biochem 2000;212:11-7.

[37] Acker T, Fandrey J, Acker H. The good, the bad and the ugly in oxygen-sensing: ROS, cytochromes and prolyl-hydroxylases. Cardiovasc Res 2006;71:195-207.

[38] Bruick RK, McKnight SL. A conserved family of prolyl-4-hydroxylases that modify HIF. Science 2001;294:1337-40.

[39] Martins Chaves M, Rocha-Vieira E, Pereira dos Reis A, de Lima e Silva R, Gerzstein NC, Nogueira-Machado JA. Increase of reactive oxygen (ROS) and nitrogen (RNS) species generated by phagocyting granulocytes related to age. Mech Ageing Dev 2000;119:1-8.

[40] Griendling KK, Sorescu D, Ushio-Fukai M. NAD(P)H oxidase: role in cardiovascular biology and disease. Circ Res 2000;86:494-501.

[41] Basset O, Deffert C, Foti M, Bedard K, Jaquet V, Ogier-Denis E, Krause KH. NADPH oxidase 1 deficiency alters caveolin phosphorylation and angiotensin II-receptor localization in vascular smooth muscle. Antioxid Redox Signal 2009;11:2371-84.

[42] Chen KC, Zhou Y, Zhang W, Lou MF. Control of PDGF-induced reactive oxygen species (ROS) generation and signal transduction in human lens epithelial cells. Mol Vis 2007;13:374-87.

[43] Hunter T. Tyrosine phosphorylation: thirty years and counting. Curr Opin Cell Biol 2009;21:140-6.

[44] Hunter T, Sun H. Crosstalk between the SUMO and ubiquitin pathways. Ernst Schering Found Symp Proc 2008;(1):1-16.

[45] Diep QN, El Mabrouk M, Cohn JS, Endemann D, Amiri F, Virdis A, Neves MF, Schiffrin EL. Structure, endothelial function, cell growth, and inflammation in blood vessels of angiotensin II-infused rats: role of peroxisome proliferator-activated receptor-gamma. Circulation 2002;105:2296-302.

[46] Diep QN, Amiri F, Touyz RM, Cohn JS, Endemann D, Neves MF, Schiffrin EL. PPARalpha activator effects on Ang II-induced vascular oxidative stress and inflammation. Hypertension 2002;40:866-71.

[47] Matzinger P. An innate sense of danger. Ann N Y Acad Sci 2002;961:341-2.

[48] Medzhitov R, Janeway C,Jr. The Toll receptor family and microbial recognition. Trends Microbiol 2000;8:452-6.

[49] Medzhitov R, Janeway C,Jr. Innate immune recognition: mechanisms and pathways. Immunol Rev 2000;173:89-97.

[50] Andrews T, Sullivan KE. Infections in patients with inherited defects in phagocytic function. Clin Microbiol Rev 2003;16:597-621.

[51] Medzhitov R, Janeway C,Jr. Innate immunity. N Engl J Med 2000;343:338-44.

[52] Medzhitov R, Janeway CA,Jr. How does the immune system distinguish self from nonself? Semin Immunol 2000;12:185,8; discussion 257-344.

[53] Janeway CA,Jr. The immune system evolved to discriminate infectious nonself from noninfectious self. Immunol Today 1992;13:11-6.

[54] Piccini A, Carta S, Tassi S, Lasiglie D, Fossati G, Rubartelli A. ATP is released by monocytes stimulated with pathogen-sensing receptor ligands and induces IL-1beta and IL-18 secretion in an autocrine way. Proc Natl Acad Sci U S A 2008;105:8067-72.

[55] Dunne A. Inflammasome activation: from inflammatory disease to infection. Biochem Soc Trans 2011;39:669-73.

[56] Martinon F, Mayor A, Tschopp J. The inflammasomes: guardians of the body. Annu Rev Immunol 2009;27:229-65.

[57] Martinon F, Tschopp J. NLRs join TLRs as innate sensors of pathogens. Trends Immunol 2005;26:447-54.

[58] Bergsbaken T, Fink SL, Cookson BT. Pyroptosis: host cell death and inflammation. Nat Rev Microbiol 2009;7:99-109.

[59] Faurschou M, Borregaard N. Neutrophil granules and secretory vesicles in inflammation. Microbes Infect 2003;5:1317-27.

[60] Vurusaner B, Poli G, Basaga H. Tumor suppressor genes and ROS: complex networks of interactions. Free Radic Biol Med 2011.

[61] Lushchak VJ. Budding Yeast Saccharomyces as a model to study modification of proteins in eukaryotes.Acta Biochimica Polonica 2006;53:679-684

[62] Mena S, Ortega A, Estrela JM. Oxidative stress in environmental-induced carcinogenesis. Mutat Res 2009;674:36-44.

[63] Berk BC. Novel approaches to treat oxidative stress and cardiovascular diseases. Trans Am Clin Climatol Assoc 2007;118:209-14.

[64] Kowaltowski AJ, Castilho RF, Vercesi AE. Mitochondrial permeability transition and oxidative stress. FEBS Lett 2001;495:12-5.

[65] Zoratti M, Szabo I. The mitochondrial permeability transition. Biochim Biophys Acta 1995;1241:139-76.

[66] Marnett LJ, Riggins JN, West JD. Endogenous generation of reactive oxidants and electrophiles and their reactions with DNA and protein. J Clin Invest 2003;111:583-93.

[67] Davies KJ. An overview of oxidative stress. IUBMB Life 2000;50:241-4.

[68] Cadenas E, Davies KJ. Mitochondrial free radical generation, oxidative stress, and aging. Free Radic Biol Med 2000;29:222-30.

[69] Davies KJ. Oxidative stress, antioxidant defenses, and damage removal, repair, and replacement systems. IUBMB Life 2000;50:279-89.

[70] Hazen SL, d'Avignon A, Anderson MM, Hsu FF, Heinecke JW. Human neutrophils employ the myeloperoxidase-hydrogen peroxide-chloride system to oxidize alpha-amino acids to a family of reactive aldehydes. Mechanistic studies identifying labile intermediates along the reaction pathway. J Biol Chem 1998;273:4997-5005.

[71] Marnett LJ, Plastaras JP. Endogenous DNA damage and mutation. Trends Genet 2001;17:214-21.

[72] Cadet J, Carvalho VM, Onuki J, Douki T, Medeiros MH, Di Mascio PD. Purine DNA adducts of 4,5-dioxovaleric acid and 2,4-decadienal. IARC Sci Publ 1999;(150):103-13.

[73] Uchida K. Cellular response to bioactive lipid peroxidation products. Free Radic Res 2000;33:731-7.

[74] Wagner JR, Hu CC, Ames BN. Endogenous oxidative damage of deoxycytidine in DNA. Proc Natl Acad Sci U S A 1992;89:3380-4.

[75] Burney S, Niles JC, Dedon PC, Tannenbaum SR. DNA damage in deoxynucleosides and oligonucleotides treated with peroxynitrite. Chem Res Toxicol 1999;12:513-20.

[76] Burney S, Caulfield JL, Niles JC, Wishnok JS, Tannenbaum SR. The chemistry of DNA damage from nitric oxide and peroxynitrite. Mutat Res 1999;424:37-49.

[77] Halliwell B, Zhao K, Whiteman M. Nitric oxide and peroxynitrite. The ugly, the uglier and the not so good: a personal view of recent controversies. Free Radic Res 1999;31:651-69.

[78] Halliwell B. Free radicals, proteins and DNA: oxidative damage versus redox regulation. Biochem Soc Trans 1996;24:1023-7.

[79] Di Micco R, Fumagalli M, Cicalese A, Piccinin S, Gasparini P, Luise C, Schurra C, Garre' M, Nuciforo PG, Bensimon A, Maestro R, Pelicci PG, d'Adda di Fagagna F. Oncogene-induced senescence is a DNA damage response triggered by DNA hyper-replication. Nature 2006;444:638-42.

[80] Bartkova J, Bakkenist CJ, Rajpert-De Meyts E, Skakkebaek NE, Sehested M, Lukas J, Kastan MB, Bartek J. ATM activation in normal human tissues and testicular cancer. Cell Cycle 2005;4:838-45.

[81] Swenberg JA, Ham A, Koc H, Morinello E, Ranasinghe A, Tretyakova N, Upton PB, Wu K. DNA adducts: effects of low exposure to ethylene oxide, vinyl chloride and butadiene. Mutat Res 2000;464:77-86.

[82] Swenberg JA, Christova-Gueorguieva NI, Upton PB, Ranasinghe A, Scheller N, Wu KY, Yen TY, Hayes R. 1,3-butadiene: cancer, mutations, and adducts. Part V: Hemoglobin adducts as biomarkers of 1,3-butadiene exposure and metabolism. Res Rep Health Eff Inst 2000;(92):191,210; discussion 211-9.

[83] Davies KJ, Pryor WA. The evolution of Free Radical Biology & Medicine: a 20-year history. Free Radic Biol Med 2005;39:1263-4.

[84] Van der Vliet A, Bast A. Effect of oxidative stress on receptors and signal transmission. Chem Biol Interact 1992;85:95-116.

[85] Sharma LK, Fang H, Liu J, Vartak R, Deng J, Bai Y. Mitochondrial respiratory complex I dysfunction promotes tumorigenesis through ROS alteration and AKT activation. Hum Mol Genet 2011.

[86] Jing Y, Liu LZ, Jiang Y, Zhu Y, Guo NL, Barnett J, Rojanasakul Y, Agani F, Jiang BH. Cadmium Increases HIF-1 and VEGF Expression through ROS, ERK and AKT Signaling Pathways and Induces Malignant Transformation of Human Bronchial Epithelial Cells. Toxicol Sci 2011.

[87] Stadtman ER. Protein oxidation and aging. Free Radic Res 2006;40:1250-8.

[88] Liochev SI, Fridovich I. The Haber-Weiss cycle -- 70 years later: an alternative view. Redox Rep 2002;7:55,7; author reply 59-60.

[89] Pastor N, Weinstein H, Jamison E, Brenowitz M. A detailed interpretation of OH radical footprints in a TBP-DNA complex reveals the role of dynamics in the mechanism of sequence-specific binding. J Mol Biol 2000;304:55-68.

[90] Roubal WT, Tappel AL. Damage to proteins, enzymes, and amino acids by peroxidizing lipids. Arch Biochem Biophys 1966;113:5-8.

[91] Stadtman ER. Cyclic oxidation and reduction of methionine residues of proteins in antioxidant defense and cellular regulation. Arch Biochem Biophys 2004;423:2-5.

[92] Dalle-Donne I, Scaloni A, Giustarini D, Cavarra E, Tell G, Lungarella G, Colombo R, Rossi R, Milzani A. Proteins as biomarkers of oxidative/nitrosative stress in diseases: the contribution of redox proteomics. Mass Spectrom Rev 2005;24:55-99.

[93] Fossel M. The long run. J Anti Aging Med 2003;6:1-2.

[94] Hayflick L. How and why we age. Exp Gerontol 1998;33:639-53.

[95] Jenner A, England TG, Aruoma OI, Halliwell B. Measurement of oxidative DNA damage by gas chromatography-mass spectrometry: ethanethiol prevents artifactual generation of oxidized DNA bases. Biochem J 1998;331 (Pt 2):365-9.

[96] Green DR, Reed JC. Mitochondria and apoptosis. Science 1998;281:1309-12.

[97] Kowaltowski AJ, Vercesi AE. Mitochondrial damage induced by conditions of oxidative stress. Free Radic Biol Med 1999;26:463-71.

[98] Green DR, Amarante-Mendes GP. The point of no return: mitochondria, caspases, and the commitment to cell death. Results Probl Cell Differ 1998;24:45-61.

[99] Kowaltowski AJ. Alternative mitochondrial functions in cell physiopathology: beyond ATP production. Braz J Med Biol Res 2000;33:241-50.

[100] Hoek JB, Harada N, Moehren G, Tomsho M, Stubbs CD. The role of calcium and phospholipase A2 in glucagon-induced enhancement of mitochondrial calcium retention. Adv Exp Med Biol 1988;232:25-36.

[101] Lenartowicz E, Bernardi P, Azzone GF. Phenylarsine oxide induces the cyclosporin A-sensitive membrane permeability transition in rat liver mitochondria. J Bioenerg Biomembr 1991;23:679-88.

[102] Kantele A, Jokiranta TS. Review of cases with the emerging fifth human malaria parasite, Plasmodium knowlesi. Clin Infect Dis 2011;52:1356-62.

[103] Figtree M, Lee R, Bain L, Kennedy T, Mackertich S, Urban M, Cheng Q, Hudson BJ. Plasmodium knowlesi in human, Indonesian Borneo. Emerg Infect Dis 2010;16:672-4.

[104] Cox-Singh J, Davis TM, Lee KS, Shamsul SS, Matusop A, Ratnam S, Rahman HA, Conway DJ, Singh B. Plasmodium knowlesi malaria in humans is widely distributed and potentially life threatening. Clin Infect Dis 2008;46:165-71.

[105] Ralph SA, van Dooren GG, Waller RF, Crawford MJ, Fraunholz MJ, Foth BJ, Tonkin CJ, Roos DS, McFadden GI. Tropical infectious diseases: metabolic maps and functions of the Plasmodium falciparum apicoplast. Nat Rev Microbiol 2004;2:203-16.

[106] Newbold C, Warn P, Black G, Berendt A, Craig A, Snow B, Msobo M, Peshu N, Marsh K. Receptor-specific adhesion and clinical disease in Plasmodium falciparum. Am J Trop Med Hyg 1997;57:389-98.

[107] Patz JA, Strzepek K, Lele S, Hedden M, Greene S, Noden B, Hay SI, Kalkstein L, Beier JC. Predicting key malaria transmission factors, biting and entomological inoculation rates, using modelled soil moisture in Kenya. Trop Med Int Health 1998;3:818-27.

[108] Amino R, Thiberge S, Blazquez S, Baldacci P, Renaud O, Shorte S, Menard R. Imaging malaria sporozoites in the dermis of the mammalian host. Nat Protoc 2007;2:1705-12.

[109] Kappe SH, Kaiser K, Matuschewski K. The Plasmodium sporozoite journey: a rite of passage. Trends Parasitol 2003;19:135-43.

[110] Vaughan AM, Aly AS, Kappe SH. Malaria parasite pre-erythrocytic stage infection: gliding and hiding. Cell Host Microbe 2008;4:209-18.

[111] Yamauchi LM, Coppi A, Snounou G, Sinnis P. Plasmodium sporozoites trickle out of the injection site. Cell Microbiol 2007;9:1215-22.

[112] Frevert U, Usynin I, Baer K, Klotz C. Nomadic or sessile: can Kupffer cells function as portals for malaria sporozoites to the liver? Cell Microbiol 2006;8:1537-46.

[113] Imwong M, Snounou G, Pukrittayakamee S, Tanomsing N, Kim JR, Nandy A, Guthmann JP, Nosten F, Carlton J, Looareesuwan S, Nair S, Sudimack D, Day NP, Anderson TJ, White NJ. Relapses of Plasmodium vivax infection usually result from activation of heterologous hypnozoites. J Infect Dis 2007;195:927-33.

[114] Mueller I, Galinski MR, Baird JK, Carlton JM, Kochar DK, Alonso PL, del Portillo HA. Key gaps in the knowledge of Plasmodium vivax, a neglected human malaria parasite. Lancet Infect Dis 2009;9:555-66.

[115] Garcia LS. Malaria. Clin Lab Med 2010;30:93-129.

[116] Malaguarnera L, Musumeci S. The immune response to Plasmodium falciparum malaria. Lancet Infect Dis 2002;2:472-8.

[117] Marsh K, Forster D, Waruiru C, Mwangi I, Winstanley M, Marsh V, Newton C, Winstanley P, Warn P, Peshu N. Indicators of life-threatening malaria in African children. N Engl J Med 1995;332:1399-404.

[118] Delmas-Beauvieux MC, Peuchant E, Dumon MF, Receveur MC, Le Bras M, Clerc M. Relationship between red blood cell antioxidant enzymatic system status and lipoperoxidation during the acute phase of malaria. Clin Biochem 1995;28:163-9.

[119] Schofield L, Tachado SD. Regulation of host cell function by glycosylphosphatidylinositols of the parasitic protozoa. Immunol Cell Biol 1996;74:555-63.

[120] Dondorp AM, Angus BJ, Chotivanich K, Silamut K, Ruangveerayuth R, Hardeman MR, Kager PA, Vreeken J, White NJ. Red blood cell deformability as a predictor of anemia in severe falciparum malaria. Am J Trop Med Hyg 1999;60:733-7.

[121] Djeu JY, Serbousek D, Blanchard DK. Release of tumor necrosis factor by human polymorphonuclear leukocytes. Blood 1990;76:1405-9.

[122] Djeu JY, Matsushima K, Oppenheim JJ, Shiotsuki K, Blanchard DK. Functional activation of human neutrophils by recombinant monocyte-derived neutrophil chemotactic factor/IL-8. J Immunol 1990;144:2205-10.

[123] Jakeman GN, Saul A, Hogarth WL, Collins WE. Anaemia of acute malaria infections in non-immune patients primarily results from destruction of uninfected erythrocytes. Parasitology 1999;119 (Pt 2):127-33.

[124] Mohan K, Ganguly NK, Dubey ML, Mahajan RC. Oxidative damage of erythrocytes infected with Plasmodium falciparum. An in vitro study. Ann Hematol 1992;65:131-4.

[125] Mohan K, Dubey ML, Ganguly NK, Mahajan RC. Plasmodium falciparum: role of activated blood monocytes in erythrocyte membrane damage and red cell loss during malaria. Exp Parasitol 1995;80:54-63.

[126] Omodeo-Sale F, Motti A, Dondorp A, White NJ, Taramelli D. Destabilisation and subsequent lysis of human erythrocytes induced by Plasmodium falciparum haem products. Eur J Haematol 2005;74:324-32.

[127] Foldes J, Matyi A, Matkovics B. The role of free radicals and antioxidative enzymes in erythrocytes and liver cells in the course of Plasmodium berghei and Plasmodium vinckei infection of mice. Acta Microbiol Immunol Hung 1994;41:153-61.

[128] Marx PA, Chen Z. The function of simian chemokine receptors in the replication of SIV. Semin Immunol 1998;10:215-23.

[129] Berger EA, Murphy PM, Farber JM. Chemokine receptors as HIV-1 coreceptors: roles in viral entry, tropism, and disease. Annu Rev Immunol 1999;17:657-700.

[130] Alkhatib G, Combadiere C, Broder CC, Feng Y, Kennedy PE, Murphy PM, Berger EA. CC CKR5: a RANTES, MIP-1alpha, MIP-1beta receptor as a fusion cofactor for macrophage-tropic HIV-1. Science 1996;272:1955-8.

[131] Dragic T, Litwin V, Allaway GP, Martin SR, Huang Y, Nagashima KA, Cayanan C, Maddon PJ, Koup RA, Moore JP, Paxton WA. HIV-1 entry into CD4+ cells is mediated by the chemokine receptor CC-CKR-5. Nature 1996;381:667-73.

[132] Alkhatib G, Broder CC, Berger EA. Cell type-specific fusion cofactors determine human immunodeficiency virus type 1 tropism for T-cell lines versus primary macrophages. J Virol 1996;70:5487-94.

[133] Rottman JB, Ganley KP, Williams K, Wu L, Mackay CR, Ringler DJ. Cellular localization of the chemokine receptor CCR5. Correlation to cellular targets of HIV-1 infection. Am J Pathol 1997;151:1341-51.

[134] Eugenin EA, Osiecki K, Lopez L, Goldstein H, Calderon TM, Berman JW. CCL2/monocyte chemoattractant protein-1 mediates enhanced transmigration of human immunodeficiency virus (HIV)-infected leukocytes across the blood-brain barrier: a potential mechanism of HIV-CNS invasion and NeuroAIDS. J Neurosci 2006;26:1098-106.

[135] Navia BA, Jordan BD, Price RW. The AIDS dementia complex: I. Clinical features. Ann Neurol 1986;19:517-24.

[136] King JE, Eugenin EA, Buckner CM, Berman JW. HIV tat and neurotoxicity. Microbes Infect 2006;8:1347-57.

[137] Gonzalez-Scarano F, Martin-Garcia J. The neuropathogenesis of AIDS. Nat Rev Immunol 2005;5:69-81.

[138] Steiner J, Haughey N, Li W, Venkatesan A, Anderson C, Reid R, Malpica T, Pocernich C, Butterfield DA, Nath A. Oxidative stress and therapeutic approaches in HIV dementia. Antioxid Redox Signal 2006;8:2089-100.

[139] Turchan J, Sacktor N, Wojna V, Conant K, Nath A. Neuroprotective therapy for HIV dementia. Curr HIV Res 2003;1:373-83.

[140] Haughey NJ, Cutler RG, Tamara A, McArthur JC, Vargas DL, Pardo CA, Turchan J, Nath A, Mattson MP. Perturbation of sphingolipid metabolism and ceramide production in HIV-dementia. Ann Neurol 2004;55:257-67.

[141] Esterbauer H, Schaur RJ, Zollner H. Chemistry and biochemistry of 4-hydroxynonenal, malonaldehyde and related aldehydes. Free Radic Biol Med 1991;11:81-128.

[142] Butterfield DA. beta-Amyloid-associated free radical oxidative stress and neurotoxicity: implications for Alzheimer's disease. Chem Res Toxicol 1997;10:495-506.

[143] Butterfield DA, Howard BJ, Yatin S, Allen KL, Carney JM. Free radical oxidation of brain proteins in accelerated senescence and its modulation by N-tert-butyl-alpha-phenylnitrone. Proc Natl Acad Sci U S A 1997;94:674-8.

[144] Gaskill PJ, Calderon TM, Luers AJ, Eugenin EA, Javitch JA, Berman JW. Human immunodeficiency virus (HIV) infection of human macrophages is increased by dopamine: a bridge between HIV-associated neurologic disorders and drug abuse. Am J Pathol 2009;175:1148-59.

[145] American Diabetes Association. Diagnosis and classification of diabetes mellitus. Diabetes Care 2011;34 Suppl 1:S62-9.

[146] Dabelea D, Pihoker C, Talton JW, D'Agostino RB,Jr, Fujimoto W, Klingensmith GJ, Lawrence JM, Linder B, Marcovina SM, Mayer-Davis EJ, Imperatore G, Dolan LM, SEARCH for Diabetes in Youth Study. Etiological approach to characterization of diabetes type: the SEARCH for Diabetes in Youth Study. Diabetes Care 2011;34:1628-33.

[147] Duncan BB, Schmidt MI, Pankow JS, Ballantyne CM, Couper D, Vigo A, Hoogeveen R, Folsom AR, Heiss G, Atherosclerosis Risk in Communities Study. Low-grade systemic inflammation and the development of type 2 diabetes: the atherosclerosis risk in communities study. Diabetes 2003;52:1799-805.

[148] Schmidt MI, Duncan BB. Diabesity: an inflammatory metabolic condition. Clin Chem Lab Med 2003;41:1120-30.

[149] Rasschaert J, Ladriere L, Urbain M, Dogusan Z, Katabua B, Sato S, Akira S, Gysemans C, Mathieu C, Eizirik DL. Toll-like receptor 3 and STAT-1 contribute to double-stranded RNA+ interferon-gamma-induced apoptosis in primary pancreatic beta-cells. J Biol Chem 2005;280:33984-91.

[150] Newsholme P, Haber EP, Hirabara SM, Rebelato EL, Procopio J, Morgan D, Oliveira-Emilio HC, Carpinelli AR, Curi R. Diabetes associated cell stress and dysfunction: role of mitochondrial and non-mitochondrial ROS production and activity. J Physiol 2007;583:9-24.

[151] Newsholme P, Keane D, Welters HJ, Morgan NG. Life and death decisions of the pancreatic beta-cell: the role of fatty acids. Clin Sci (Lond) 2007;112:27-42.

[152] Newsholme P, Bender K, Kiely A, Brennan L. Amino acid metabolism, insulin secretion and diabetes. Biochem Soc Trans 2007;35:1180-6.

[153] Bender K, Newsholme P, Brennan L, Maechler P. The importance of redox shuttles to pancreatic beta-cell energy metabolism and function. Biochem Soc Trans 2006;34:811-4.

[154] Kruman I, Guo Q, Mattson MP. Calcium and reactive oxygen species mediate staurosporine-induced mitochondrial dysfunction and apoptosis in PC12 cells. J Neurosci Res 1998;51:293-308.

[155] Bosch RR, Janssen SW, Span PN, Olthaar A, van Emst-de Vries SE, Willems PH, Martens JMG, Hermus AR, Sweep CC. Exploring levels of hexosamine biosynthesis pathway intermediates and protein kinase C isoforms in muscle and fat tissue of Zucker Diabetic Fatty rats. Endocrine 2003;20:247-52.

[156] Buse MG, Robinson KA, Gettys TW, McMahon EG, Gulve EA. Increased activity of the hexosamine synthesis pathway in muscles of insulin-resistant ob/ob mice. Am J Physiol 1997;272:E1080-8.

[157] Brownlee M. Biochemistry and molecular cell biology of diabetic complications. Nature 2001;414:813-20.

[158] Coughlan MT, Yap FY, Tong DC, Andrikopoulos S, Gasser A, Thallas-Bonke V, Webster DE, Miyazaki J, Kay TW, Slattery RM, Kaye DM, Drew BG, Kingwell BA, Fourlanos S, Groop PH, Harrison LC, Knip M, Forbes JM. Advanced Glycation End Products Are Direct Modulators of {beta}-Cell Function. Diabetes 2011;60:2523-32.

[159] Iborra RT, Machado-Lima A, Castilho G, Nunes VS, Abdalla DS, Nakandakare ER, Passarelli M. Advanced Glycation in macrophages induces intracellular accumulation of 7-ketocholesterol and total sterols by decreasing the expression of ABCA-1 and ABCG-1. Lipids Health Dis 2011;10:172.

[160] Madian AG, Myracle AD, Diaz-Maldonado N, Rochelle NS, Janle EM, Regnier FE. Determining the Effects of Antioxidants on Oxidative Stress Induced Carbonylation of Proteins. Anal Chem 2011.

[161] Gabriely I, Yang XM, Cases JA, Ma XH, Rossetti L, Barzilai N. Hyperglycemia induces PAI-1 gene expression in adipose tissue by activation of the hexosamine biosynthetic pathway. Atherosclerosis 2002;160:115-22.

[162] Dandona P, Aljada A, Mohanty P, Ghanim H, Hamouda W, Assian E, Ahmad S. Insulin inhibits intranuclear nuclear factor kappaB and stimulates IkappaB in mononuclear cells in obese subjects: evidence for an anti-inflammatory effect? J Clin Endocrinol Metab 2001;86:3257-65.

[163] Eizirik DL, Colli ML, Ortis F. The role of inflammation in insulitis and beta-cell loss in type 1 diabetes. Nat Rev Endocrinol 2009;5:219-26.

[164] Fernandez-Real JM, Pickup JC. Innate immunity, insulin resistance and type 2 diabetes. Trends Endocrinol Metab 2007.

[165] Feve B, Bastard JP, Vidal H. Relationship between obesity, inflammation and insulin resistance: new concepts. C R Biol 2006;329:587,97; discussion 653-5.

[166] Das UN. Obesity, metabolic syndrome X, and inflammation. Nutrition 2002;18:430-2.

[167] Steinberg GR. Inflammation in obesity is the common link between defects in fatty acid metabolism and insulin resistance. Cell Cycle 2007;6:888-94.

[168] Steinberg GR, Jorgensen SB. The AMP-activated protein kinase: role in regulation of skeletal muscle metabolism and insulin sensitivity. Mini Rev Med Chem 2007;7:519-26.

[169] Zulet MA, Puchau B, Navarro C, Marti A, Martinez JA. Inflammatory biomarkers: the link between obesity and associated pathologies. Nutr Hosp 2007;22:511-27.

[170] Saltiel AR, Kahn CR. Insulin signalling and the regulation of glucose and lipid metabolism. Nature 2001;414:799-806.

[171] Chiang SH, Baumann CA, Kanzaki M, Thurmond DC, Watson RT, Neudauer CL, Macara IG, Pessin JE, Saltiel AR. Insulin-stimulated GLUT4 translocation requires the CAP-dependent activation of TC10. Nature 2001;410:944-8.

[172] Saltiel AR. New perspectives into the molecular pathogenesis and treatment of type 2 diabetes. Cell 2001;104:517-29.

[173] Hotamisligil GS, Peraldi P, Budavari A, Ellis R, White MF, Spiegelman BM. IRS-1-mediated inhibition of insulin receptor tyrosine kinase activity in TNF-alpha- and obesity-induced insulin resistance. Science 1996;271:665-8.

[174] Paris M, Bernard-Kargar C, Vilar J, Kassis N, Ktorza A. Role of glucose in IRS signaling in rat pancreatic islets: specific effects and interplay with insulin. Exp Diabesity Res 2004;5:257-63.

[175] Hotamisligil GS, Budavari A, Murray D, Spiegelman BM. Reduced tyrosine kinase activity of the insulin receptor in obesity-diabetes. Central role of tumor necrosis factor-alpha. J Clin Invest 1994;94:1543-9.

[176] Nathan C. Epidemic inflammation: pondering obesity. Mol Med 2008;14:485-92.

[177] Bastard JP, Maachi M, Lagathu C, Kim MJ, Caron M, Vidal H, Capeau J, Feve B. Recent advances in the relationship between obesity, inflammation, and insulin resistance. Eur Cytokine Netw 2006;17:4-12.

[178] Drevon CA. Fatty acids and expression of adipokines. Biochim Biophys Acta 2005;1740:287-92.

[179] Trayhurn P, Wood IS. Signalling role of adipose tissue: adipokines and inflammation in obesity. Biochem Soc Trans 2005;33:1078-81.

[180] Onat A, Ayhan E, Hergenc G, Can G, Barlan MM. Smoking inhibits visceral fat accumulation in Turkish women Relation of visceral fat and body fat mass to atherogenic dyslipidemia, inflammatory markers, insulin resistance, and blood pressure. Metabolism 2009.

[181] Steinberg GR, Kemp BE. Adiponectin: starving for attention. Cell Metab 2007;6:3-4.

[182] Bastard JP, Maachi M, Van Nhieu JT, Jardel C, Bruckert E, Grimaldi A, Robert JJ, Capeau J, Hainque B. Adipose tissue IL-6 content correlates with resistance to insulin activation of glucose uptake both in vivo and in vitro. J Clin Endocrinol Metab 2002;87:2084-9.

[183] Kauf TL, Coates TD, Huazhi L, Mody-Patel N, Hartzema AG. The cost of health care for children and adults with sickle cell disease. Am J Hematol 2009.

[184] Adams-Graves P, Ostric EJ, Martin M, Richardson P, Lewis JB,Jr. Sickle cell hospital unit: a disease-specific model. J Healthc Manag 2008;53:305,15; discussion 316-7.

[185] Aliyu ZY, Kato GJ, Taylor J,4th, Babadoko A, Mamman AI, Gordeuk VR, Gladwin MT. Sickle cell disease and pulmonary hypertension in Africa: a global perspective and review of epidemiology, pathophysiology, and management. Am J Hematol 2008;83:63-70.

[186] Hebbel RP. Adhesion of sickle red cells to endothelium: myths and future directions. Transfus Clin Biol 2008;15:14-8.

[187] Eaton WA, Hofrichter J. Hemoglobin S gelation and sickle cell disease. Blood 1987;70:1245-66.

[188] Reiter CD, Wang X, Tanus-Santos JE, Hogg N, Cannon RO,3rd, Schechter AN, Gladwin MT. Cell-free hemoglobin limits nitric oxide bioavailability in sickle-cell disease. Nat Med 2002;8:1383-9.

[189] Gladwin MT, Schechter AN, Ognibene FP, Coles WA, Reiter CD, Schenke WH, Csako G, Waclawiw MA, Panza JA, Cannon RO,3rd. Divergent nitric oxide bioavailability in men and women with sickle cell disease. Circulation 2003;107:271-8.

[190] Hebbel RP. The systems biology-based argument for taking a bold step in chemoprophylaxis of sickle vasculopathy. Am J Hematol 2009;84:543-5.

[191] Wu CJ, Krishnamurti L, Kutok JL, Biernacki M, Rogers S, Zhang W, Antin JH, Ritz J. Evidence for ineffective erythropoiesis in severe sickle cell disease. Blood 2005;106:3639-45.

[192] Taylor JG 6, Nolan VG, Mendelsohn L, Kato GJ, Gladwin MT, Steinberg MH. Chronic hyper-hemolysis in sickle cell anemia: association of vascular complications and mortality with less frequent vasoocclusive pain. PLoS ONE 2008;3:e2095.

[193] Muller-Eberhard U, Javid J, Liem HH, Hanstein A, Hanna M. Plasma concentrations of hemopexin, haptoglobin and heme in patients with various hemolytic diseases. Blood 1968;32:811-5.

[194] Sultana C, Shen Y, Johnson C, Kalra VK. Cobalt chloride-induced signaling in endothelium leading to the augmented adherence of sickle red blood cells and transendothelial migration of monocyte-like HL-60 cells is blocked by PAF-receptor antagonist. J Cell Physiol 1999;179:67-78.

[195] Houston M, Estevez A, Chumley P, Aslan M, Marklund S, Parks DA, Freeman BA. Binding of xanthine oxidase to vascular endothelium. Kinetic characterization and oxidative impairment of nitric oxide-dependent signaling. J Biol Chem 1999;274:4985-94.

[196] Wood KC, Hsu LL, Gladwin MT. Sickle cell disease vasculopathy: a state of nitric oxide resistance. Free Radic Biol Med 2008;44:1506-28.

[197] Endemann DH, Schiffrin EL. Endothelial dysfunction. J Am Soc Nephrol 2004;15:1983-92.

[198] Cai H, Harrison DG. Endothelial dysfunction in cardiovascular diseases: the role of oxidant stress. Circ Res 2000;87:840-4.

[199] Griendling KK, FitzGerald GA. Oxidative stress and cardiovascular injury: Part II: animal and human studies. Circulation 2003;108:2034-40.

[200] Griendling KK, Sorescu D, Lassegue B, Ushio-Fukai M. Modulation of protein kinase activity and gene expression by reactive oxygen species and their role in vascular physiology and pathophysiology. Arterioscler Thromb Vasc Biol 2000;20:2175-83.

[201] Griendling KK, Ushio-Fukai M. Reactive oxygen species as mediators of angiotensin II signaling. Regul Pept 2000;91:21-7.

[202] Higashi Y, Noma K, Yoshizumi M, Kihara Y. Endothelial Function and Oxidative Stress in Cardiovascular Diseases. Circ J 2009.

[203] Higashi Y, Noma K, Yoshizumi M, Kihara Y. Endothelial Function and Oxidative Stress in Cardiovascular Diseases. Circ J 2009.

[204] Kato GJ, Hebbel RP, Steinberg MH, Gladwin MT. Vasculopathy in sickle cell disease: Biology, pathophysiology, genetics, translational medicine, and new research directions. Am J Hematol 2009;84:618-25.

[205] Wood KC, Hebbel RP, Lefer DJ, Granger DN. Critical role of endothelial cell-derived nitric oxide synthase in sickle cell disease-induced microvascular dysfunction. Free Radic Biol Med 2006;40:1443-53.

[206] De Caterina R, Libby P, Peng HB, Thannickal VJ, Rajavashisth TB, Gimbrone MA,Jr, Shin WS, Liao JK. Nitric oxide decreases cytokine-induced endothelial activation. Nitric oxide selectively reduces endothelial expression of adhesion molecules and proinflammatory cytokines. J Clin Invest 1995;96:60-8.

[207] Libby P. Inflammation in atherosclerosis. Nature 2002;420:868-74.

[208] Boger RH, Bode-Boger SM, Szuba A, Tsao PS, Chan JR, Tangphao O, Blaschke TF, Cooke JP. Asymmetric dimethylarginine (ADMA): a novel risk factor for endothelial dysfunction: its role in hypercholesterolemia. Circulation 1998;98:1842-7.

[209] Boger RH, Bode-Boger SM, Phivthong-ngam L, Brandes RP, Schwedhelm E, Mugge A, Bohme M, Tsikas D, Frolich JC. Dietary L-arginine and alpha-tocopherol reduce vascular oxidative stress and preserve endothelial function in hypercholesterolemic rabbits via different mechanisms. Atherosclerosis 1998;141:31-43.

[210] Achan V, Broadhead M, Malaki M, Whitley G, Leiper J, MacAllister R, Vallance P. Asymmetric dimethylarginine causes hypertension and cardiac dysfunction in humans and is actively metabolized by dimethylarginine dimethylaminohydrolase. Arterioscler Thromb Vasc Biol 2003;23:1455-9.

[211] Dayoub H, Achan V, Adimoolam S, Jacobi J, Stuehlinger MC, Wang BY, Tsao PS, Kimoto M, Vallance P, Patterson AJ, Cooke JP. Dimethylarginine dimethylaminohydrolase regulates nitric oxide synthesis: genetic and physiological evidence. Circulation 2003;108:3042-7.

[212] Hill JM, Zalos G, Halcox JP, Schenke WH, Waclawiw MA, Quyyumi AA, Finkel T. Circulating endothelial progenitor cells, vascular function, and cardiovascular risk. N Engl J Med 2003;348:593-600.

[213] Szmitko PE, Fedak PW, Weisel RD, Stewart DJ, Kutryk MJ, Verma S. Endothelial progenitor cells: new hope for a broken heart. Circulation 2003;107:3093-100.

[214] Finkel T, Holbrook NJ. Oxidants, oxidative stress and the biology of ageing. Nature 2000;408:239-47.

6

Mathematical Modeling of IL-2 Based Immune Therapy on T Cell Homeostasis in HIV

Priti Kumar Roy[1,*], Sonia Chowdhury[1],
Amarnath Chatterjee[1] and Sutapa Biswas Majee[2]
*[1]Centre for Mathematical Biology and Ecology, Department of Mathematics,
Jadavpur University, Kolkata,
[2]NSHM College of Pharmaceutical Technology,
NSHM Knowledge Campus, Kolkata
India*

1. Introduction

The past few years there have been witnessed the initiation of new or more effective therapies for the treatment of HIV disease. But it is the established reality for the treatment procedure of HIV disease; mathematical modeling is very essential and supportive, in accepting the dynamics of HIV infection and also for the purpose of specific antiviral treatment strategies. Mathematical models have been constructed to explore the co- relation between disease progression, generation of HIV specific immune response in primary stage, depletion of CD4[+] T cell population, leading to severe impairment and dysregulation of host immune system and emergence of numerous opportunistic infection. Mathematical model accompanied with definite biological interpretation and relevance can provide a clear representation of host-pathogen interaction dynamics. Human Immunodeficiency Virus (HIV) targets the immune cells mainly CD4 positive T lymphocytes (CD4[+]T, a type of white blood cells), which is the main component of immune system. CD4[+]T cells or " helper" T cells also send signals to the second group of immune response cells (CD8[+]T cell or CTL) in the body, the precursor Cytotoxic T Lymphocytes (CTL_p) to induce HIV-specific CTL response through the generation of functionally active effector CTL (CTL_e). HIV infection can be finally eradicated through co-ordinated interplay between CD4[+]T cells and CTLs when infected CD4[+]T cells are killed by CTLs. Thus, if CTL population can be maintained at a high level, the HIV-infected individuals can remain healthy for a longer period of time due to slower disease progression. The safest and cheapest therapeutic intervention aims to keep the CD4[+]T cell population together with CTL count at a positive value, both of which will bring down the viremia to very low levels.

From an immunological standpoint, progression of HIV can be characterized by continual reduction of CD4[+]T lymphocyte subset levels in peripheral compartment and lymphoid tissue as well, with greater reduction being observed in the former. Dysfunctional lymphocytes with high propensity for apoptosis and loss of proper cell cycle control account

*Research is supported by the Government of India, Ministry of Science and Technology, Mathematical Science office, No. SR/S4/MS: 558/08.

for deviation from T cell homeostasis in an HIV-infected individual. HIV antigen activates immune system, increases cell turnover and induces apoptosis of uninfected $CD4^+T$ and $CD8^+T$ cells leading to complete impairment of immune system (Sereti et al., 2004).

Immune activation and subsequent sensitivity to apoptotic stimuli can be reverted back by introduction of potent antiretroviral agents. Successful therapy with Highly Active Anti Retroviral Therapy (HAART) efficiently suppresses viral replication but with only partial immune reconstitution. Moreover, complete eradication of viral population from the system is practically not feasible with HAART alone, even if continued for a long time. Viral relapse is known to occur as soon as the therapy is discontinued (Roy & Chatterjee, 2011). Thus arises the need of addition of new therapeutic modalities in the form of administration of immunomodulatory agent, IL-2, to the armamentarium of antiretroviral agents promoting complete immune reconstitution.

IL-2 is a very well characterized T-cell growth factor determining proliferation and differentiation of whole T cell compartment. Following antigen-activation, IL-2 is produced by both $CD4^+$ and $CD8^+T$ (in comparatively lesser quantities) cell subsets, in the peripheral lymphoid tissues of spleen and lymph nodes, in an autocrine and paracrine fashion respectively (Smith, 2001), (Banerjee, 2008).

Infection by HIV affects $CD4^+T$ and $CD8^+T$ cells in a differential manner with selective depletion of the $CD4^+T$ cells whereas expansion of $CD8^+T$ cells is maintained till late stages of infection (Marchettia et al., 2004). Though IL-2 is produced by $CD4^+$ and $CD8^+T$ cells, it exerts differential effects on $CD4^+T$ cells, with preferential expansion and prolonged survival of peripheral naïve and recall subsets, but not effector and memory phenotype (Sereti et al., 2004), (Marchettia et al., 2004). IL-2 does not target progenitor cells of the bone marrow or thymus (Smith, 2001), (De, 2001). Net outcome of IL-2 therapy is rejuvenation of T cell pool marked by decreases in T cell turnover, proliferation and activation. IL-2 therapy also increases T cell responsiveness to suboptimal levels of endogenous IL-2 by increasing expression of its receptor, CD25, on $CD4^+$ T cells (Sklar et al., 2007). $CD8^+$ cells seem to follow different homeostatic dynamics, more or less independent of immunoregulatory activity of IL-2. Apart from its regulatory activity on specific cellular populations, IL-2 can also augment the production of IL-2 itself (Bortolin et al., 2001). In contrast, HAART alone results in selective rescue of $CD4^+$ memory cells, with no change in naïve compartment (Franzetti et al., 2005). Thus, IL-2 immunotherapy broadens HAART-induced immune recovery.

The degree of $CD4^+T$ cell recuperation after IL-2 administration depends on the nadir $CD4^+$ T cell count and the dose and duration of IL-2 therapy (Paredes et al., 2002). IL-2 can be given either intravenously or subcutaneously at a low dose intermittently but it is recommended that it should never be given alone. It should always be administered as an adjuvant to HAART for maximum biological and clinical benefits. It may be stopped as soon as $CD4^+T$ cell count is "normalized" to pre-infection levels and immune activation is reduced (De, 2001). Improvement in immunological parameters of the host such as expansion of $CD4^+T$ cells may continue for several months even after IL-2 administration has been interrupted (Bortolin et al., 2001). The potential of IL-2 to reverse the HIV-mediated T cell homeostasis imbalances by altering the in vivo dynamics of T-lymphocytes and regulatory cytokines, with transient or almost no change in HIV viral load, offers the appealing prospect of obtaining major immune reconstitution in the treatment of HIV disease.

Several mathematical models have been developed to describe the behavior of the HIV, when it interacts with the human immune system and causes a decline in the CD4$^+$T cells count (Bonhoeffer et al., 1997), (Perelson & Nelson, 1999), (Wodarz et al., 2000), (Gumel et al., 2002), (Roy & Chatterjee, 2010). In their research they expand a innovative thinking, impact of drag in a HIV individual integrating with their model dynamics. Perelson et al. utilized clinical data from HIV infected patients and fitted them to their mathematical model and subsequent numerical simulations to prove the clinical manifestations of AIDS such as long latency period, depletion of CD4$^+$T cells and low level of free virus in the whole body.

Now a days most of the authors developed their work by including various aspects of HIV specific antiviral immune response dominated by CTLs because of its significant role in controlling virus replication and disease progression. A simple mathematical model was developed by Wodarz et al. (Wodarz et al., 1999) to study the co-relation between HIV and immune system during the natural course of infection and in the background of different antiviral treatment regimes. They have suggested the need for an efficient CTL memory response for effective containment of viral replication. CTL memory is adversely affected during long-term infection due to depletion of CD4$^+$T cell pool in the system. From analytical and numerical analysis in their mathematical model, (Roy & Chatterjee, 2011) has been shown that when the immune response are high, less medication is needed to control and regulate infection. Their mathematical model also reflect that optimal treatment is reduces the period of time while the immune response of the uninfected T cell takes over.

Discrete and continuous time delay or time lag is assumed to exist in the various stages of HIV progression (Herz et al., 1996), (Calshaw et al., 2000), (Roy & Chatterjee, 2011), and (Roy & Chatterjee, 2010) which have been incorporated into the mathematical model with firm biological explanations. It is well known that, delay differential equations cause a stable steady state to lose its stability and cause oscillations. For avoiding the side effects due to chemotherapy, various mathematical models have been formulated in control therapeutic approach (Fleming et al., 1975), (Gumel et al., 2002).

In the present paper, the reconstitution dynamics of CD4$^+$T cells and effect on CTLs in HIV-infected individuals has been studied in presence of HAART and IL-2, where the basic model as proposed by Wodarz and Nowak has been modified (Wodarz and Nowak). They have suggested the need for an efficient CTL memory response for effective containment of viral replication. CTL memory is adversely affected during long-term infection due to depletion of CD4$^+$T cell pool in the system. Mathematical modeling of such dynamics will help in delineating the interplay between T lymphocyte subsets in the course of HIV infection and thereby establishing optimum conditions for effective immune -based therapy associated with HAART. In this research article delay induced system in the same mathematical model of HIV has been investigated to understand the effect of combination therapy of HAART and IL-2. Attempts have also been made to apply the principles of optimal control theory to the proposed mathematical model for rational administration of IL-2 adjuvanated HAART in an effort to successfully eradicate the virus from the host system and cure the patient completely.

2. Presentation of the mathematical model

In this research article we develop a viral dynamical model of Wodarz et. al (Wodarz et al., 1999) by introducing IL-2 therapy in presence of HAART.

The model is given below,

$$\dot{x}(t) = \lambda - \beta(1 - \eta_1 u_1)x(t)y(t) - dx(t) + \gamma x(t)$$
$$\dot{y}(t) = \beta(1 - \eta_1 u_1)x(t)y(t) - ay(t) - py(t)z(t)$$
$$\dot{w}(t) = cx(t)y(t)w(t) - cq_1y(t)w(t) - bw(t) + \gamma_1 w(t)$$
$$\dot{z}(t) = cq_2y(t)w(t) - hz(t), \tag{1}$$

with initial conditions: $x(0) > 0, y(0) > 0, w(0) > 0, z(0) > 0$.

Here x represents uninfected CD4$^+$T cells, and y, w, z are infected CD4$^+$T cells, Cytotoxic T lymphocyte precursors (CTL_p), CTL effector cells respectively. Here λ represents the rate of production of CD4$^+$T cells from bone marrow and these immature cells migrate to thymus and they are matured to immunocompetent T cells. The natural death rate of uninfected CD4$^+$T cell is d and β is the rate at which uninfected CD4$^+$T cell become infected. Natural death rate of infected cell is a. The clearance rate of infected cells by CTL effector is p. CTL_p are assumed to proliferate in response to antigenic stimulation and then differentiate into CTL memory. The rate of proliferation of CTL_p population is c and they decay at a rate b. Since the differentiation rate of precursor CTL (CTL_p) not at all same as the proliferation rate of effector CTL (CTL_e), thus we consider q_1 and q_2 as multiplicative capacity of differentiated precursor CTL and proliferated effector CTL respectively. We also assume that the removal rate of effector CTL is h.

Here we introduce IL-2 therapy in presence of HAART. We also consider that the RTI reduces the infection rate β by $(1 - \eta_1 u_1)$ where η_1 represents the drug efficacy parameter and u_1 is the control input doses of the drug RTI. By introducing interleukin protein it enhances the growth of uninfected T cell and also in a smaller quantity, increases growth of CTL_p. Here γ and γ_1 are the activation rates of uninfected T cell and CTL_p population respectively.

3. General analysis of the mathematical model

Figure 1 shows that, due to introducing of cocktail drug therapy (HAART and IL-2), uninfected CD4$^+$ T cell moves to its stable position. Further infected CD4$^+$ T cell population moves to a very lower levels, and ultimately goes towards extinction. Thus effector CTL population attains a lower steady state, where as CTL precursor enhanced due to effect of IL-2.

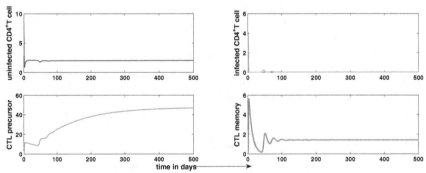

Fig. 1. Solution trajectory of the non-delayed system. All parameter values are taken from Table 1.

3.1 Equilibria and their existence

The system (1) with the initial condition possesses the following positive equilibrium $E_1(x_1, 0, 0, 0)$, $E_2(x_2, y_2, 0, 0)$ and $E^*(x^*, y^*, w^*, z^*)$.

Where, $x_1 = \frac{\lambda}{d-\gamma}$, $x_2 = \frac{a}{\beta(1-\eta_1 u_1)}$, $y_2 = \frac{\beta(1-\eta_1 u_1)\lambda + a(\gamma - d)}{a\beta(1-\eta_1 u_1)}$ and $x^* = \frac{\lambda}{d + \beta(1-\eta_1 u_1)y^* - \gamma}$,

$y^* = \frac{-\{(d-\gamma)cq_1 + \beta(1-\eta_1 u_1)(b-\gamma_1) - c\lambda\} + \sqrt{\{(d-\gamma)cq_1 + \beta(1-\eta_1 u_1)(b-\gamma_1) - c\lambda\}^2 - 4acq_1\beta(1-\eta_1 u_1)(b-\gamma_1)(d-\gamma)}}{2cq_1\beta(1-\eta_1 u_1)}$,

$w^* = \frac{h\beta(1-\eta_1 u_1)x^* - ha}{cpq_2 y^*}$, $z^* = \frac{\beta(1-\eta_1 u_1)x^* - a}{p}$.

During initial stages of infection when the virus enter in the system but not yet attack any CD4$^+$T cell, then infection free steady state E_1 exists, if $d > \gamma$, entail that death rate of uninfected CD4$^+$T cells is greater than the rate of production of uninfected cells under the influence of IL-2.

E_2 exists if $x_1 > x_2$, i.e at early stages of infection when T cells have become infected but CTL response is yet to develop and it indicates a very crucial situation. It exists when uninfected cell population at initial stage of infection is greater than steady state value of uninfected T cell population in presence of infection but without any immune response.

E^* exists if the following conditions holds, (i) $\frac{\gamma - d}{\beta(1-\eta_1 u_1)} < y^* < y_2$, (ii) $(b - \gamma_1)(d - \gamma) < 0$.

From the above two conditions we can say that (i) if infected cell population (y^*) at coexistence equilibrium point lies between these two threshold values and (ii) product of two terms $(b - \gamma_1)(d - \gamma)$, i.e. difference between death rate and production rate of CTL_p in presence of IL-2 $(b - \gamma_1)$ and difference between death rate and production rate of uninfected CD4$^+$T cell in presence of IL-2, $(d - \gamma)$ is negative.

3.2 Stability analysis of the system:

Here we study the nature of stability of the system (1) around different equilibrium points. From our mathematical study we have the following three propositions.

Proposition 1 : The system (1) is locally asymptotically stable around E_1 if the following condition holds,

$$(i) \gamma < d$$
$$(ii) \gamma_1 < b$$
$$(iii) \frac{\beta(1-\eta_1 u_1)\lambda + a(\gamma - d)}{a\beta(1-\eta_1 u_1)} < 0.$$

Proof :
The s/eigenvalues of the above upper triangular jacobian matrix are

$$\xi_1 = \gamma - d$$
$$\xi_2 = \frac{\beta(1-\eta_1 u_1)\lambda}{d-\gamma} - a$$
$$\xi_3 = \gamma_1 - b$$
$$\xi_4 = -h.$$

All the characteristic roots corresponding to E_1 will be negative if above proposed conditions are satisfied. Hence the system is locally asymptotically stable around E_1. Whenever E_1 is locally asymptotically stable E_2 does not exists.

Proposition 2: System (1) is locally asymptotically stable around E_2 if $y_2 < \frac{\beta(1-\eta_1 u_1)(b-\gamma_1)}{c(a-q_1\beta(1-\eta_1 u_1))}$ holds.

Proof :
By the same way we can prove this proposition.

Proposition 3: The system is locally asymptotically stable around E^* under R-H criterion for the following parameter values in Table 1.

Parameters	Definition	Values assigned
λ	Constant rate of production of $CD4^+T$ Cells	10.0 cells/ day
d	Death rate of Uninfected $CD4^+T$ cells	0.01 cells/ day
β	Rate of infection	0.001 cells/ day
a	Death rate of infected cells	0.24 cells/ day
p	Clearance rate of infected cells by CTL_e	0.002 / day
c	Rate of proliferation of CTL_p	0.6 /day
b	Decay rate of CTL_p	0.01 /day
h	Decay rate of CTL_e	0.02/day
γ	activation rate of uninfected $CD4^+T$ cell by IL-2	0.5/day
γ_1	activation rate of CTL_p by IL-2	0.1/day
q_1	multiplication capacity of differentiated precursor CTL	0.5
q_2	multiplication capacity of proliferated effector CTL	0.3

Table 1. Variables and parameters used in the models (1), (2), (16, 17). All parameter values are taken from (Wodarz et al., 1999), (Calshaw et al., 2000), (Roy & Chatterjee, 2010), (Bonhoeffer et al., 1997), (Nowak and Bangham, 1996).

4. Delay induced system

In this section we proposed and analyzed the mathematical model (1), incorporating delay in activation of uninfected $CD4^+T$ cell populations through IL-2 therapy. It should be mentioned here that delay-differential equations demonstrate in a complex dynamics rather than ordinary-differential equations in view of the fact that a time lag could cause a stable equilibrium to become unstable and hence the population may be fluctuated. For better understanding and also for realistic emulation of the delay induced system, we thus introduced a time delay in the production of CTL in our model (1). We also initiated another discrete time delay due to the account of the time lag in CTL_p activation. Thus we have the following delay differential equation model in the form of:

$$\dot{x}(t) = \lambda - \beta(1 - \eta_1 u_1)x(t)y(t) - dx(t) + \gamma x(t - \tau_1)$$
$$\dot{y}(t) = \beta(1 - \eta_1 u_1)x(t)y(t) - ay(t) - py(t)z(t)$$
$$\dot{w}(t) = cx(t)y(t)w(t) - cq_1y(t)w(t) - bw(t) + \gamma_1 w(t - \tau_2)$$
$$\dot{z}(t) = cq_2y(t)w(t) - hz(t), \tag{2}$$

with initial conditions $x(\theta) = x_0 > 0, y(\theta) = 0, w(\theta) = 0, z(\theta) = 0$ for $\theta \in [-max\{\tau_1, \tau_2\}, 0]$.

4.1 Stability analysis of the delay induced system

We further paying our attention to investigate the local asymptomatic stability of the infected steady state E^* for the delay induced system (Equation 2). Now linearizing the system (2)

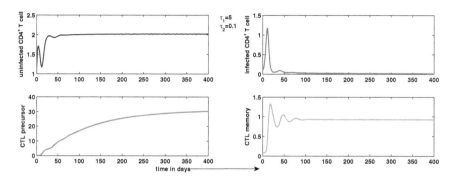

Fig. 2. Solution trajectory of the delayed system. Here $\tau_1 = 5, \tau_2 = 0.1$, and all other parameter values are same as Table 1.

about E^* we get,

$$\frac{dT}{dt} = FT(t) + GT(t - \tau_1) + HT(t - \tau_2). \tag{3}$$

Here F, G, H are 4x4 matrices given below,

$$F = \begin{pmatrix} -d - \beta(1 - \eta_1 u_1)y^* & -\beta(1 - \eta_1 u_1)x^* & 0 & 0 \\ \beta(1 - \eta_1 u_1)y^* & \beta(1 - \eta_1 u_1)x^* - a - pz^* & 0 & -py^* \\ cy^*w^* & cx^*w^* - cq_1w^* & cx^*y^* - cq_1y^* - b & 0 \\ 0 & cq_2w^* & cq_2y^* & -h \end{pmatrix}$$

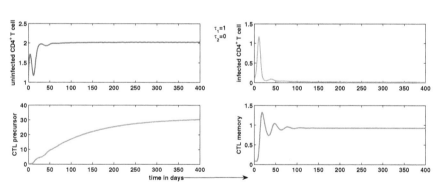

Fig. 3. Solution trajectory of the delayed system. Here $\tau_1 = 1, \tau_2 = 0$, and all other parameter values are same as Table 1.

$$G = \begin{pmatrix} \gamma & 0 & 0 & 0 \\ 0 & 0 & 0 & 0 \\ 0 & 0 & 0 & 0 \\ 0 & 0 & 0 & 0 \end{pmatrix}$$

$$H = \begin{pmatrix} 0 & 0 & 0 & 0 \\ 0 & 0 & 0 & 0 \\ 0 & 0 & \gamma_1 & 0 \\ 0 & 0 & 0 & 0 \end{pmatrix}$$

The characteristic equation of system (2) is given by,

$$\triangle(\zeta) = | \zeta I - F - e^{-\zeta \tau_1} G - e^{-\zeta \tau_2} H | = 0.$$

This equation can be written as,

$$\psi(\zeta, \tau_1, \tau_2) = \zeta^4 + A_1 \zeta^3 + A_2 \zeta^2 + A_3 \zeta + A_4 \zeta + e^{-\zeta \tau_1}[B_1 \zeta^3 + B_2 \zeta^2 + B_3 \zeta + B_4]$$
$$e^{-\zeta \tau_2}[C_1 \zeta^3 + C_2 \zeta^2 + C_3 \zeta + C_4] + e^{-\zeta(\tau_1 + \tau_2)}[D_1 \zeta^2 + D_2 \zeta + D_3] = 0. \qquad (4)$$

The coefficients are given below,

$$m_{11} = -d - \beta(1 - \eta_1 u_1)y^*, \quad m_{12} = -\beta(1 - \eta_1 u_1)x^*, \quad m_{21} = \beta(1 - \eta_1 u_1)y^*,$$
$$m_{22} = \beta(1 - \eta_1 u_1)x^* - a - pz^*, \quad m_{24} = py^*, \quad m_{31} = cy^* w^*, \quad m_{32} = cx^* w^* - cq_1 w^*,$$
$$m_{33} = cx^* y^* - cq_1 y^* - b, \quad m_{42} = cq_2 w^*, m_{43} = cq_2 y^*, m_{44} = -h,$$

where,

$$A_1 = m_{44} - m_{33} - m_{22} - m_{11},$$

$$A_2 = m_{33}m_{44} + m_{11}m_{44} + m_{22}m_{44} + m_{22}m_{33} + m_{11}m_{33} + m_{22}m_{11} - m_{12}m_{21} - m_{24}m_{42},$$

$$A_3 = -m_{11}m_{33}m_{44} - m_{22}m_{33}m_{44} - m_{11}m_{22}m_{44} + m_{12}m_{21}m_{44} - m_{24}m_{32}m_{43},$$
$$+ m_{24}m_{33}m_{42} + m_{11}m_{24}m_{42} + m_{11}m_{24}m_{42} - m_{11}m_{22}m_{33} + m_{12}m_{21}m_{33},$$

$$A_4 = m_{11}m_{22}m_{33}m_{44} - m_{12}m_{21}m_{33}m_{44} + m_{11}m_{24}m_{32}m_{43} - m_{12}m_{24}m_{31}m_{43}$$
$$- m_{11}m_{24}m_{33}m_{42},$$

$$B_1 = -\gamma,$$

$$B_2 = \gamma(m_{44} + m_{33}m_{22}),$$

$$B_3 = \gamma(-m_{33}m_{44} - m_{22}m_{44} - m_{22}m_{33} + m_{24}m_{42}),$$

$$B_4 = \gamma(m_{22}m_{33}m_{44} + m_{24}m_{32}m_{43} - m_{24}m_{33}m_{42}),$$

$$C_1 = -\gamma_1,$$

$$C_2 = \gamma_1(m_{44} + m_{22}m_{11}),$$

$$C_3 = \gamma_1(-m_{22}m_{44} - m_{11}m_{44} - m_{22}m_{11} + m_{24}m_{42}),$$

$$C_4 = \gamma_1(m_{11}m_{22}m_{44} - m_{12}m_{21}m_{44} - m_{11}m_{24}m_{42}),$$

$$D_1 = \gamma \gamma_1,$$

$$D_2 = \gamma \gamma_1(-m_{22}m_{44}),$$

$$D_3 = \gamma \gamma_1(m_{22}m_{44}).$$

The characteristic equation (4) is a transcendental equation in ζ. It is known that E^* is locally asymptotically stable if all the roots of the corresponding characteristic equation have negative real parts and unstable if purely imaginary roots are appears. As we know that the transcendental equation has infinitely many complex roots (Calshaw et al., 2000), so in presence of τ_1, τ_2, analysis of the sign of roots is very complicated. Thus, we begin our analysis by setting one delay which is equal to zero and then deduce the conditions for stability, when both time delays are non zero.

Case I :- When $\tau_1 = \tau_2 = 0$:
In absence of both the delays the characteristics equation (4) becomes,

$$\zeta^4 + \zeta^3(A_1 + B_1 + C_1) + \zeta^2(A_2 + B_2 + C_2 + D_1) + \zeta(A_3 + B_3 + C_3 + D_2)$$
$$+ (A_4 + B_4 + C_4 + D_3) = 0. \tag{5}$$

Employing Routh Hurwitz criteria for sign of roots we have the same results as in non delayed system analysis.

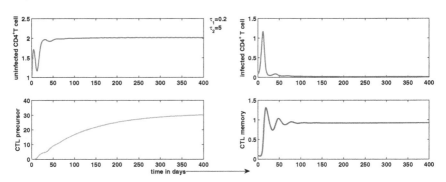

Fig. 4. Solution trajectory of the delayed system. Here $\tau_1 = 0.2, \tau_2 = 5$, and all other parameter values are same as Table 1.

Case II :- When $\tau_1 > 0, \tau_2 = 0$:

In this case we consider no delay in CTL precursor immune response i.e $\tau_2 = 0$, then the characteristic equation becomes,

$$\zeta^4 + \zeta^3(A_1 + C_1) + \zeta^2(A_2 + C_2) + \zeta(A_3 + C_3) + (A_4 + C_4)$$
$$+ e^{-\zeta \tau_1}[B_1\zeta^3 + \zeta^2(B_2 + D_1) + \zeta(B_3 + D_2) + (B_4 + D_3)] = 0. \tag{6}$$

For $\tau_1 > 0$, (6) has infinitely many roots. Using Rouche's theorem and continuity of τ_1, the transcedental equation has roots with positive real parts if and only if it has purely imaginary roots. Let $i\theta$ be a root of equation (6) and hence we get,

$$\theta^4 - \theta^2(A_2 + C_2) + (A_4 + C_4) = \cos\theta\tau_1[\theta^2(B_2 + D_1) - (B_4 + D_3)]$$
$$+ \sin\theta\tau_1[\theta^3 D_1 - \theta(B_3 + D_2)]$$
$$\theta(A_3 + C_3) - \theta^3(A_1 + C_1) = \cos\theta\tau_1[\theta^3 D_1 - \theta(B_3 + D_2)]$$
$$- \sin\theta\tau_1[\theta^2(B_2 + D_1) - (B_4 + D_3)]. \tag{7}$$

Squaring and adding above two equations,

$$\theta^8 + \theta^6[(A_1 + C_1)^2 - 2(A_2 + C_2) - D_1^2]$$
$$+ \theta^4[(A_2 + C_2)^2 + 2(A_4 + C_4) - 2(A_3 + C_3)(A_1 + C_1) - (B_2 + D_1)^2$$
$$+ 2D_1(B_3 + D_2)] + \theta^2[(A_3 + C_3)^2$$
$$- 2(A_2 + C_2)(A_4 + C_4) + 2(B_2 + D_1)(B_4 + D_3) - (B_3 + D_2)^2]$$
$$+ [(A_4 + C_4)^2 - (B_4 + D_3)^2] = 0. \tag{8}$$

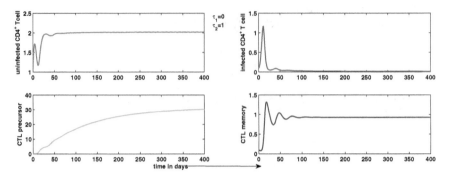

Fig. 5. Solution trajectory of the delayed system. Here $\tau_1 = 0, \tau_2 = 1$, and all other parameter values are same as Table 1.

Simplifying and substituting $\theta^2 = l$ in equation (8) we get the following equation,

$$l^4 + \alpha_1 l^3 + \alpha_2 l^2 + \alpha_3 l + \alpha_4 = 0. \tag{9}$$

Where,

$$\alpha_1 = (A_1 + C_1)^2 - 2(A_2 + C_2) - D_1^2,$$
$$\alpha_2 = (A_2 + C_2)^2 + 2(A_4 + C_4) - 2(A_3 + C_3)(A_1 + C_1) - (B_2 + D_1)^2 + 2D_1(B_3 + D_2),$$
$$\alpha_3 = (A_3 + C_3)^2 - 2(A_2 + C_2)(A_4 + C_4) + 2(B_2 + D_1)(B_4 + D_3) - (B_3 + D_2)^2,$$
$$\alpha_4 = (A_4 + C_4)^2 - (B_4 + D_3)^2.$$

It may be noted that the equation (9) will have negative real part if and only if Routh-Hurwitz criterion is satisfied and hence equation (6) will have no purely imaginary root. From the above analysis we have the following proposition.

Proposition 4 : In the delay induced system (2), the infected steady state E^* will be locally asymptotically stable for all $\tau_1 > 0$ if the following conditions are satisfied: $\alpha_1 > 0, \alpha_4 > 0, \psi = \alpha_1\alpha_2 - \alpha_3 > 0, \psi\alpha_3 - \alpha_1^2\alpha_4 > 0.$

Case III :- When $\tau_1 = 0, \tau_2 > 0$:
In absence of τ_1, the characteristic equation (4) have the following form,

$$\xi^4 + \xi^3(A_1 + B_1) + \xi^2(A_2 + B_2) + \xi(A_3 + B_3) + (A_4 + B_4)$$
$$+ e^{-\xi\tau_2}[C_1\xi^3 + \xi^2(C_2 + D_1) + \xi(C_3 + D_2) + (C_4 + D_3)] = 0. \tag{10}$$

Similarly as in case II we substitute $\xi = i\theta$ and we get,

$$\theta^4 - \theta^2(A_2 + B_2) + (A_4 + B_4) = \cos\theta\tau_2[\theta^2(C_2 + D_1) - (C_4 + D_3)]$$
$$+ \sin\theta\tau_2[\theta^3 C_1 - \theta(C_3 + D_2)]. \tag{11}$$

$$\theta(A_3 + B_3) - \theta^3(A_1 + B_1) = \cos\theta\tau_2[\theta^3 C_1 - \theta(C_3 + D_2)]$$
$$- \sin\theta\tau_1[\theta^2(C_2 + D_1) - (C_4 + D_3)]. \tag{12}$$

Squaring and adding, and then substituting $\theta^2 = s$ we have,

$$s^4 + \delta_1 s^3 + \delta_2 s^2 + \delta_3 s + \delta_4 = 0. \tag{13}$$

Where,

$$\delta_1 = (A_1 + B_1)^2 - 2(A_2 + B_2) - C_1^2$$
$$\delta_2 = (A_2 + B_2)^2 + 2(A_4 + B_4) - 2(A_3 + B_3)(A_1 + B_1) - (C_2 + D_1)^2 + 2C_1(C_3 + D_2)$$
$$\delta_3 = (A_3 + B_3)^2 - 2(A_2 + B_2)(A_4 + B_4) + 2(C_2 + D_1)(C_4 + D_3) - (C_3 + D_2)^2$$
$$\delta_4 = (A_4 + B_4)^2 - (C_4 + D_3)^2.$$

From the above analysis we have the following proposition.

Proposition 5 : In the delay induced system (2), the infected steady state E^* will be locally asymptotically stable for all $\tau_2 > 0$ if the following conditions are satisfied $\delta_1 > 0$, $\delta_4 > 0$, $\varphi = \delta_1 \delta_2 - \delta_3 > 0$, $\varphi \delta_3 - \delta_1^2 \delta_4 > 0$. If $\delta_4 < 0$ then we have the following proposition,

Proposition 6 : Equation (13) admits at least one positive root if $\delta_4 < 0$ is satisfied.

If θ_0 be a positive root of (13), then equation (10) will have a purely imaginary root $\pm i\theta_0$ corresponding to τ_2. Now we evaluate the critical value of τ_2 for which the deley induced system (2) remain stable. From equation (11,12),

$$\tau_2^* = \frac{a\cos\phi(\theta_0)}{\theta_0}. \tag{14}$$

Where,

$$\phi(\theta_0) = [\{\theta^2(C_2 + D_1) - (C_4 + D_3)\}\{\theta^4 - \theta^2(A_2 + B_2) + (A_4 + B_4)\}$$
$$+ \{\theta^3 C_1 - \theta(C_3 + D_2)\}\{\theta(A_3 + B_3) - \theta^3(A_1 + B_1)\}]$$
$$\div [\{\theta^2(C_2 + D_1) - (C_4 + D_3)\}^2 + \{\theta^3 C_1 - \theta(C_3 + D_2)\}^2]. \tag{15}$$

From the above analysis we construct the following theorem.

Theorem 1 :

If $\delta_4 < 0$ is satisfied, then the steady state E^* is locally asymptotically stable for $\tau_2 < \tau_2^*$ and becomes unstable for $\tau_2 > \tau_2^*$. When $\tau_2 = \tau_2^*$ a Hopf bifurcation occurs.

Case IV :- $\tau_1 > 0, \tau_2 > 0$

In this case we studied the stability of the steady state E^* in presence of both delays. If all the roots of equation (10) have negative real parts for $\tau > 0$ i.e when the system is locally asymptotically stable then there exists a τ_1^* depending upon τ_2 such that all roots of equation (4) have negative real parts whenever $\tau_1 < \tau_1^*$. Considering all the cases we have the following theorem .

Theorem 2 : Whenever $\delta_4 < 0$ holds then for $\tau_2 < \tau_2^*$, there exists a τ_1^* depending upon τ_2 the steady state E^* is locally asymptotically stable for $\tau_1 < \tau_1^*$ and $\tau_2 < \tau_2^*$.

Special Remarks of the Delay Induced System in view of Numerical Analysis:
Though it is eventually true from our analytical results that for a longer value of delay the

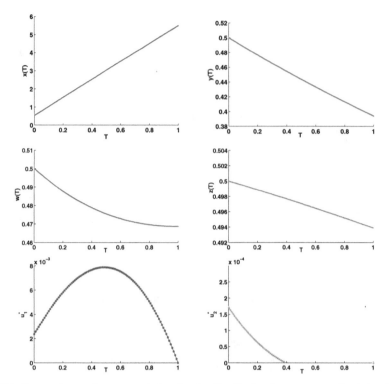

Fig. 6. This figure shows the system behavior for the Optimal treatment schedule of the control variable $u_1(t)$ and $u_2(t)$ for $R = 0.1$, $P = 0.5$, and $\eta_1 = 0.5$, $\eta_2 = 0.1$, $\eta_3 = 0.01$. All other parameter values are same as Table 1.

system become unstable (Theorem 1 and Theorem 2), however it is essential to mention here that in our delay induced system, numerical analysis reveal, when $\tau_1 = 0$ and $\tau_2 = 1$, its reflect from solution trajectory, there are no such oscillations in Figure, which may conclude that delay does affect the stability of the system.

Further we change the values of both delays τ_1, and τ_2, and varied them from 1 to 20, we also observe that no significant changes does arise in each case for which we can express that delay affect the stability of the system. Thus, in a nutshell we can say that incorporation of time delay into the existing model to account for time lag in activation of CTL_p did not exhibit any biologically significant interpretation.

5. The optimal control problem

In this section our main object is to minimize the infected CD4$^+$T cells population as well as minimize the systemic cost of drug treatment. Here we formulate an optimal control problem. We also want to maximize the level of healthy CD4$^+$T cells. So in our basic model (1), we use control variables $u_1(t), u_2(t)$ represents the drug dose satisfying $0 \leq u_1(t) \leq 1$ and $0 \leq u_2(t) \leq 1$. Here $u_1(t) = 1, u_2(t) = 1$ events are represents the maximal use of chemotherapy and $u_1(t) = 0, u_2(t) = 0$ represents no treatment.

Here we consider that the RTI reduces the infection rate by $(1 - \eta_1 u_1)$, where η_1 represents the drug efficacy and u_1 is the control input doses of the drug RTI. We also consider the enrichment of uninfected T cell and CTL responses through IL-2 treatment is given by $\eta_2 u_2$, and $\eta_3 u_2$, where u_2 as a control input of IL-2 treatment and η_2, η_3 are the drug efficacy of IL-2 for uninfected T cell and precursor CTL responses.

In this section our main aim is to minimize the cost as well as minimize the infected CD4$^+$T cell and maximize the uninfected CD4$^+$T cell. Thus we construct the optimal control problem where the state system is

$$\dot{x} = \lambda - dx - \beta(1 - \eta_1 u_1(t))xy + (1 - \eta_2 u_2(t))\gamma x$$
$$\dot{y} = \beta(1 - \eta_1 u_1(t))xy - ay - pyz$$
$$\dot{w} = cxyw - cq_1 yw - bw + (1 - \eta_3 u_2(t))\gamma_1 w$$
$$\dot{z} = cq_2 yw - hz, \tag{16}$$

and the control function is defined as

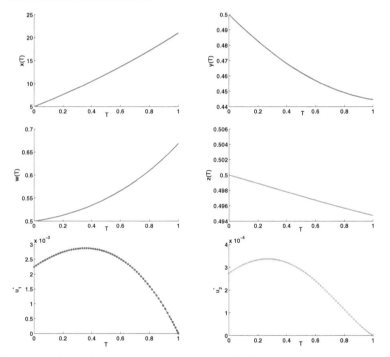

Fig. 7. This figure shows the system behavior for the Optimal treatment schedule of the control variable $u_1(t)$ and $u_2(t)$ for $R = 10$, $P = 50$, and $\eta_1 = 0.1$, $\eta_2 = 0.1$, $\eta_3 = 0.01$. All other parameter values are same as Table 1.

$$J(u_1, u_2) = \int_{t_0}^{t_f} [y(t) - x(t) - w(t) + Ru_1^2 + Pu_2^2]dt. \tag{17}$$

Where the parameter R and P respectively the weight on the benefit of the cost.

Here the control function $u_1(t)$ and $u_2(t)$ are bounded, Lebesgue integrable function (Swan, 1984).

In this problem we are seeking the optimal control pair $(u_1{}^*, u_2{}^*)$ such that
$J(u_1{}^*, u_2{}^*) = \min\{J(u_1, u_2) : (u_1, u_2) \in U\}$.

Here U is the control set defined by
$U = \{u = (u_1, u_2) : \ u_1, u_2$ are the measurable, $0 \le u_1(t) \le 1, \ 0 \le u_2(t) \le 1, \ t \in [t_0, t_f]\}$.

To determine the optimal control $u_1{}^*$ and $u_2{}^*$, we use the "Pontryagin Minimum Principle" (Pontryagin et al., 1986). To solve the problem we use the Hamiltonian given by

$$H = y(t) - x(t) - w(t) + Ru_1^2 + Pu_2^2 + \xi_1\{\lambda - dx - \beta(1 - \eta_1 u_1(t))xy + (1 - \eta_2 u_2(t))\gamma x\}$$
$$+ \xi_2\{\beta(1 - \eta_1 u_1(t))xy - ay - pyz\} + \xi_3\{cxyw - cq_1 yw - bw + (1 - \eta_3 u_2(t))\gamma_1 w\}$$
$$+ \xi_4\{cq_2 yw - hz\}. \tag{18}$$

By using the "Pontryagin Minimum Principle" and the existence condition for the optimal control theory (Fleming et al., 1975) we obtain the theorem.

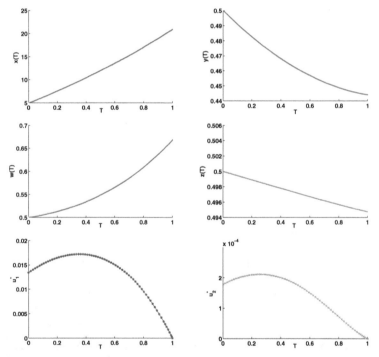

Fig. 8. This figure shows the system behavior for the Optimal treatment schedule of the control variable $u_1(t)$ and $u_2(t)$ for $R = 10$, $P = 50$, and $\eta_1 = 0.6$, $\eta_2 = 0.1$, $\eta_3 = 0.01$. All other parameter values are same as Table 1.

Theorem: The objective cost function $J(u_1, u_2)$ over U is minimum for the optimal control $u^* = (u_1{}^*, u_2{}^*)$ corresponding to the interior equilibrium (x^*, y^*, w^*, z^*). Also there exist adjoint function $\xi_1, \xi_2, \xi_3, \xi_4$ satisfying the equation (18) and (19).

Proof: By using Pontryagin Minimum principle (Fleming et al., 1975) the unconstrained optimal control variable $u_1{}^*$ and $u_2{}^*$ satisfy

$$\frac{\partial H}{\partial u_1{}^*} = \frac{\partial H}{\partial u_2{}^*} = 0. \tag{19}$$

Since

$$\begin{aligned} H = &[Ru_1^2 - \xi_1(1 - \eta_1 u_1(t))\beta xy + \xi_2(1 - \eta_1 u_1(t))\beta xy] + [Pu_2^2 + \xi_1(1 - \eta_2 u_2)\gamma x \\ &+ \xi_3(1 - \eta_3 u_2)\gamma_1 w] + \text{other terms without } u_1 \text{ and } u_2, \end{aligned} \tag{20}$$

then we obtain $\frac{\partial H}{\partial u_i{}^*}$ for $u_i{}^*$ where $(i = 1, 2)$, and hence equation with zero becomes,

$$\frac{\partial H}{\partial u_1{}^*} = 2Ru_1{}^* + \eta_1 \beta x^* y^*(\xi_1 - \xi_2) = 0$$

$$\frac{\partial H}{\partial u_2{}^*} = 2Pu_2{}^* - \xi_1 \eta_2 \gamma x^* - \xi_3 \eta_3 \gamma_1 z^* = 0.$$

Thus we obtain the optimal control $u_1{}^*$ and $u_2{}^*$ corresponding to the interior equilibrium (x^*, y^*, w^*, z^*) as,

$$u_1{}^* = \frac{\beta \eta_1 x^* y^*(\xi_2 - \xi_1)}{2R}$$

$$u_2{}^* = \frac{(\xi_1 \eta_2 \gamma x^* + \xi_3 \eta_3 \gamma_1 z^*)}{2P}. \tag{21}$$

According to Pontryagin minimum Principle (Pontryagin et al., 1986) we know that,

$$\frac{d\xi}{dt} = -\frac{\partial H}{\partial x}, \tag{22}$$

and

$$H(x(t), u^*(t), \xi(t), t) = \min_{u \in U} H(x(t), u(t), \xi(t), t). \tag{23}$$

The above equations are the necessary conditions satisfying the optimal control $u(t)$ and again for the system (16, 17) the adjoint equations are

$$\frac{d\xi_1}{dt} = -\frac{\partial H}{\partial x}, \quad \frac{d\xi_2}{dt} = -\frac{\partial H}{\partial y}, \quad \frac{d\xi_3}{dt} = -\frac{\partial H}{\partial w}, \quad \frac{d\xi_4}{dt} = -\frac{\partial H}{\partial z}.$$

Taking the partial derivative of H we get,

$$\frac{d\xi_1}{dt} = 1 + \xi_1\{d_1 + (1 - \eta_1 u_1(t))\beta y - (1 - \eta_2 u_2(t))\gamma\} - \xi_2(1 - \eta_1 u_1(t))\beta y - \xi_3 cyw$$

$$\frac{d\xi_2}{dt} = -1 + \xi_1(1 - \eta_1 u_1(t))\beta x - \xi_2\{(1 - \eta_1 u_1(t))\beta x - a - pz\} - \xi_3\{cxw - cq_1 w\} - \xi_4 cq_2 w$$

$$\frac{d\xi_3}{dt} = 1 - \xi_3\{cxy - cq_1 y - b + (1 - \eta_3 u_2(t))\gamma_1\} - \xi_4 cq_2 y$$

$$\frac{d\xi_4}{dt} = \xi_2 py + \xi_4 h. \tag{24}$$

Hence the optimality of the system consists of the state system along with the adjoint system. Also it depends on the initial conditions and the transversality condition which satisfy $\xi_i(t_f) = 0$ and $x(0) = x_0$, $y(0) = y_0$, $w(0) = w_0$, $z(0) = z_0$.

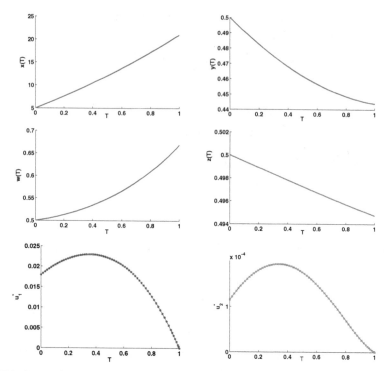

Fig. 9. This figure shows the system behavior for the Optimal treatment schedule of the control variable $u_1(t)$ and $u_2(t)$ for $R = 10$, $P = 50$, and $\eta_1 = 0.8$, $\eta_2 = 0.4$, $\eta_3 = 0.1$. All other parameter values are same as Table 1.

6. Conclusion

In this research article we have considered a mathematical model of immune system representing the response of a HIV infected individual in presence of HAART and IL-2. We have studied how the immune system recovers by applying IL-2 as an immune activator along with HAART. We have also observed the effect of delay in activation of uninfected $CD4^+T$ populations through IL-2 therapy. We have noticed the control therapy, which is more effective with respect to cost and also less side effect. Here analytical as well as numerical approaches have been observed. We have also noticed that, the rational behind concomitant administration of IL-2 with HAART is to augment host immune responses through prevention of destruction of the immunity system without stimulation of HIV replication. In the beginning of our research article, our mathematical model of HIV dynamics in presence of HAART and IL-2 suggest the existence of three equilibrium conditions : $E_1(x_1,0,0,0)$, $E_2(x_2,y_2,0,0)$ and $E^*(x^*,y^*,w^*,z^*)$. Our analytical studies first indicates the infection free steady state or uninfected equilibrium, where $CD4^+T$ cells are healthy and no infected cell population exists and there is no HIV-specific CTL immune response. The second equilibrium condition is not a very desirable one since there is no immune response even in presence of HIV antigen. The third equilibrium state or infected steady state is said to be exist at certain limiting values of infected cell population in presence of HAART and IL-2. We also studied the stability of the system for different equilibrium points. Further a time delay has been introduced into the existing model to account for the activation of immune response through infected $CD4^+T$ cells. In that study, we noticed that delay induced system has no useful delay effect which changes its stability. From optimal control studies, several interesting results have been obtained. As weight factors (R and P) increase from 0.1 to 10 and 0.5 to 50 respectively, there is a significant increase in the uninfected cell population with very little effect on the count of infected cells. The increase in the weight factors does not produce proportionate increase in the precursor CTL population and increase in effectiveness of HAART or IL-2 as denoted by η, is not manifested by remarkable change in precursor CTL number. The CTL effector population is found to decrease in all the cases. Thus, optimal control approach will help in designing an innovative cost-effective safe therapeutic regimen of HAART and IL-2 where the uninfected cell population will be enhanced with simultaneous decrease in the infected cell population. Moreover, successful immune reconstitution can also be achieved with increase in precursor CTL population. Mathematical modeling of viral dynamics thus enables maximization of therapeutic outcome even in case of multiple therapies with specific goal of reversal of immunity impairment.

From our above discussion of the results, it is clear that, though incorporation of time delay into the existing model (1) to account for time lag in activation of CTL_p did not exhibit any biologically significant interpretation, however, adoption of optimal control strategy in optimization of therapeutic regime of combination therapy of HAART and IL-2 was found to be really satisfactory in terms of enhancing the life expectancy of HIV-afflicted patients by improving the uninfected T cell count.

7. References

Wodarz, D.; Nowak, M.A. (1999). Specific therepy regimes could lead to long term immunological control to HIV, *Proc. Natl. Acad. Sci. USA*, Vol. 96, No. 25, pp. 14464-14469.

Srivastava, P.K.; Banerjee, M.; Chandra, P. (2010). A primary infection model for HIV and immune response with two discreat time delays, *Differ Equ Dyn Syst*, Springer.

Pontryagin, L.S.; Boltyanskii, V.G.; Gamkrelidze, R. V.; Mishchenko, E. F. (1986). Mathematical Theory of Optimal Processes, *Gordon and Breach Science Publishers*, Vol. 4.

Culshaw, R.V.; Ruan, S. (2000). A delay -differentianal equation model of HIV-1 infection of $CD4^+T$-cells, *Math. Biosci.*, Vol. 165, pp. 425-444.

Fleming, W.; Rishel, R. (1975). Deterministic and Stochastic optimal controls, *Springer-Verlag*, Chapter 3, pp. 545-562.

Swan, G. M. (1984). Application of Optimal Control Theory in Biomedicine, *CRC Press*.

Sereti, I.; Anthony, K.B.; Martinez-Wilson H.; Lempicki R. Adelsberger, J.; Metcalf, J.A.; Hallahan; C.W.; Follmann, D.; Davey, R.T.; Kovacs, J.A.; & Lane H.C. (2004). IL-2 induced CD4+ T-cell expansion in HIV-infected patients is associated with long-term decreases in T-cell proliferation, *Blood* , 104, pp. 775-780.

Smith, K.A. (2001). Low-dose daily interleukin-2 immunotherapy: accelerating immune restoration and expanding HIV-specific T-cell immunity without toxicity AIDS, *suppl* 1, vol. 15, pp. S28-S35.

Banerjee, S. (2008). Immunotherapywith Interleukin-2: A Study Based On Mathematical Modeling, *Int. J. Appl. Math. Comput. Sci.*, vol. 18, pp. 389-398.

Marchettia, G.; Meroni, L.; Molteni, C.; Bandera, A.; Franzetti, F.; Galli, M.; Moroni, M.; Clericib, M.; & Gori, A. (2004). Interleukin-2 immunotherapy exerts a differential effect on CD4 and CD8 T cell dynamics, *AIDS*, vol.18, pp. 211-216.

De, Paoli P. (2001). Immunological effects of Interleukin-2 therapy in human immune-deficiency virus-positive subjects Clin. Diagn. Lab., *Immunol.*, vol. 8, pp. 671-677.

Sereti, I.; Sklar, P.; Ramchandani, M.S.; Read, S.W.; Aggarwal, V.; Imamichi, H.; Natarajan, V.; Metcalf, J.A.; Davey, R.T.; Kovacs, J.A.; DerSimonian, R.; & Lane, H.C. (2007). CD4+ T Cell Responses to Interleukin-2 Administration in HIV-Infected Patients Are Directly Related to the Baseline Level of Immune Activation, *J. Infect. Dis.*, vol.196 , pp. 677-683.

De, Paoli P.; Bortolin, M. T; Zanussi, S.; Monzoni, A.; Pratesi, C; $ Giacc M. (2001). Changes in thymic function in HIV-positive patients treated with highly active antiretroviral therapy and interleukin-2, *Clin Exp Immunol*, vol. 125, pp.440-446.

Marchettia, G.; Franzetti, F.; & Gori, A. (2005). Partial immune reconstitution following highly active antiretroviral therapy: can adjuvant interleukin-2 fill the gap?, *J. Antimicrob. Chemother.*, vol. 55, pp. 401-409.

Paredes, R.; deQuiros, J.C.L.B.; Fernandez-Cruz, Z.; Clotet, $ Lane, H.C. (2002). Potential role of interleukin-2 in patients with HIV infection, *AIDS Rev.*, vol. 4, pp. 36-40.

Roy Priti Kumar; Chatterjee Amar Nath. (2011). Effect of HAART on CTL Mediated Immune Cells: An Optimal Control Theoretic Approach, *Electrical Engineering and Applied Computing, Springer*, Vol. 90, pp.595-607.

Roy Priti Kumar; Chatterjee, A. N. (2011). Delay Model of HIV with Cure Rate During Long Term Disease Progression, *Electrical Engineering and Applied Computing, Springer*, Vol. 90, pp. 699-713.

Roy Priti Kumar; Chatterjee, A. N. (2010). T-cell Proliferation in a Mathematical Model of CTL Activity Through HIV-1 Infection, *Lecture Notes in Engineering and Computer Science, WCE, UK*, Vol. 1, pp. 615-620.

Roy Priti Kumar; Chatterjee, A. N. (2010). Delay effect in a Mathematical model of HIV infected T-cell against killing by CTL, *Bull. Cal. Math. Soc.*, Vol. 102(6), pp. 513-524.

Perelson, A.S; Nelson, P.W. (1999). Mathematical Analysis of HIV-1 Dynamics in Vivo, *SIAM Review*, Vol. 41, pp. 3-41.

Wodarz, D.; May, R.M.; Nowak, M.A. (2000). The role of antigen independent persistance of memory cytotoxic T lymphocytes, *Int Immunol*, Vol. 12, pp.467.

Bonhoeffer, S.; Coffin, J.M.; Nowak, M.A. (1997). Human Immunodeficiency Virus Drug Therapy and Virus Load, *Journal of Virology*, Vol. 71, pp. 3275–3278.

Nowak, M.A.; Bangham, C.R.M. (1996). A delay -differentianal equation model of HIV-1 infection of CD4+T-cells, *Science*, Vol. 272(5258), pp. 74-79.

Kirschner, D. (1996). Using mathematics to underdtand HIV immune dynamics, *Notice of the AMS*.

Gumel, A. B.; Zhang, X. W.; Shivkumar, P. N.; Garba, M. L.; Sahai, B. M. (2002). A new mathematical model for assessing therapeutic strategies for HIV infection, *J. Theo. Medicin*, Vol. 4(2), pp. 147-155.

Herz, A. V. M.; Bonhoeffer, S.; Anderson, R. M.; May, R. M.; Nowak, M. A. (1996). Viral dynamicsin vivo; limitations on estimates of intracellular delay and virus decay, *Proc. Natl. Acad. Sci. USA*, Vol. 93, pp. 7247-7251.

7

Worldwide Trends in Infectious Disease Research Revealed by a New Bibliometric Method

Hiromi Takahashi-Omoe[1] and Katsuhiko Omoe[2]
[1]National Institute of Science and Technology Policy (NISTEP)
[2]Iwate University
Japan

1. Introduction

Infectious diseases cause serious public health problems and their threat has been increasing. This is because these diseases are now spreading geographically much faster than at any time in history as a result of the highly mobile, interdependent, and interconnected society (World Health Organization [WHO], 2007). In addition, it is distressing that outbreaks of emerging infectious diseases such as severe acute respiratory syndrome, Nipah virus infection, and West Nile fever have been occurring at an unprecedented rate of one or more per year in animal and human populations since the 1970s (Brown, 2004; WHO, 2007). As a recent example, the 2009 H1N1 pandemic caused by a new subtype of influenza virus inflicted damage on people around the world. Because of these reasons, infectious disease research has been promoted primarily by developed countries to provide effective countermeasures against the diseases.

Infectious disease research has become more sophisticated and diversified. For example, the identification of natural reservoirs of emerging disease pathogens requires an interdisciplinary approach among microbiology, ecology, zoology, and other fields. The risk analysis of epidemic norovirus infection requires data regarding not only the virological properties of the virus but also wastewater management and hygienic conditions. In studies on influenza in Japan, a variety of basic and applied research approaches such as analysis of pathogenesis, vaccine development, clinical investigation of prepandemic vaccines, and surveys of the route of virus transmission via migratory birds have been conducted (Figure 1) (Takahashi-Omoe & Omoe, 2009). Toward building further strategies for infectious disease research at domestic and international levels, the real trends in such studies should be grasped systematically.

As a measure to grasp trends in various research fields including infectious disease research, quantitative surveys of research articles, as an application of bibliometrics, have been conducted using scientific literature databases such as the Web of Science® (Thomson Reuters), Scopus™ (Elsevier B.V.), and PubMed (National Library of Medicine). The results of surveys provide the information needed for decision makers, public policymakers, researchers, and business leaders (Statistics Canada, 1998).

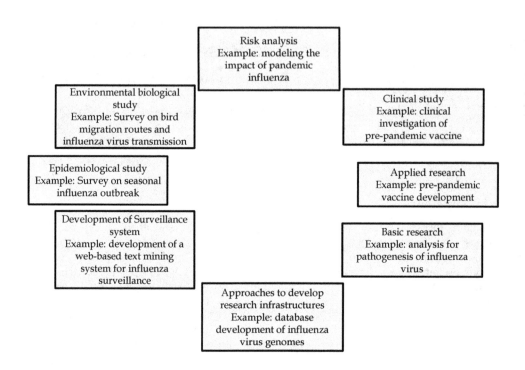

Fig. 1. An example of studies on influenza in Japan.

Regarding quantitative surveys in infectious disease research, in addition to specific diseases such as acquired immune deficiency syndrome (AIDS; caused by the human immunodeficiency virus [HIV]) (Patra & Chand, 2006; Uthman, 2008), tuberculosis (Ramos et al., 2008), and malaria (Garg et al., 2009), infectious diseases in general (Bliziotis et al., 2005; Ramos et al., 2004; Ramos et al., 2009) have been targeted. These studies demonstrated that the US, EU, and other specific world regions or nations showed a gradual increase in the publication of research articles, contributing to an increased grasp of general trends in infectious disease research in the world. However, the studies did not adequately demonstrate the real research trends in the non-English-speaking world because of limitations regarding journal selection for surveys of research articles. Previous studies were more likely to survey research articles in journals registered in the "Infectious Disease Category" of the Science Citation Index Expanded™ in the Web of Science® (the SCI Infectious Disease Category) (Thomson Reuters, 2011) and articles in international English-language journals, resulting in an underestimation of articles in non-English or regional journals that were published in the EU and Asia. Such limitations of bibliometric studies have been discussed in previous reports about the trends in infectious disease research

(Ramos et al., 2004), microbiology (Vergidis et al., 2005), and public health (Soteriades & Falagas, 2006). For example, Ramos et al. reported that European countries such as Germany, France, Italy and Spain had a long tradition of scientific publication in their own languages and might be penalized in comparative studies relying on the SCI (Ramos et al., 2004). Vergidis et al. also noted that journal selection based on the SCI particularly affected the survey results for Eastern Europe and Japan because scientists in these regions tended to publish their findings in regional journals more than scientists in others regions (Vergidis et al., 2005).

To improve on previous bibliometric analyses, we previously developed a method using 100 journals specializing in infectious disease research (infectious disease journals) (Takahashi-Omoe et al., 2009). These 100 journals, which were selected on the basis of keywords that exhaustively covered various infectious disease research fields, are published in various countries and written in various languages. Using these journals, we succeeded in surveying actual research trends in Asia between 1998 and 2006 without underestimating the number of articles in non-English and regional journals in comparison with surveys based on journals registered in the SCI Infectious Disease Category. This method using 100 journals has demonstrated the prospect for a more exhaustive survey of infectious disease research with less bias among nations and regions, although it is not perfect in comprehensiveness, similar to other bibliometric methods.

In this chapter, the features and usability of a new method using these 100 journals are being introduced, and the latest worldwide trends in infectious disease research is being presented as a practical application of the method.

2. Development of a survey method for infectious disease research

The 100 infectious disease journals used in this survey method were selected as described in section 2.1. The journals were assessed by their usability by comparison with journals registered in the SCI Infectious Disease Category as described in section 2.3.

2.1 Selection of 100 infectious disease journals

At the inception of selecting infectious disease journals, the Scopus™ database (as of 2011, the SciVerse Scopus, Elsevier B.V.; registered in January 2008) was used as a source. This is an abstract and citation database of the scientific literature that includes over 18,000 peer-reviewed journals.

On the basis of the Scopus™ database, infectious disease journals were screened using English keywords directly linked to disease control in detection, prevention, diagnosis, and medical care (A–E) (Figure 2). The keywords were chosen to select journals specifically focusing on infectious disease (A), general infectious diseases or infectious diseases belonging to specific categories (B), the field of clinical microbiology (C), the development of medicines (D), and overall technology development for disease control (E). In addition, related journals in the field of public health were selected on the basis of the author's experience (F).

In parallel, non-English journals were screened using Japanese, Chinese, French, German, Italian, Spanish, and Turkish keywords corresponding to the keywords in A–E. To screen

Korean journals, English keywords were used because almost all journal titles (89 of 91 journals) were registered in English or both English and Korean (in Roman letters) in the Scopus™ database. In the survey with English and non-English keywords, an approach based on both partial matching (for a search of journal titles that contain the keywords) and complete matching (for a search of titles that perfectly matches the keywords) was introduced to capture journal titles involving inflected forms of the keywords.

Through this screening, 264 candidates were selected, of which 240 were selected by English keywords and 24 by non-English words. The 264 journals were published in 30 countries and written in 12 languages: English, Japanese, Chinese, Korean, French, German, Italian, Spanish, Turkish, Polish, Russian, and Croatian. The list of journals can be found in our previous report (Takahashi- Omoe et al., 2009).

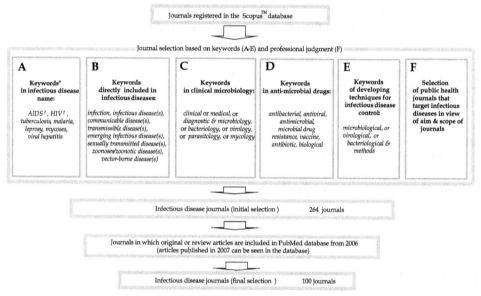

Fig. 2. Framework for selecting 100 infectious disease journals. *All keywords in A (excluding HIV); infection, infectious disease, communicable disease, sexually transmitted disease, and zoonosis in B; and antibacterial, antiviral, antimicrobial, vaccine, and antibiotic in D were translated into French, German, Italian, Spanish, Turkish, Chinese (in Roman letters), and Japanese (in Roman letters) to select journals written in non-English languages. †Journals regarding research on AIDS and HIV were selected according to the "Infectious Disease Category" of the Science Citation Index Expanded™ because several journals specializing in social-scientific and policy studies on patients could not be excluded by only the keywords "AIDS" and "HIV."

Subsequently, 100 of the 264 journals were selected on the basis of the usability of the PubMed database for indexing them. This was done to emphasize the further usability of the present survey method; the PubMed database is freely accessible and widely used, and the selected journals have continued in print through 2006 and beyond. The 100 journals listed in Table 1 were published in 18 countries and written in English and 7 non-English

AIDS

AIDS Patient Care and STDs

The AIDS Reader

AIDS Research and Human Retroviruses

AIDS Reviews

American Journal of Infection Control

The American Journal of Tropical Medicine and Hygiene

Annals of Tropical Medicine and Parasitology

Antimicrobial Agents and Chemotherapy

Annals of Clinical Microbiology and Antimicrobials

Antiviral Chemistry & Chemotherapy

Antiviral Research

Antiviral Therapy

Biologicals

BMC Infectious Diseases

Canada communicable disease report

Clinical and Vaccine Immunology

Clinical Infectious Diseases

Clinical Microbiology and Infection

Clinical Microbiology Reviews

Communicable Diseases Intelligence

Comparative Immunology, Microbiology and Infectious Diseases

Current HIV Research

Current Infectious Disease reports

Current Opinion in Infectious Diseases

Diagnostic Microbiology and Infectious Disease

Emerging Infectious Diseases

EnfermedadesInfecciosasy MicrobiologíaClínica

Epidemiologyand Infection

European Journal of Clinical Microbiology & Infectious Diseases

Expert Review of Vaccines

FEMS Immunology and Medical Microbiology

Genetic Vaccines and Therapy

HIV Clinical Trials

HIV Medicine

Human Vaccines

Indian Journal of Leprosy

Indian Journal of Medical Microbiology

Infection

Infection and Immunity

Infection Control and Hospital Epidemiology

Infectious Disease Clinics of North America

Infectious Diseases in Obstetrics and Gynecology

Infectious Disorders Drug Targets

International Journal of Antimicrobial Agents

International Journal of Hygiene and Environmental Health

International Journal of Infectious Diseases

International Journal of Medical Microbiology

International Journal of STD & AIDS

The International Journal of Tuberculosis and Lung Disease

Journal of Acquired Immune Deficiency Syndromes (1999)

The Japanese Journal of Antibiotics

Japanese Journal of Infectious Diseases

Nihon Hansenby? Gakkai zasshi (Japanese Journal of Leprosy)

Nihon Ishinkin Gakkai zasshi (Japanese Journal of Medical Mycology)

The Journal of Antibiotics

The Journal of Antimicrobial Chemotherapy

Journal of Clinical Microbiology

Journal of Clinical Virology

Journal of Communicable Diseases

The Journal of Hospital Infection

Journal of Immune Based Therapies and Vaccines

The Journal of Infection

Journal of Infection and Chemotherapy

The Journal of Infectious Diseases

Journal of Medical Microbiology

Journal of Medical Virology

Journal of Microbiological Methods

Wei mian Yu gan ran za zhi (Journal of Microbiology, Immunology, and Infection)

Journal of Vectorborne Diseases

Journal of Viral Hepatitis

Journal of Virological Methods

Kansenshogakuzasshi (The Journal of the Japanese Association for Infectious Diseases)

Kekkaku (Tuberculosis)

The Lancet Infectious Diseases

Leprosy Review

Malaria Journal

Médecine et Maladies Infectieuses

Medical Microbiology and Immunology

Medical Mycology

Microbes and Infection

Microbial Drug Resistance

Mycoses

The Pediatric Infectious Disease Journal

Problemy Tuberkuleza Boleznei Legkikh

Reviews in Medical Virology

Scandinavian Journal of Infectious Diseases

Sexually Transmitted Diseases

Sexually Transmitted Infections

Surgical Infections

The Brazilian Journal of Infectious Diseases

Transplant Infectious Disease

Travel Medicine and Infectious Disease

Tropical Medicine & International Health

Tuberculosis

Tuberkulozve Toraks

Vaccine

Vector-borne and Zoonotic Diseases

Zhonghua jie he he hu xi za zhi (Chinese Journal of Tuberculosis and Respiratory Diseases)

Zhonghua shi yan he lin chuang bing du xue za zhi (Chinese Journal of Experimental and Clinical Virology)

Table 1. List of the 100 infectious disease journals.

languages: Japanese, Chinese, French, German, Spanish, Turkish, and Russian. Forty-eight of the journals matched the journals in the SCI Infectious Disease Category. The remaining 52 journals were newly selected and included 15 Asian journals, comprising 3 journals written in Japanese, 2 in Chinese, 7 in English, and 3 in both English and Japanese or Chinese. The breakdown of the 100 journals corresponding to categories A to F is given in Figure 1: 21 were in A, 35 in B, 16 in C, 17 in D, 2 in E, and 3 in F (94 journals). Six of the journals belonged to 2 categories: 2 in A and B, 2 in B and C, 1 in B and D, and 1 in C and D.

2.2 Survey method using the 100 infectious disease journals

Using the 100 journals described in section 2.1 and the PubMed database, a method was developed to survey the actual number of research articles per infectious disease journal, publication year, and country where the first author of the article originated.

In this method, original articles and reviews were surveyed as research articles (hereafter, the term "research articles" includes both original articles and reviews); the former group was considered as an indicator of research activity, and the latter group was considered an appreciation of research results. As it was considered that highly valued scientists were given more opportunities to write reviews, meaning that their research results had attracted a good opinion and had relatively good qualities, reviews were also targeted in addition to original research articles. On the basis of the concept that the number of reviews might be indicative of research quality, the number of reviews was surveyed separately from the number of original articles.

The "Limits" function of the PubMed database was integrated into this survey method. The function contains tags for limiting the journal name (*[Jour]*), affiliation of author (*[ad]*), publication date (*[PPDAT]* for print date and *[EPDAT]* for electronic publication date), and publication type (*[pt]*). Concerning the publication date, the print date for journals that had both print and electronic versions was prioritized. Detailed information whether each infectious disease journal was surveyed on the basis of the print publication date or electronic publication date can be found in our previous report (Takahashi-Omoe et al., 2009).

For example, the following text to search for research articles published on *"AIDS"* during 2006 and first author of which lived in Japan was applied: *AIDS [Jour] AND journal article [pt] AND Japan [ad] AND 2006 [PPDAT]*.

2.3 Usability of the survey method

2.3.1 Method of usability analysis

To ascertain whether the 100 newly selected journals could survey a wide range of infectious disease research articles, the 100 journals and the journals of the SCI Infectious Disease Category were compared from the viewpoint of the difference in the proportion of Asian research articles relative to the world total. A usability analysis of the 100 journals intended for Asian articles was appropriate because research articles in non-English or regional journals published in the EU and Asia tend to be underestimated as described in the "Introduction."

The actual number of research articles in the 100 journals in 1998–2006 was surveyed using the PubMed database. The target Asian countries were Japan, China, India, Taiwan, Korea,

Singapore, Malaysia, Indonesia, Vietnam, Thailand, and the Philippines. The world total number of articles was also surveyed. Articles registered in the SCI category were surveyed in a manner similar to those in the 100 journals.

2.3.2 Results of the usability analysis

Concerning the proportion of Asian articles relative to the world total, it was revealed that a survey of the 100 journals revealed a consistently higher percentage than the SCI Infectious Disease Category in 1998-2006. The total number of Asian research articles accounted for 12% of the world total in the survey of the 100 journals (actual numbers of Asian and worldwide research articles were 14,156 and 118,158, respectively, as described in this paragraph) (Table 2) and 6.9% in the survey of SCI Infectious Disease Category (4,621 and 66,518, respectively) (Table 3). Each year during the study period, the proportion of original articles of Asian origin relative to the world total was approximately 8.6%-14.2% in the 100 journals and 4.7%-9.3% in the SCI category, and that of reviews of Asian origin was approximately 4.2%-6.9% in the 100 journals and 1.0%-3.9% in the SCI category (Table 2 and 3).

From these findings, it was demonstrated that a survey method using the 100 journals could identify more research articles and avoid underestimation of the numbers of articles in regional and non-English journals. Therefore, this method was considered beneficial to grasp the overall trends in infectious disease research in comparison with previous bibliometric studies based on journals registered in the SCI Infectious Disease Category.

Year/original articles or reviews	1998/ OR	1998/ RV	1999/ OR	1999/ RV	2000/ OR	2000/ RV	2001/ OR	2001/ RV	2002/ OR	2002/ RV
Total number of articles in Asian countries	830	48	1079	54	1330	60	1389	74	1516	66
Total number of articles in the world	9,661	1,013	10,430	1,237	10,764	1,442	10,919	1,484	11,032	1,405
Proportion of Asian articles relative to the world total (%)	8.6	4.7	10.3	4.4	12.4	4.2	12.7	5.0	13.7	4.7

Year/original articles or reviews	2003/ OR	2003/ RV	2004/ OR	2004/ RV	2005/ OR	2005/ RV	2006/ OR	2006/ RV	1998-2006/ OR	1998-2006/ RV	1998-2006/ OR+RV
Total number of articles in Asian countries	1605	107	1825	96	1847	99	2010	105	13452	705	14156
Total number of articles in the world	12,239	1,584	12,896	1,580	13,246	1,580	14,121	1,525	105,308	12,850	118,158
Proportion of Asian articles relative to the world total (%)	13.1	6.8	14.2	6.1	13.9	6.3	14.2	6.9	12.8	5.5	12.0

Table 2. Total number of articles in Asian countries and the world, and the proportion of Asian articles relative to the world total in 100 infectious disease journals in 1998-2006. OR is original articles, and RV is reviews.

Year/original articles or reviews	1998/ OR	1998/ RV	1999/ OR	1999/ RV	2000/ OR	2000/ RV	2001/ OR	2001/ RV	2002/ OR	2002/ RV
Total number of articles in Asian countries	259	7	365	14	438	20	450	25	472	28
Total number of articles in the world	5,489	697	5,847	805	6,256	919	6,262	976	6,243	864
Proportion of Asian articles relative to the world total (%)	4.7	1.0	6.2	1.7	7.0	2.2	7.2	2.6	7.6	3.2

Year/original articles or reviews	2003/ OR	2003/ RV	2004/ OR	2004/ RV	2005/ OR	2005/ RV	2006/ OR	2006/ RV	1998-2006/ OR	1998-2006/ RV	1998-2006/ OR+RV
Total number of articles in Asian countries	480	26	617	38	629	33	698	21	4,412	209	4,621
Total number of articles in the world	6,615	932	7,039	981	7,163	1,043	7,510	877	58,424	8,094	66,518
Proportion of Asian articles relative to the world total (%)	7.3	2.8	8.8	3.9	8.8	3.2	9.3	2.4	7.6	2.6	6.9

Table 3. Total number of articles in Asian countries and the world, and the proportion of Asian articles relative to the world total in the SCI Infectious Disease Category during 1998–2006. OR is original articles, and RV is reviews.

3. Worldwide trends in infectious disease research

As the method using 100 infectious disease journals was demonstrated to be beneficial as described in section 2.3.2, worldwide trends in infectious disease research were subsequently surveyed using the method.

3.1 Survey method

The number of research articles in the 100 infectious disease journals in 2001–2010 was surveyed on country-by-country and year-by-year bases and analyzed for relative comparisons among countries, yearly change, and the relationship between socioeconomic as well as science and technology factors.

Specifically, in a similar manner as described in section 2.2, the actual number of research articles was surveyed using the "Limits" function of the PubMed database. The targeted countries were the US, EU countries (the UK, France, Germany, Italy, Spain, and the Netherlands), and Asian countries (Japan, China, and India). These 6 EU and 3 Asian countries were selected on the basis of the higher production of infectious disease research articles in the areas, which has been previously reported (the EU and Asian top countries) (Ramos et al., 2009; Takahashi-Omoe et al., 2009). In addition, the US was reported to produce the most articles in the SCI Infectious Disease Category in 1995–2002 (Bliziotis et al., 2005). Therefore, a survey for these 10 countries was considered appropriate to grasp the worldwide trends in infectious disease research.

In the case of the UK, articles from England, Wales, Scotland, and Northern Ireland were grouped together, and the following limitation was set in the affiliation field of the PubMed database: UK[ad] OR United Kingdom[ad] OR Great Britain[ad] OR (England[ad] NOT New England[ad]) OR (Wales[ad] NOT New South Wales[ad]) OR Scotland [ad] OR (N Ireland[ad] OR Northern Ireland[ad]). For example, the following text was applied to search for research articles published on *"AIDS"* in 2010 and the first author of which lived in the UK: *AIDS [Jour] AND journal article [pt] AND (UK[ad] OR United Kingdom[ad] OR Great Britain[ad] OR (England[ad] NOT New England[ad]) OR (Wales[ad] NOT New South Wales[ad]) OR Scotland [ad] OR (N Ireland[ad] OR Northern Ireland[ad])) AND 2010 [PPDAT].*

As a further analysis of worldwide trends, the number of research articles registered in the 100 journals in 2001–2010 was weighted according to socioeconomic factors (the population and gross domestic product [GDP]) and science and technology factors (the number of researchers in research and development [R&D] and health expenditure per capita) of each country. Annual data for the population, GDP, number of researchers in R&D, and health expenditure of 10 countries were obtained from the World Bank. Detailed information about these socioeconomic and science and technology factors can be found in the World Bank database (The World Bank, 2011). Specifically, researchers in R&D are defined as professionals engaged in the conception or creation of new knowledge, products, processes, methods, or systems and in the management of the projects concerned, including postgraduate PhD students engaged in R&D. Health expenditure is derived from a sum of public and private health expenditures as a ratio of total population and covered the provision of health services (preventive and curative), family planning activities, nutrition activities, and emergency aid designated for health but did not include provision of water and sanitation.

Using the non-parametric correlation statistical test (Spearman's Rank Correlation test), the numbers of research articles were analyzed in relation to the socioeconomic and science and technology factors. Statistical analyses were performed using SPSS Statistics (version 17.0; SPSS Japan Inc., Tokyo, Japan).

3.2 Survey result

3.2.1 Leading countries in the number of research articles

The total number of infectious disease research articles throughout the world in the 100 infectious disease journals was 148,435 in 2001–2010 (Table 4). Among 10 countries, the US published the most infectious disease research articles (41,055 articles, 27.7% of the world total). This total far outpaced that of the second leading country, the UK (10,893 articles, 7.3%). France and Japan were the third and fourth most productive countries (7,711 [5.2%] and 7,582 articles [5.1%], respectively).

When original articles and reviews were viewed separately, the US remained the top country in terms of research article production, being responsible for 26.8% and 34.9% of original articles and reviews in the world, respectively (Table 5). The UK was a distant second, publishing 6.9% of original articles and 11.1% of reviews. Japan had a relatively higher percentage of original articles (5.4%) and was third in productivity, followed by France (5.2% of original articles). Interestingly, Spain and China produced an equal percentage of original articles (3.5%). Regarding reviews, it was remarkable that Asian countries had relatively lower percentages than the EU countries. In particular, the number of reviews originating from China totaled 118, which was 0.7% of the world total and the lowest proportion among the 10 countries.

At the domestic level, the proportion of reviews among the total number of articles was highest in the UK (16.4%), followed by the US (13.7%) and Germany (12.2%). Five EU countries had proportions exceeding 10%, whereas all 3 Asian countries had proportions less than 10%, including Japan (6.6%).

Countries	Original articles	Reviews	Original articles & reviews
World	132,282	16,153	148,435
US	35,425	5,630	41,055
UK	9,106	1,787	10,893
France	6,884	827	7,711
Germany	5,457	756	6,213
Italy	4,129	484	4,613
Spain	4,587	464	5,051
The Netherland	3,172	353	3,525
Japan	7,081	501	7,582
China	4,618	118	4,736
India	3,337	187	3,524

Table 4. Total number of research articles originating from the US, EU, and Asian countries in 100 infectious disease journals in 2001–2010. The numeric data show the number of original articles and reviews.

	Relative to the domestic total number		Relative to the total number of OR, RV, or OR+RV of the world		
	OR /OR+RV	RV /OR+RV	OR/OR	RV/RV	OR+RV /OR+RV
US	86.3	13.7	26.8	34.9	27.7
UK	83.6	16.4	6.9	11.1	7.3
France	89.3	10.7	5.2	5.1	5.2
Germany	87.8	12.2	4.1	4.7	4.2
Italy	89.5	10.5	3.1	3.0	3.1
Spain	90.8	9.2	3.5	2.9	3.4
The Netherlands	90.0	10.0	2.4	2.2	2.4
Japan	93.4	6.6	5.4	3.1	5.1
China	97.5	2.5	3.5	0.7	3.2
India	94.7	5.3	2.5	1.2	2.4

Table 5. Relative comparison of the number of articles originating from the US, EU, and Asian countries in 100 infectious disease journals in 2001–2010. The numeric data indicate percentages. OR: original articles, RV: reviews.

3.2.2 Yearly change in the number of research articles

As shown in Figure 3, the number of original articles across the world increased from 2001 to 2010. By contrast, the numbers from the US and the UK did not remarkably change, regardless of their high numbers. The increase in the total number of original articles across the world resulted from the increase in articles from China as shown in Fig. 4, or perhaps other countries that were not surveyed in this study.

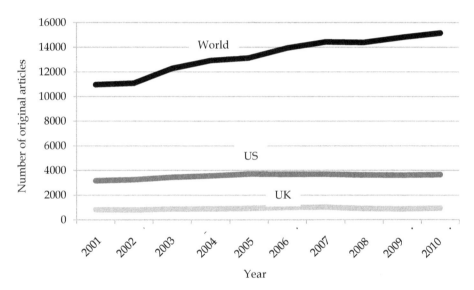

Fig. 3. Number of original articles in 100 infectious disease journals originating from the world, US, and UK in 2001–2010.

As noted previously, the number of original articles originating from China remarkably increased during this same period (Figure 4). The number in 2010 was more than 3-fold higher than that in 2001, including remarkable growth in the number of articles over the last 5–6 years. The concrete number of original articles from China exceeded that from Germany in 2008 (616 vs. 539 articles), Japan in 2009 (733 vs. 711 articles), and France in 2010 (809 vs. 764 articles).

Concerning the number of reviews, no noticeable increase was revealed in the world or the US and UK totals during the study period (Figure 5). The number from France showed a 2-fold increase in 2002–2006, but a slight decline since 2007. By contrast, the numbers from China and India remarkably increased from 2001 to 2010 (approximately 8.3-fold and 5.7-fold), but their numbers were lower than other countries (Figure 6). In addition, the number from Italy relatively increased among 10 countries (approximately 2.3-fold).

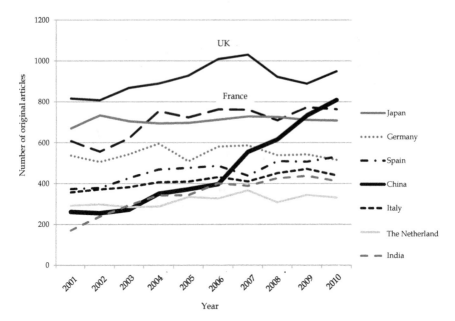

Fig. 4. Number of original articles in 100 infectious disease journals originating from the EU and Asian countries in 2001–2010.

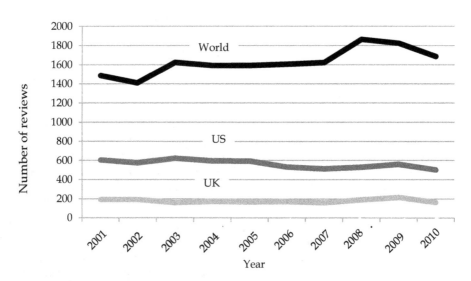

Fig. 5. Number of reviews in 100 infectious disease journals originating from the world, US, and UK in 2001–2010.

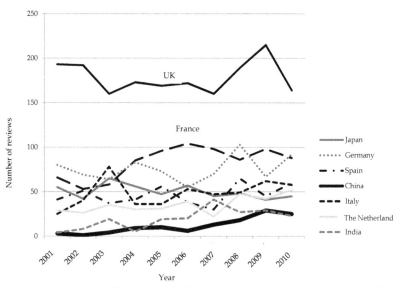

Fig. 6. Number of reviews in 100 infectious disease journals originating from the EU and Asian countries in 2001–2010.

3.2.3 Research productivity from the socioeconomic viewpoint

As a further analysis of publications of infectious disease research, the number of research articles was compared among 10 countries in terms of socioeconomic factors, the population, and GDP of each country.

Regarding the population, the ratio of the number of original articles to the population of individual countries exhibited a median value of 9 publications/1 million population/year (range, 0.3–19.3) in 2001–2009. Using population-adjusted ratios, the Netherlands (median value of 19.3) and the UK (14.9) were the most productive countries (Figure 7). The ratio of the number of reviews exhibited a median value of 0.9 publications/1 million population/year (range, 0–2.8). Using population-adjusted ratios, the UK ranked first (2.8), followed by the Netherlands (2.0) and the US (1.9). No statistically significant correlation were found between the average population and the number of original articles (Spearman's correlation coefficient = 0.213, p = 0.554) or reviews (Spearman's correlation coefficient = −0.097, p = 0.789) in the 10 countries in 2001–2009.

Regarding the ratio of the number of original articles to the GDP, the median value was 3.2 publications/10 billion GDP/year (range, 1.5–4.8) in 2001–2009. According to GDP-adjusted ratios for original articles, the Netherlands (4.8), India (4.2), and the UK (4.1) were highly productive (Figure 8). The ratio of the number of reviews exhibited a median value of 0.4 publications/10 billion GDP/year (range, 0–0.8) in 2001–2009. According to GDP-adjusted ratios for reviews, the UK (0.8) and the Netherlands (0.5) were most productive. A statistical correlation was found between the average GDP and the number of original articles (Spearman's correlation coefficient = 0.778, p = 0.008), but no statistically significant correlation between the average GDP and the number of reviews was observed (Spearman's correlation coefficient = 0.576, p = 0.082) in the 10 countries.

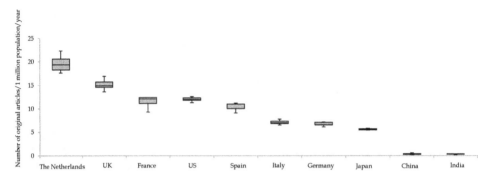

Fig. 7. Publication of original articles in 100 infectious disease journals by population in 2001–2009. Upper horizontal lines, dots, and lower horizontal lines in the boxes represent the first, second (median), and third quartiles, respectively. Whiskers represent the extension of values up and down.

In summary, we demonstrated that the Netherlands and the UK were most productive among the 10 countries when adjusting the production of original articles and reviews according to socioeconomic factors such as the population and GDP of each country.

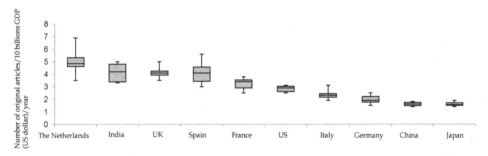

Fig. 8. Publication of original articles in 100 infectious disease journals by GDP in 2001–2009. Upper horizontal lines, dots, and lower horizontal lines in the boxes represent the first, second (median), and third quartiles, respectively. Whiskers represent extension of values up and down.

3.2.4 Research productivity from the science and technology viewpoint

In addition to socioeconomic factors, science and technology factors, represented by the number of researchers in R&D and health expenditure per capita, were applied to analyze the research productivity of each country.

The ratio of the number of original articles to the number of researchers in R&D exhibited a median value of 0.3 publications/number of researchers per 100 thousand people/year (range, 25.1–1.2) in 2001–2007. Using the number of researchers-adjusted ratios, India (median value of 25.1) was the most productive country (Figure 9). The ratio of the number of reviews exhibited a median value of 0.3 publications/number of researchers per 100 thousand people/year (range, 0.1–1.4) in 2001–2007. When adjusting the production of reviews according to the number of researchers, India ranked first (1.4), followed by the US (1.3). There were statistically significant correlations between the average number of researchers and original articles (Spearman's correlation coefficient = 0.802, p = 0.005) and reviews (Spearman's correlation coefficient = 0.806, p = 0.005) in the 10 countries in 2001–2007.

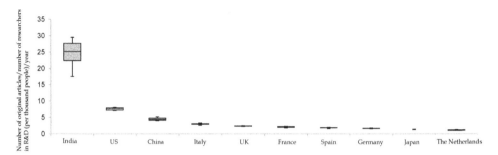

Fig. 9. Publication of original articles in 100 infectious disease journals according to the number of researchers in R&D in 2001–2007. Upper horizontal lines, dots, and lower horizontal lines in the boxes represent the first, second (median), and third quartiles, respectively. Whiskers represent the extension of values up and down. The survey period was 2001–2007 because data for the 10 countries were not fully gained from the World Bank data source in 2008–2009.

Concerning the ratio of the number of original articles to the health expenditure per capita, the median value was 2.3 publications/10 dollars health expenditure per capita/year (range, 0.8–113.2). For health expenditure-adjusted ratios, India (113.2) and China (45.5) were highly productive (Figure 10).

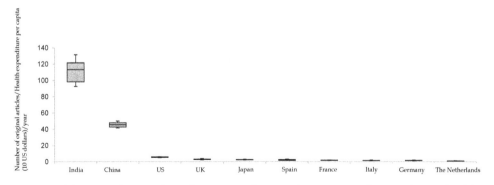

Fig. 10. Publication of original articles in 100 infectious disease journals according to health expenditure per capita in 2001–2009. Upper horizontal lines, dots, and lower horizontal lines in the boxes represent the first, second (median), and third quartiles, respectively. Whiskers represent the extension of values up and down.

The ratio of the number of reviews exhibited a median value of 0.2 publications/10 dollars health expenditure per capita/year (range, 0.1–6.3). When adjusting the production of reviews according to the health expenditure per capita, India (6.3) and China (1.2) were the most productive countries. There was no statistical correlation between the average of the health expenditure per capita and the number of original articles (Spearman's correlation coefficient = 0.407, p = 0.243), but a statistical correlation between the average of the health expenditure per capita and the number of reviews was observed (Spearman's correlation coefficient = 0.697, p = 0.025) for the 10 countries.

Generally, India was the most productive according to science and technology factors such as the number of researchers and health expenditure of each country. The US and China were ranked in the top three for both researcher- and health expenditure-adjusted ratios.

3.3 General overview of worldwide trends in infectious disease research

Through a bibliometric analysis using the 100 infectious disease journals described previously, 5 features were highlighted as the worldwide research trends in 2001–2010.

3.3.1 Vigorous infectious disease research around the world

We demonstrated that increasing numbers of infectious disease research articles were published around the world. This result was similar to previous bibliometric data reported by Bliziotis et al., although their study targeted journals registered in the SCI Infectious Disease Category and published in 1995–2002 (Bliziotis et al., 2005). It can be said that infectious disease research has been evidently vigorous without the influence of survey methods.

3.3.2 US as the leading country in infectious disease research

Our survey demonstrated that the US was the leading country in infectious disease research, as the US produced the highest percentage of total research articles (27.7% of the world total). The UK ranked second (7.3% of the world), but its output was dwarfed by that of the US. Ramos et al. also reported these 2 countries as the leading countries (Ramos et al., 2009) based on their study on journals registered in the SCI Infectious Disease Category covering the period of 2002–2007 (Bliziotis et al., 2005). These results from surveys based on 100 infectious journals and journals in the SCI Infectious Disease Category demonstrated that the US and the UK had an undisputed lead in infectious disease research productivity.

3.3.3 The Netherlands, India, and China as productive countries in the field of infectious disease research according to socioeconomic and science and technology factors

The US and the UK dominated the field of infectious disease research according to the global share of research articles, but the Netherlands, India, and China were considered productive countries when adjusting the production of original articles for socioeconomic factors and science and technology factors.

3.3.4 Developing infectious disease research in China

According to our findings, the productivity of infectious disease research in terms of a noticeable increase in the number of produced original articles was observed for China.

Significantly, China overtook France and Japan regarding the number of original articles in 2010 and 2009, respectively. However, China had the lowest proportion of reviews among the 10 countries. This trend might indicate that infectious disease research in China was developing and that it has not come to be well recognized.

3.3.5 More appreciated outputs of infectious disease research from the US and the top EU countries

Through this method, it became clear that the US and the top EU countries produced relatively higher proportions of reviews than the top Asian countries. Even Japan, which produced the most research articles in Asia, produced fewer reviews than the UK, France, and Germany. It could be speculated that the research output from the US and the top EU countries was more appreciated than those from top Asian countries.

4. Conclusion

This chapter presented the recent worldwide trends in infectious disease research as a practical application of a method using 100 infectious disease journals. The trends in 2001–2010 included vigorous research, with the US and the UK being the most active countries. Given the research productivity based on socioeconomic and science and technology factors, the Netherlands, India, and China had relatively high productivity. The developing research in China and more appreciated research outputs from the top EU countries were also significant. Based on these survey results, further content analysis of infectious disease research articles may be necessary to build future research strategies for effective disease control.

5. Acknowledgment

The study introduced in this chapter was supported by Japan Grants-in Aid for Scientific Research (KAKENHI) (research project number 23580435).

6. References

Bliziotis, I.A.; Paraschakis, K.; Vergidis, P.I.; Karavasiou, A.I. & Falagas, M.E. (2005). Worldwide trends in quantity and quality of published articles in the field of infectious diseases. *BMC Infectious Diseases*, Vol.5, No.16, ISSN 1471-2334

Brown, C. (2004). Emerging zoonoses and pathogens of public health significance–an overview. *Revue scientifique et technique (International Office of Epizootics)*, Vol.23, No.2, pp. 435-42, ISSN 0253-1933

Elsevier B.V. (2011). SciVerse Scopus, Available from
http://www.info.sciverse.com/scopus/about

Garg, K.C.; Kumar, S.; Madhavi, Y. & Bahl, M. (2009). Bibliometrics of global malaria vaccine research. *Health Information and Libraries Journal* Vol.26, pp.22-31, ISSN 1471-1834

Patra, S.K. & Chand, P. (2007). HIV/AIDS research in India: A bibliometric study. *Library & Information Science Research* Vol.29, pp.124-134, ISSN 0740-8188

Ramos, J.M.; Gutiérrez, F.; Masía, M. & Martín-Hidalgo, A. (2004). Publication of European union research on infectious diseases (1991-2001): A bibliometric evaluation.

European Journal of Clinical Microbiology & Infectious Diseases, Vol.23, pp.180-184, ISSN 0934-9723

Ramos, J.M.; Masía, M.; Padilla, S. & Gutiérrez, F. (2009). A bibliometric overview of infectious diseases research in European countries (2002-2007). *European Journal of Clinical Microbiology & Infectious Diseases*, Vol.28, pp.713-716, ISSN 0934-9723

Ramos, J.M.; Padilla, S.; Masía, M. & Gutiérrez, F. (2008). A bibliometric analysis of tuberculosis research indexed in PubMed, 1997-2006. *International Journal of Tuberculosis and Lung Disease*, Vol.12, pp.1461-1468, ISSN 1027-3719

Soteriades, E.S. & Falagas M.E. (2006). A bibliometric analysis in the fields of preventive medicine, occupational and environmental medicine, epidemiology, and public health. *BMC Public Health*, Vol.6, No.301, ISSN 1471-2458

Statistics Canada (1998). *Bibliometric analysis of scientific and technological research: A user's guide to the methodology*, Canada, Available from
http://www.statcan.gc.ca/pub/88f0006x/88f0006x1998008-eng.pdf

Takahashi-Omoe, H. & Omoe, K. (2009). Regulatory and scientific framework for zoonosis control in Japan–contributing to International Health Regulations (2005). *Revue scientifique et technique (International Office of Epizootics)*,Vol.28, pp.957-973, ISSN 0253-1933

Takahashi-Omoe, H.; Omoe, K. & Okabe, N. (2009). New journal selection for quantitative survey of infectious disease research: application for Asian trend analysis. *BMC Medical Research Methodology*, Vol.9, No.67, ISSN 1471-2288

Thomson Reuters (2011). Science Sitation Index Expanded, Available from
http://science.thomsonreuters.com/cgi-bin/jrnlst/jloptions.cgi?PC=D

Uthman, O.A. (2008). HIV/AIDS in Nigeria: a bibliometric analysis. *BMC Infectious Diseases*, Vol. 8, No.19, ISSN 1471-2334

Vergidis, P.I.; Karavasiou, A.I.; Paraschakis, K.; Bliziotis, I.A.; Falagas M.E. (2005). Bibliometric analysis of global trends for research productivity in microbiology. *European Journal of Clinical Microbiology & Infectious Diseases*, Vol. 24, pp.342-345, ISSN 0934-9723

World Bank. (2011). Data, Inficators, Available from http://data.worldbank.org/indicator

World Health Organization. (2007). *The World Health Report 2007, A Safer Future: Global Public Health Security in the 21st Century*, Geneva, Switzerland, Available from
http://www.who.int/whr/2007/whr07_en.pdf

Part 2

Immuno-Kinetics and Vaccination

8

Immunological Pathogenesis of Septic Reactions and Elimination of Triggers and Mediators of Inflammation

Irina Shubina, Natalia Anisimova, Elena Gromova,
Irina Chikileva and Mikhail Kiselevsky
NN Blokhin Russian Cancer Research Center
Russia

1. Introduction

Modern intensive therapy is armed with very sophisticated methods, however sepsis is still one of the most challenging issues of medicine. Death rate in patients caused by sepsis remains high and reaches about 30-80% (Yegenaga I. et al., 2004). This problem is especially important in oncology, as every sixth septic patient has a diagnosis of cancer; and the death risk of such patients is 30% higher (Angus D.C. et al., 2001).

The established bacteriologic paradigm of sepsis implies an infectious component for its development. The priority in the pathogenesis of this disease has been assigned to microorganisms, and therefore sepsis is regarded primarily as an infective disease. However, over the last decades there have appeared tendencies for an essential revision in the understanding of mechanisms of sepsis development; inflammatory reactions of the organism are now regarded as important as infection. In particular, according to a current definition, approved by American College of Chest Physicians/Society of Critical Care Medicine (ACCP/SCCM) Consensus Conference, "sepsis is a systemic inflammatory response syndrome developing in response to an invasion of different pathogenic microorganisms, which is diagnosed if an infective agent and two or more signs of the systemic inflammatory response are present" (USA, Chicago, 1991).

Systemic inflammatory response syndrome (SIRS) includes the whole set of the clinical manifestations of systemic inflammatory response (SIR), which is a generalized form of inflammatory reaction and is formed as a result of an excessive immune cell activation that produce different types of mediators (cytokines, leukotrienes, thromboxanes, etc.). SIRS is a necessary component of sepsis, however, it is not the same, as SIRS may be induced by different non-infective causes such as trauma, pancreatitis, etc. Thus, signs of systemic infection are necessary to prove diagnosed sepsis. Besides, it should be taken into account that bacteremia is not pathognomonic to sepsis. The rate of diagnosed bacteremia even in the most serious cases does not exceed 45% if accurate techniques of blood sampling and modern microbiologic methods are applied. Detection of microorganisms in the patient's peripheral blood with no clinical and laboratory test conclusion of SIRS may be considered as transitory bacteremia that is not necessarily caused by septic process. Some authors recommend differentiating localized focus of infection from true sepsis even if it is associated with the symptoms of systemic inflammatory reaction. In about half of cases (30-60%) when clinical symptoms of sepsis were evident, it was impossible to isolate live microorganisms from the blood or find the focus of infection.

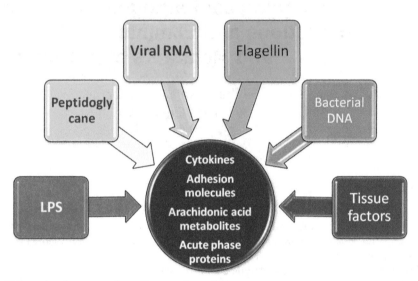

Fig. 1. Triggering factors and mediators of sepsis.

The disease status that demonstrates the whole set of septic symptoms but lack of infection is regarded like pseudosepsis or sepsis-like syndrome. Trigger factors initiating systemic inflammatory response might be derivatives of microorganisms (exo- or endotoxins) rather than microorganisms themselves, or even factors of non-infective origin including endogeneous factors (such as tissue factors, elastin, thrombin, etc.), which appear primarily during organ or tissue damage (Fig. 1) as a result of traumas, burns, etc.

Clinical symptoms of sepsis as well as organ or multi-organ dysfunction syndrome (MODS) may develop in response to endo- and exotoxins of microorganisms in the absence of bacteremia (septicemia) or localized focus of infection. The macroorganism reaction to bacterial products displays totally the whole symptom complex that is characteristic for bacterial sepsis. LPS poisoning does not only induce clinical presentations of sepsis and septic (endotoxic shock), but leads to pathomorphologic changes characteristic for septic conditions (Angus D.C. et al., 2001).

Present understanding of sepsis states that it is a systemic inflammatory response of the macroorganism, which develops as a result of interaction of the immune system with bacteria or their toxins and is mediated by the over-expression of a complex of humoral factors: cytokines and other substances (platelet activation factor, metabolites of arachidonic acid, endotelin-1, and complement components). Local tissue damage during SIRS arises from the release of active oxygen forms, proteases and escalation of cytokine synthesis. Such vision of sepsis pathogenesis suggests that new diagnostic and prognostic markers of this condition should be identified in patient's immunologic parameters. Following this concept, new therapeutic strategies of inactivation or elimination of SIR triggers and mediators are being developed.

2. Bacterial toxins: triggers of inflammation

Infective agents have various factors of virulence which can affect protective reactions of the body. In septic and inflammatory conditions cascade of events initiated by microbes and their products may develop out of control. Immune effectors recognize pathogens, firstly, by innate immunity receptors detecting different pathogen-associated molecular patterns that include various components of microbial cell wall (such as, LPS –lipopolysaccharide, peptidoglycan, lipoteichoic acid, mannan, flagellin, bacterial DNA, viral double-helical RNA, glucan and intracellular components, etc.)

Bacterial toxins, primarily LPS of gram-negative bacteria, have significant impact on activating mechanisms of inflammation and may induce or potentiate systemic inflammatory response in the absence of microbial cells. In particular, it was shown that in humans LPS in the minimal dose (4 ng/kg) initiates release of inflammatory mediators, alterations of hemostasis and fall of the blood pressure resulting from the decrease of the cardiac output and vascular resistance. Sepsis-like conditions were described in volunteers after injections of high endotoxin doses as well as in patients receiving therapies based on LPS-immunomodulators (Laurenzi L. et al., 2004, Zucker T. et al., 2004). Sepsis-like syndrome is observed in patients after cardiac surgery, closed injury, and in patients resuscitated after cardiac arrest.

One of the major mechanisms of infection is penetration of normal microflora and substances including endotoxins into blood circulation from the natural organism biocoenoses, mainly from the bowels (Annane D. et al., 2005). Translocation of bacteria and their toxins into the bloodstream might be caused by changes in the mucous intestine tunic (Moore F.A. , 1999). Nevertheless, impairment of the intestine permeability most often has a secondary origin and results from the SIR to trauma, surgical stress, burn, high-dose antibiotic therapy and other damaging factors (Deitch E.A.&Bridges R.M. , 1987, Balzan S.et al., 2007). In cancer patients, risk of bacterial toxin translocation increases due to disorders of the intestine mucous barrier function caused by the major disease and especially, by anti-tumor aggressive therapy. An additional unfavorable factor is older age of patients because of the age-related changes in the intestines permeability. These patients, despite of the widely accepted view about immunity involution and down-regulation of immune reactions in the elderly, demonstrate an enhanced response to bacterial toxins. For example, patients over 65 have a more significant drop of the blood pressure after injections of minimal LPS doses (2 ng/kg) compared with younger individuals. The phenomenon is apparently linked to the systemic chronic inflammatory reaction of the elderly, associated with a higher initial level of pro-inflammatory factors.

When LPS enters blood circulation, it partly links to the LPS-binding protein (LBP) and the newly formed complex interacts with CD14-positive cells, such as macrophages.   LPB potentiates LPS transport to receptors of macrophages (CD14) and stimulates functional activity of these innate immunity effectors (Takeshita S. et al., 2002). The endotoxin-shipping function in the blood also refers to the soluble circulating macrophage CD14-receptors. A number of studies showed an increase in these markers in patients with sepsis, including cancer patients (Myc A. et al., 1997, Nijhuis C. S. et al., 2003).

Our data show that LPS serum concentration increases in patients with sepsis aggravated by organ failure or MODS. Particularly, in contrast to healthy volunteers, whose blood almost lacks LPS, patients with kidney or hepatic failure with no symptoms of SIRS showed moderate increase of LPS serum concentrations (0,1-0,2 IU/ml), while patients with sepsis and septic shock had markedly increased blood serum concentrations of this bacterial toxin – median parameter in the group was 0,55 IU/ml, sometimes reaching 6,25 IU/ml (Fig. 2).

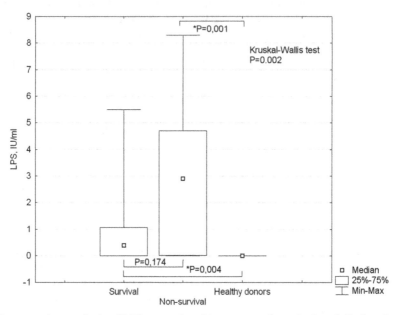

Fig. 2. Comparative analysis of LPS serum level in groups of survival and died patients with sepsis and in healthy volunteers.

A high LPS concentration in peripheral blood is generally associated with a drop of LPB level. In patients with sepsis the ratio of blood serum concentrations LPS/LPB is on average ten-fold higher than in healthy individuals. Therefore, dynamic growth of LPS concentration and decrease of LPB level in sepsis may be considered as negative prognostic factors.

3. Cytokines

Over the last years, a lot of data have been accumulated that discuss the role of endogenic bioregulators of different origin (cytokines, kinins, phospholipids, arachidonic acid metabolites, etc.) in development of structural and functional alterations leading to systemic inflammatory reactions and sepsis. Immune mediators – cytokines have an absolutely important role in inflammation pathogenesis. Their high biologic activity and a small difference between effective and toxic concentrations make them key factors both in natural physiologic processes and pathologic conditions. As it was mentioned earlier, a triggering mechanism of SIRS, besides bacteria and/or their toxins, might be a trauma, including surgical intervention. With no microbial components it may also initiate an inflammatory cascade, leading to cellular damage and organ dysfunctions. Different endogenous factors, so-called alarmins, which are activated by tissue damage (for example, necrotic cells, RNA, urine acid crystals, etc.), may bind leucocyte receptors and induce systemic inflammatory response or "sepsis with no infective agent". A term "alarmin" was suggested by J. Oppenheim for endogenous stress molecules that provide signals about tissue and cell damage (Oppenheim J.J.& Yang D., 2005).

Thus, excessive concentrations of these endogenous modulators provoke development of pathophysiologic abnormalities leading to organ failure or MODS. However, despite numerous studies looking at prognostic or diagnostic significance of cytokine concentrations in the serum of patients with purulent and septic complications, there is still disagreement on the topic. Serum cytokine low levels are registered in the peripheral blood of many patients regardless clinical symptoms of sepsis or septic shock. At the same time, some authors report data of increased concentrations of several cytokines such as interleukin(IL)-8, tumor necrosis factor (TNF)α, IL-6 in the peripheral blood of patients with sepsis (Calandra T.et al., 1990, Anderson R.&Schmidt R., 2010, Gaïni S. et al., 2006).

Risk of SIRS development is extremely high in cancer patients, as the necessary extensive surgery stimulates release of pro-inflammatory cytokines that may promote development of systemic inflammatory response (Hildebrand F. et al., 2005, Lenz A. et al., 2007). Some authors suggested diagnostic and prognostic significance of TNFα serum level (Calandra T., 1990). The results showed both increased as well as similar to the control group concentrations of TNFα in serum of patients with severe sepsis. An unfavorable course of the septic process was observed in the cases of low basic TNFα level or its negative dynamics (TNFα level dropped from 30,4 ± 2,7 pg/ml to 15,8 ± 6,3 pg/ml). Originally high TNFα in the blood of septic patients (1020,7 ± 30,1 pg/ml) was considered as a "cytokine cascade out of control". They also presented data demonstrating that intensive therapy in the group of patients with originally high TNFα concentration leaded to its significant decrease (from 680,4 ± 32,7 pg/ml to 450 ± 16,7 pg/ml), which was associated with favorable prognosis. TNFα level varied in a wide range from 50 to 3500 pg/ml in patients with septic shock. Median TNFα level was 180 pg/ml in the group of survived patients; and 330 pg/ml in the group of the deceased. On the basis of these data, contradictory conclusions were made about prognostic significance of pro-inflammatory cytokine serum levels in general and TNFα, in particular. However, many researchers agree that both high and low TNFα serum levels in critical conditions may be regarded as a poor prognostic parameter (Martin C.et al., 1994, Quinn J.V.&Slotman G.J., 1999).

According to our data, only the concentration of IL-6 was significantly increased in the peripheral blood of cancer patients with sepsis (Table 1). The highest mediator levels were observed in patients with septic shock. A probable cause of the pro-inflammatory cytokine increase in the patients' blood could be its overproduction by the resident macrophages, in particular, by the hepatic Kupffer cells. Besides TNFα, IL-6 is one of the probable markers of severity of an infective or non-infective stress. It induces production of a wide range of proteins of the acute phase that regulate inflammation process. In septic shock, the cytokine may directly affect organs and tissues; in particular, it may suppress myocardium. Various studies investigated the role of this cytokine in pathogenesis of septic shock, MODS and other systemic processes and its prognostic significance; however, their conclusions are somewhat contradictory (Anderson R.&Schmidt R., 2010, Pinsky M.R., 2004).

Groups	IL-6	IL-8	IL-10	INFγ	TNFα	TNF β	IL-1β	IL-4	IL-17
Cancer patients with sepsis	203*	17	48	0	4	4	1	6	31
	61÷494	6÷130	31÷163	0÷16	0÷30	4÷26	0÷28	3÷13	0÷73
healthy volunteers	0	3	80	2	0	0	0	10	9
	0÷1	0÷11	0÷108	0÷16	0÷0	0÷9	0÷0	2÷12	6÷19

* – significant difference compared to the control group of healthy volunteers (P<0.01)

Table 1. Cytokine profile of cancer patients with sepsis compared to healthy volunteers (median, 25th ÷75th quartiles), pg/ml.

On the whole, the above data suggest that determination of free cytokine serum concentrations in the peripheral blood of patients with septic complications presents little information, except for IL-6, which is statistically significantly increased in patients with sepsis, and, especially, with septic shock. Therefore IL-6 is the only serum cytokine, which concentration might be recommended as a marker for sepsis. A possible reason of low importance of the cytokine profile determination in sepsis may be due to the fact that commercially available kits are designed to evaluate concentrations of free (soluble) cytokines only. It is a serious obstacle for the estimation of the total cytokine concentrations secreted into the blood circulation. Even if free cytokines are not detected in the blood, their receptor-bound complexes may be circulating. As a result, "hidden cytokinemia" – high cytokine concentrations non-detectable by conventional methods – may take place.

Therefore, low levels of serum cytokines do not necessarily reflect the true mediator concentrations in blood serum and may result not only from insufficient activity of immune effectors of cancer patients, but also from specific binding with increased concentrations of cytokine soluble receptors. A number of studies reported on the statistically significant increase of concentrations of soluble cytokine receptors: TNF receptors (sTNF-R I and sTNF-R II) (Zhang B.et al., 1998), IL-1 – sIL-1 RII (Müller B., 2002) and decrease of soluble IL-6 receptor (sIL-6 R) (Frieling J.T.M.et al., 1995, Zeni F. et al., 1995) in patients with sepsis. However, other researchers presented different results (Barber M.D.et al, 1999).

The data of our studies showed that only sTNF-RI (p55) serum level was significantly more enhanced in cancer patients with sepsis compared with control group of healthy volunteers. However, the comparative analysis of cytokine and their soluble receptor concentrations in the blood of survived and deceased patients with sepsis showed that simultaneous increase of IL-6, IL-8, IL-10, sTNF-RI, sIL-1RII and sIL-6R was associated with poor prognosis. Probably, the mentioned facts result from the so-called "cytokine storm" and reflect the extreme imbalance of the immune system in sepsis leading to the fatal outcome. This suggestion is supported by the increased level of both pro-inflammatory cytokines (IL-6, IL-8) and anti-inflammatory IL-10 in the patients died from sepsis

Comparative studies of immunocompetent cell potential for cytokine secreting presented more precise data. The level of spontaneous production of these endogenous bioregulators characterizes the original physiologic activity of the blood cells. The intensity of the stimulated cytokine production helps to determine the potential reactivity in response to a possible infection.

The obtained data from our studies showed that blood cells of septic cancer patients with spontaneous overproduction of certain cytokines (IL-6, IL-8) are mostly non-responsive to any stimulation. The observation suggests that immune effectors in this group of patients are over-stimulated.

The inflammatory reaction in response to trauma or infection is induced mainly by innate immunity and develops rapidly at the early stage. Endogenous inflammation mediators synthesized by immune cells in response to microbial components or tissue factors are released within few minutes and may peak within 1-3 hours in peripheral blood. These factors play a major role in the formation of the protective response to infection (they enhance bactericidal activity of phagocytes, promote recruitment of leukocytes to the infection site, stimulate hemopoiesis, and cause fever). However, inflammatory over-reaction leads to an excessive release of inflammatory mediators both of peptide (cytokines) and lipid nature (metabolites of membrane lipids –leukotrienes, thromboxanes, platelet activation factor). These substances, besides protective functions, are highly toxic and may cause hemodynamic imbalance, metabolic and pathologic alterations that are characteristic for sepsis and septic shock. Activation of anti-inflammatory factors, as well as of inhibitors of inflammatory mediators (prostaglandin E2, IL-1Ra, IL-10 and TGF-β), takes place during SIRS and is considered as compensatory anti-inflammatory syndrome, a protective response limiting tissue damage by endogenous pro-inflammatory factors. On the other hand, prevalence of anti-inflammatory mediators may lead to immune suppression and anergy of immune cells (Keel M.&Trentz O., 2005). Evidently, both hyper- and hypo-inflammatory phases may follow each other or develop independently from each other, according to the original reactivity of the organism. Both conditions of hyper- and hyporeactivity are equally dangerous and may cause fatal outcome.

4. Functional activity of leukocytes

So far a lot of data have been collected to characterize immune status of cancer patients with suppurative septic complications (Martin C., 1994, Quinn J.V.&Slotman G.J., 1999, Anderson R.&Schmidt R., 2010, Pinsky M.R. et al., 2004, Zhang B. et al, 1998, Frieling J.T.M.et al., 1995). Although most of the studies look at parameters of humoral immunity, particularly, at assessment of cytokine profile, a higher interest has been seen in studying functions of immune competent cells over the last years. Special attention is aimed at effectors of innate immunity (natural killers, granulocytes and monocytes), which play a key role in pathogenesis of sepsis (Zeerleder S., 2005). A number of authors show an increasing suppression of cellular immunity with septic background that reveals as decreased function of immune competent cells due to high rate of immunosuppressive agents (IL-10) and decrease of regulatory peptides (IL-12). On the other hand, there are data that prove enhanced production of pro-inflammatory cytokines (IL-8, TNFα, IL-6, IL-1β) in cancer patients, which level is many times higher than that in healthy individuals (Rigato O.et al., 1996, Kumar A.T. et al., 2009). The logic consequence of this phenomenon may be higher cellular functioning, mostly - innate immunity effector cells function. In the environment of bacteriemia and bacterial toxicity these cells are responsible for natural resistance to infectious agents. However their super activation triggers cascade hyperproduction of inflammatory mediators which initiate SIRS (Angus D.C. et al., 2001, Hildebrand F. et al., 2005).

The results of our studies showed that cancer patients with sepsis have a significant increase of natural killer (NK) cells activity as compared with cancer patients having no sepsis or healthy volunteers. These data comply with results of other authors who demonstrated an enhanced function of NK in patients with sepsis (Giamarellos-Bourboulis E.J.et al., 2006, Yoneda O. et al., 2000). The observed phenomenon seemed to be associated with the enhanced rate of IL-12 in blood serum of patients with severe sepsis or septic shock due to the fact that IL-12 stimulates NK and T-killer cells cytotoxicity as a result of secreting molecules involved in cytolytic reactions (gransymes A and B) (Zeerleder S., et al. 2005).

Neutrophils are the first line of protection against acute infections and play an important role in pathogenesis of sepsis (Segal A.W. , 2005). On the one hand they are major players in eliminating infectious microorganisms, on the other hand – an excessive release of oxidants and proteases by neutrophils leads to damaging organs and tissues. Neutrophils are involved both in inflammatory processes and natural immunity effects migrating to the site of infection or inflammation to eliminate infectious agents. Besides that they produce signals about invasion of a foreign agent to alert effectors of innate immunity. These signals induce activation of other cells, such as, monocytes/ macrophages as well as epithelial and mast cells and trombocytes. On activation neutrophils generate various chemotaxic factors attracting macrophages. Because of their common origin neutrophils and macrophages have common functions (phagocytosis, similar behavioral kinetics in infectious and inflammatory process, anti-microbial and immunomodulating functions). Activated neutrophils releasing chemokines stimulate and recruit to the inflammation site monocytes and macrophages and may effect on macrophage differentiation into pro- or anti-inflammatory subtype (type I or type II macrophages). In addition to release of pro-inflammatory cytokines neutrophils also secrete reactive oxygen radicals that induce acute tissue destruction, such as lung destruction in acute reactive distress syndrome (ARDS) or pneumonia (Kumar V. et al., 2010). Besides phagocytosis and secretion of anti-bacterial molecules neutrophils form so-called extra-cellular traps. Extra-cellular traps are formed from the decondensated chromatin and the contents of some granule, as well as from the cytoplasmic proteins and can interact both with gram-negative and gram-positive bacteria leading to destruction of virulent factors and killing bacteria. However the excessive reaction of innate immunity following bacterial infection may lead to immune suppression in the end. Part of this condition is impairment of neutrophil phagocytic activity, which is the major component determining the status of anti-infectious defense (Kumar V. et al., 2010, Giamarellos-Bourboulis E.J. et al., 2010, Volk H.D. et al., 1999).

Patients with sepsis and the background of neutrophil sequestration can often develop complications in tissues, such as ARDS, and excessive activation of neutrophils is associated with lung destruction (Kumar V. et al., 2010, Giamarellos-Bourboulis E.J. et al., 2010).

There is a number of data that demonstrate long-term cellular over-production of pro-inflammatory cytokines (IL-8, TNFα, IL-6, IL-1β) in cancer patients with sepsis, which can effect neutrophil functions (Martin C. et al., 1994, Zhang B. et al., 1998, Frieling J.T.M. et al., 1995, Barber M.D. et al., 1999, Rigato O. et al., 1996, Segal A.W., 2005). The results revealed that in most cases the phagocytotic activity of neutrophils of cancer patients with sepsis (phagocytic index and phagocytic number) were higher than those of healthy volunteers (in 2,6 and 6,3 times, respectively) (Fig. 3a,b, Fig.4 a,b). This phenomenon may be the results of increased production of pro-inflammatory cytokines, in particular IL-8: key cytokine involved in recruitment of neutrophiles into the inflammation site and stimulating their function (Hammond M.E. et al., 1995).

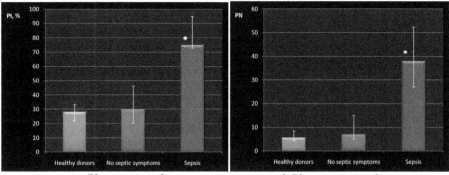

a Phagocytic index   b Phagocytic number

*– values that have reliable difference from those of healthy volunteers   (p<0,05).

Fig. 3. Parameters of phagocytosis rate of blood granulocytes in cancer patients with sepsis and patients with no septic symptoms in comparison with healthy volunteers (median, 25%÷75%).

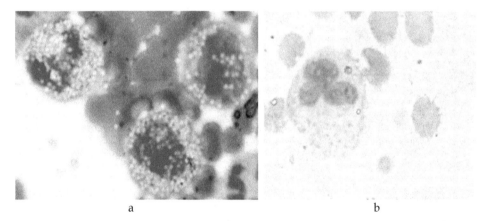

a   b

Fig. 4. Microphotos of neutrophils in peripheral blood of healthy volunteers (a) and cancer patient with sepsis (b) after incubation with latex particles (t=40 min).

Patients with sepsis have a significant increase in activation of oxygen dependent mechanisms of phagocytes as compared to those of patients with no complications or healthy volunteers (5-fold and 15-fold, respectively) that points to a high rate of activation of intracellular bactericidal systems when there is septic process (Fig. 5).

Hydrogen peroxide combined with myeloperoxidase (enzyme of primary neutrophil granules) and halogen ions forms an effective bactericidal system that kills bacteria by halogenation of the cellular wall (Zychlinsky A. et al., 2003). But phagocytes release these endogenous active substances into the inter-cellular medium so that they also destroy self-tissues and thus they become involved in developing organ dysfunction or MODS (Thomas S. et al., 2004).

Previous studies suggest that the basis for MODS in critical conditions is the impairment of vessel endothelium, which was the result of active function of immune competent cells induced by microbial products. Therefore super-activation of effectors of innate immunity (neutrophils, natural killers) may be considered as an important link in pathogenesis of organ or multi-organ dysfunction syndrome.

Excessive reaction of innate immune system after contact with bacterial infection can lead to immune suppression. A part of this condition is the disorder in phagocytic function of neutrophils, which to a high extent determines anti-infectious defense (Volk H.D. et al., 1999, Alves-Filho J.C. et al., 2010, Giamarellos-Bourboulis EJ et al., 2010).

One of the results of the developing immune suppression in patients with sepsis can be decreased number of lymphocytes that is associated with their sequestration in the inflammation site or their apoptotic death as a result of the excessive production of pro-apoptotic factors. Clinical studies showed marked T-cell lymphopenia with its maximum within a few days. Absolute and relative number of CD4+ and CD8+ T-lymphocytes reduces. At the same time percentage of B-lymphocytes in the peripheral blood goes up (Murphy R.&DeCoursey T. E., 2006, Holub M. et al., 2000). Essential alterations were observed in NK examination (Emoto M. et al., 2002, Kerr A.R., et al., 2005).

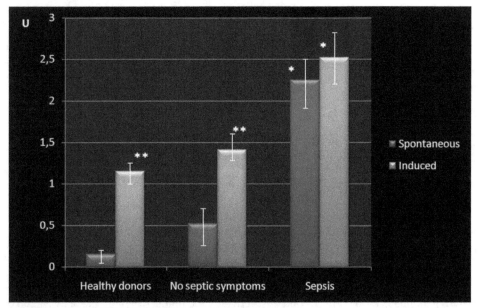

*– values that have reliable difference from control (p<0,05);

**– results of the induced NB-test reliably different from the results of spontaneous NB-test (p<0,05).

Fig. 5. Rate of metabolic activity of neutrophils in peripheral blood of cancer patients in comparison with those of healthy volunteers in spontaneous and induced NB-test (nitrone blue test) (median, 25%÷75%).

Peripheral blood NK number enhances at the early stage of sepsis in patients with sepsis (Giamarellos-Bourboulis E.J. et al., 2006), while in patients with septic shock their relative number decreases (Holub M. et al., 2000).

5. Apoptosis of the immune cells after trauma

Apoptosis of various immune cells is an important part of immune suppression development in response to an emergency situation (trauma, burns, infection). Suppression of active immunity due to the death of monocytes, macrophages and lymphocytes can enhance risk of opportunistic infections. Moreover, a higher rate of apoptosis in lymphoid tissues and parenchyma organs may lead to disorders in cellular homeostasis and the following inadequate response of the organism as a whole including development of MODS.

Clinical and experimental studies of trauma and burns showed that enhanced production of endogenous mediators of inflammation (heat shock proteins, free oxygen radicals, NO, TNF, IL-1 and IL-6) could activate signaling pathways of apoptosis in different immune cells. Increased expression of apoptotic markers on T-cells (Fas и FasL) was observed in patients who underwent surgery that makes reason for lymphopenia leading to a higher risk of post-surgical infections. However, some authors reported about decrease of apoptotic marker on leukocytes in sepsis and SIRS (Härter L. et al., 2003, Sayeed M.M., 2004, Papathanassoglou E.D.E. et al., 2005, Jimenez M.F., et al. 1997, Lee WL & Downey GP. , 2001). The expression level of this marker on neutrophils correlates with the severity of the inflammation (Fialkow L. et al., 2006). Apparently, alterations in apoptosis regulation as the process responsible for the elimination of fading cells play an essential role in pathogenesis of sepsis and multi-organ dysfunction syndrome (Pierozan P. et al.,2006, Mahidhara R. et al, 2000).

6. Platelets in sepsis

Platelets may be considered as a linking chain between innate immunity and homeostasis. Activated platelets can form clusters in blood circulation system that leads to thromboses and their sequestration in microcirculation often leads to dessiminated inter-vessel blood coagulation.

Systemic capillary thrombosis in situation of inter-vessel blood coagulation is one of the reasons for multi-organ dysfunction. Moreover, extended and long-term activation of the coagulation system results in exhausted factors of coagulation and platelet function, which causes increased bleeding.

7. Immunoglobulins

Imbalance of humoral immunity that develops in sepsis presents quantitative and qualitative changes in serum immunoglobulins. A lot of authors report about reduction of immunoglobulins A, G, M and their subtype levels in SIRS (Kyles B.D.M.& Baltimore J., 2005, Tabata N. et al., 1995). The results of a prospective study (Dietz S. et al., 2010) of 543 patients with sepsis demonstrated that half of them had physiological normal IgG level in peripheral blood (6,1-11,9 g/dL). However intra-venous infusion of immunoglobulins in patients with systemic inflammatory processes is widely used (Berlot G. et al, 2007, Jenson H.B., 1998, Pildal J.& Gotzsche P.C., 2008). On the other hand, some authors state that there was no reliable increase of survival in patients with sepsis after treatment with exogenous immunoglobulins (Alejandria M.M. et al., 2002, Werdan K., 1999).

8. Immunological imbalance in patients with sepsis

At present there is a standpoint of the massive inflammatory reaction as a result of systemic release of cytokines that is the basic cause for MODS (Goris J.A. et al., 1985). A MODS is the result of endothelial cell damage, impairment of vessel penetrative capacity, micro circular disorders with developing cellular hypoxia and finally, cell apoptosis with the release of immune or necrotic proteins. Kidneys and gastro-intestinal tract are highly sensitive to micro-circular disorders, which lead to necrosis of renal tubules that enhances concentration of serum creatinine, develops oliguria or anuria and necrosis of intestine fringes. Excessive inflammatory reaction may change to areactivity that leads to immune suppression (and even to immunological paralysis) and joining secondary infection. Pathological morphological analysis often cannot detect correspondence between histological results and the grade of organ dysfunction registered in patients who died from sepsis. The number of dead tissue cells of heart, kidneys, liver and lungs can be insignificant to reflect the marked organ dysfunctions. Apparently, most symptoms of organ dysfunctions in patients with sepsis can be due to "cell hibernation" or "cell stunning" in the way it happens in myocardial ischemia (Sawyer DB & Loscalzo J., 1985). Reactions that are observed in septic conditions can be also seen in other pathological processes that are not directly linked to effects of microbes or their products, such as trauma, shock, advanced surgical interventions. Therefore the correct definition of sepsis is crucial because different approach to understanding sepsis leads to different treatment strategy (primarily, anti-bacterial) and directly effects the outcome. Biological response to microbial components at the beginning of SIRS and sepsis is considered to be immunological reaction of the body in order to reduce the number of pathogens. However unrestricted and excessive production of pro- and anti-inflammatory mediators plays the major role in pathogenesis of sepsis and MODS. Therefore treatment of sepsis should involve control of mediators of inflammatory cascade. Microbial components (such as endotoxin, etc.) and other mediators of inflammation (cytokines, chemokines, leukotriens, thromboxanes, platelet activating factor) that induce systemic inflammatory syndrome should be eliminated at the early stage of sepsis. Some authors proposed restriction of excessive activation of immune system of patients with sepsis by inhibiting various elements of inflammatory cascade. Monoclonal antibodies against LPS and TNF and other biological regulatory factors were offered to achieve the desired effect. However randomized clinical studies did not show clinical effectiveness of such agents (Vincent J.-L.&Abraham E., 2006). Another promising approach is the use of selective haemosorption with LPS-absorbers that allow elimination of a large part of bacterial toxins and inflammatory mediators from patient's peripheral blood.

9. Haemosorption with LPS-adsorber for elimination of triggers and mediators of inflammation in patients with sepsis and SIRS

Endotoxin (lipopolysaccharide, LPS) is well known as the main biological substance causing Gram-negative septic shock. The lack of clinical success in anti-endotoxin therapies with antibodies determined the development of extracorporeal methods aimed at reducing the circulating endotoxin level by adsorption. Theoretically such procedures could prevent progression of the systemic inflammatory reaction due to the elimination of inflammation trigger factors and mediators (cytokines, bacterial exo- and endotoxins) from the patient's body. The necessity of eliminating a wide spectrum of substances characterized by different physical and chemical features from blood stipulates the application of non-selective and non-specific methods such as haemosorption. In current clinical practice some devices for haemosorption are used as specific (LPS) adsorbers. Launched in 2006 the Alteco® LPS Adsorber (Alteco Medical AB, Sweden; class IIa medical device) is based on a tailor-made synthetic peptide which is non-toxic and adsorbs endotoxin selectively in a recommended single 2-h treatment with a blood flow of 100–200 ml/min and activated clotting time of ≥180 s (information provided by the manufacturer).

Data available confirmed an effective reduction in the LPS level in the patients' blood after this procedure (Yaroustovsky M, 2009, Andersen T.H., 2009). In particular, Kulabukhov VV et al. demonstrated almost total elimination of LPS from the patient's blood (from 1.44 EU/ml before treatment to 0.03 EU/ml post treatment) (Kulabukhov VV., 2008). This effect was accompanied by a reduction in procalcitonin and inflammatory cytokines levels. Also, an obvious improvement was observed in the patient's haemodynamics.

The same results were shown in the work of T. Ala-Kokko et al.(T. Ala-Kokko, 2009). The mean total duration of vasopressor infusion was 46 h shorter in the treatment group compared with the control group (95% CI, 104–12 h, p = 0.165), with an average vasopressor requirement period of 17.4 ± 6.8 h (95% CI, 5.8–23.8 h) following the start of adsorption treatment. The level of LPS decreased in all cases except in one study patient and all were without vasopressors at 24 h. The decrease in the Sequential Organ Failure Assessment (SOFA) score was 3.4 ± 1.7 from baseline to 24 h after the treatment. The average period of hospital stay was 3.4 days shorter in the treatment group (95% CI, 21.7–14.8 days, p = 0.881).

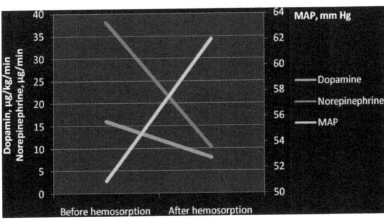

Fig. 6. Inverse correlation of MAP dynamics and vasopressor requirement before and after haemosorption by Alteco.

We studied LPS adsorbers for treating 7 patients with sepsis or septic shock. During the course of extracorporeal detoxification a number of clinical parameters were estimated.

These were temperature, mean arterial pressure (MAP), central venous pressure (CVP), the percentage of available haemoglobin saturated with oxygen (SaO_2), the fraction of inspired oxygen (FiO_2), the partial pressure of oxygen in arterial blood (PaO_2), PaO_2/FIO_2 ratio (an index to characterize the acute respiratory distress syndrome), severe hypoxaemia (insufficient oxygen content in blood), the biochemical parameters of blood (lactate, procalcitonin (PCT)), and concentrations of LPS and cytokines in blood. The requirement for vasopressors (Dopamine, Norepinephrine) was also evaluated.

Data shown in Table 2 and Figure 6 unambiguously demonstrated a pronounced tendency towards the oxygen saturation of haemoglobin (SaO_2) and normalization of the oxygen index (decreasing FiO2 on 22%). This was associated with a rise in MAP and a decrease in CVP. Normalization of cardio-vascular system function led to a reduction in the requirement for vasopressors.

Parameters	Before hemosorption	After hemosorption	p
CVP, mm Hg	16±5.0	12±4.1	>0.05
SaO_2 ,%	87±6.1	94±5.9	>0.05
FiO_2 ,%	77±32.3	55±15.4	<0.05*
PaO_2/FIO_2	160±70.9	200±54.1	<0.05*
PCT ng/ml	22±14.3	12±6.0	>0.05
Lactate, mmol/l	4.3±1.3	4.5±3.2	>0.05

* Significant difference

Table 2. Clinical parameters before/after haemosorption by Alteco.

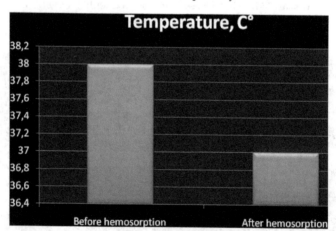

Fig. 7. The body temperature values for patients before and after haemosorption by Alteco.

The significant increase in the respiratory index (PaO2/FiO2) after haemosorption evidenced the improvement of oxygen diffusion through the alveoli-capillary membrane.

As a result, normalization of integral indices, such as body temperature and blood PCT level, was observed (Fig.7).

The level of LPS, the key trigger signal for system inflammatory reaction, decreased by a factor of 2 to 3 versus control after haemosorption (Fig.8).

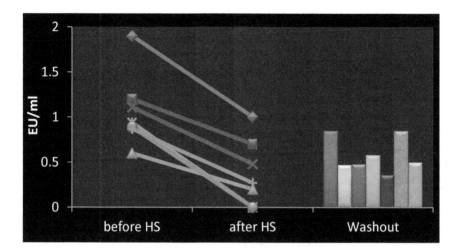

Fig. 8. LPS level in the blood of patients with sepsis before and after haemosorption by Alteco.

As hypercytokinaemia determines the development of SIRS, it seems to be possible that reducing cytokine levels (IL-8, IL-1β, IL-6, IL-10 etc) in blood may block the generalization of this pathological process or interrupt the cascade of cytokine storm. We studied the influence of haemosorption on the cytokine content in blood (Fig. 9).

Equal portions of sorbent were suspended in equal volumes of physiological solution (0.9% NaCl) and put onto the shaker during temperature control. High levels of some cytokines (IL-6, IL-8, IL-12, INFγ and TNF) were indicated in the supernatant (Fig.9).

We also investigated washouts from a sorbent after the termination of the haemosorption procedure. There were no well-developed specific conditions for the extraction and quantitative estimation of the characteristics of the sorbent.

This approach was especially informative in cases in which the level of analyte was higher in the blood after haemosorption than before the treatment (see examples in Fig. 9). Moreover, an increase in the concentration of some soluble cytokine receptors (sIL-1 II R, sIL-6 R) was observed in patient blood after haemosorption (Fig. 10).

We assumed that this phenomenon was determined by the release of cytokines from their complexes with receptors or proteins during the course of haemosorption.

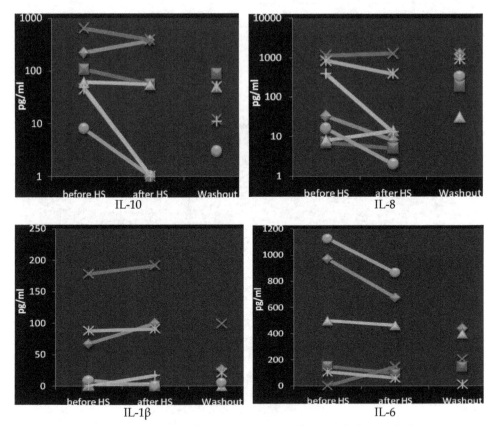

Fig. 9. The levels of cytokines in the blood of patients with sepsis before and after haemosorption by Alteco.

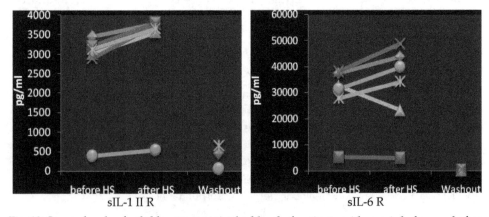

Fig. 10. Serum levels of soluble receptors in the blood of patients with sepsis before and after haemosorption by Alteco.

Our results indicated that low levels of serum cytokines revealed by ELISA did not reflect the real content of these mediators of inflammation in the blood of patients with septic complications. Perhaps a high secretion of cytokines was accompanied by an increase in the expression of congruent receptors, which bound a significant quantity of free cytokines in ligand-receptor complexes capable of dissociation. We showed that extracorporeal detoxification using the Alteco device allowed the elimination not only of free cytokines, but also the majority of bound endogenous bioregulators from cytokine/receptor complexes. Removal of the trigger factor (LPS) along with a wide range of pro- and anti-inflammatory cytokines, and possibly with other inflammation mediators (leukotrienes, thromboxanes, C-reactive protein) led to the interruption of the systemic inflammatory reaction, which was regarded as positive clinical effect of haemosorption for extracorporeal detoxification. Correlation analysis demonstrated a close connection between the concentrations in blood of LPS and TNFα (p= 0.050), LPS and IL-8 (p= 0.050). During the study, a 28-day survival of 9 critical patients was 96%, only 1 patient died after the procedure.

Taking into account a high correlation of normalized clinical parameters and the dynamics of LPS level and the serum profile of cytokines, the testing parameters (serum levels of IL-6, TNFα, IL-8) could be considered additional indicators of patient's status during the course of treatment, including methods of extracorporeal detoxification.

We assumed that changes in serum concentrations of cytokines after haemosorption might influence the functional activity of immune cells. Neutrophils and natural killers (NK) play a crucial role in pathogenesis of organ and multi-organ failures in case of sepsis. Our results demonstrated a pronounced tendency towards normalization of the functional activity of these innate immunity effectors after haemosorption by Alteco. Thus, phagocytic number (PN) and phagocytic index (PI) decreased after haemosorption in 1.3 – 2.1 times and 2.1 – 2.6 times, respectively. A reduction in spontaneous neutrophil activity was also observed. This parameter indicates the intensity of oxygen-dependent phagocytosis associated with the release of free radicals destroying the adjacent cells including endothelium. Moreover, the decrease was observed in the super-aggressive non-specific reaction of NK: index of cytotoxic activity (ICA) reduced after haemosorption from 75-90% to 54-58% (normal for healthy volunteers). This effect of normalizing functional activity of neutrophils and NK is likely connected with the elimination of LPS molecules and cytokines from peripheral blood.

Stimulation of immune cells for a long period could lead to exhaustion of their killing activity, resulting in the circulation of leukocytes that are unable to provide defence functions, such as termination of phagocytosis and killing transformed cells. These "ballast" cells do not express apoptosis receptor CD95 on their surface membrane, and consequently they cannot be eliminated from system circulation.

It was shown previously that prolongation of life of leukocytes could produce tissue and organ damage in case of SIRS and sepsis. A change in apoptosis regulation may influence pathogenesis of sepsis and multi-organ failure. We demonstrated the increase in CD45+CD95+ cell number (from 21-24% to 38-40%) after haemosorption. After the treatment, the number of CD45+CD66b+CD95+ neutrophils was higher by 32-42%, which correlated with an increase in the number of phagocytes able to terminate oxygen-dependent phagocytosis. Correlation analysis revealed a strong connection between these parameters (p=0.0086).

Therefore, reduction of the functional activity of leukocytes (PN, PI, ICA) to the level of that of healthy individuals and simultaneous increase in CD95+ leukocyte level could be considered a favourable prognostic factor.

The obtained results demonstrated that the LPS adsorber could effectively eliminate a wide range of the factors from peripheral blood (such as LPS, cytokines, etc.), which mediate all the stages of systemic inflammatory reaction in the body. Significant improvement of the performance status of patients with sepsis was observed after extracorporeal detoxification with LPS adsorber. This was the normalization of cardio-respiratory functions and reduction in hyperthermia and vasopressor requirement, normalization of MAP and concentration of gases in peripheral blood.

10. Conclusion

The discussed data and information show that cancer patients with sepsis have an enhanced serum level of LPS as compared to healthy volunteers. There is a close link between a decreased serum level of LPB along with the 10-fold reduction of LPB/LPS ratio and poor prognosis in cancer patients with sepsis. A characteristic cytokine profile of septic condition demonstrated that IL-6, IL-18 and soluble receptor sTNF RI concentrations significantly exceeded those of healthy volunteers and therefore high serum concentrations of IL-6, IL-8, IL-10, sTNF RI, sIL-1 RII, and sIL-6 R could be suggested as markers of sepsis for cancer patients.

In conclusion, triggers and mediators of inflammation secreted by immune cells play a crucial role in pathogenesis of SIRS and sepsis. Management of the inflammatory cascade should be considered an essential part of the complex approach to the treatment of systemic suppurative septic complications.

11. References

Alejandria M.M., Lansang M.A., Dans L.F., Mantaring J.B.V. Intravenous immunoglobulin for treating sepsis and septic shock. Cochrane Database Syst Rev. 2002;CD001090.

Alves-Filho J.C., Spiller F., Cunha F.Q. Neutrophil paralysis in sepsis. Shock. 2010;34 (Suppl 1):15-21.

Andersen T.H., Jensen T.H., Andersen L.W. Adjunctive therapy of severe sepsis and septic shock in adults Current Anaesthesia & Critical Care Volume 20, Issues 5-6, 2009, P. 254-258

Anderson R., Schmidt R. Clinical biomarkers in sepsis. Front Biosci (Elite Ed). 2010 1;2:504-520.

Anderson R., Schmidt R. Clinical biomarkers in sepsis. Front Biosci (Elite Ed). 2010 1;2:504-20.

Angus D.C., Linde-Zwirble W.T., Lidicker J., Clermont G., Carcillo J., Pinsky M.R. Epidemiology of severe sepsis in the United States: analysis of incidence, outcome, and associated costs of care. Crit Care Med. 2001; 29: 1303–1310.

Annane D, Bellissant E, Cavaillon J-M. Septic shock. Lancet. 2005; 365: 63-78.

Balzan S., Quadros C. D. A., Cleva R.D., Zilberstein B., Cecconello I. Bacterial translocation: Overview of mechanisms and clinical impact Issue J Gastroenterol Hepatol. 2007; 22(4): 464–471.

Barber M.D., Fearon K.C., Ross J.A. Relationship of serum levels of interleukin-6, soluble interleukin-6 receptor and tumour necrosis factor receptors to the acute-phase protein response in advanced pancreatic cancer. Clin Sci (Lond). 1999 ;96(1):83-87.

Barber M.D., Fearon K.C., Ross J.A. Relationship of serum levels of interleukin-6, soluble interleukin-6 receptor and tumour necrosis factor receptors to the acute-phase protein response in advanced pancreatic cancer. Clin Sci (Lond). 1999 ;96(1):83-87.

Berlot G., Bacer B., Piva M., Lucangelo U., Viviani M. Immunoglobulins in sepsis Adv In Sepsis. 2007; 6 (2): 41-46.

Calandra T., Baumgartner J.D., Grau G.E., Wu M.M., Lambert P.H., Schellekens J., Verhoef J., Glauser M.P. Prognostic values of tumor necrosis factor/cachectin, interleukin-1, interferon-alpha, and interferon-gamma in the serum of patients with septic shock. J Infect Dis. 1990;161(5):982-987.

Deitch EA, Bridges RM. Effect of stress and trauma on bacterial translocation from the gut. J Surg Res 1987; 42 (5): 536–42

Dietz S., Lautenschlaeger C., Mueller-Werdan U., Werdan K. Low levels of immunoglobulin G in patients with sepsis or septic shock: a signum mali ominis? Crit Care. 2010; 14(Suppl 1): P26.

Emoto M., Miyamoto M., Yoshizawa I., Emoto Y., Schaibe U.E., Kita E., Kaufmann S.H.E. Critical role of NK cells rather than Vα14+NKT cells in lipopolysaccharide-induces lethal shock in mice. J Immunol. 2002; 169:1426-1432.

Fialkow L., Filho L.F., Bozzetti M.C., Milani A.R., Filho E.M.R., Ladniuk R.M., Pierozan P., de Moura R.M.,Prolla J.C., Vachon E., Downey G.P. Neutrophil apoptosis: a marker of disease severity in sepsis and sepsis-induced acute respiratory distress syndrome Crit Care. 2006; 10(6): R155.

Frieling J.T.M., Van Deuren M., Wijdenes J. Circulating interleukin-6 receptor in patients with sepsis syndrome. J Infect Dis 1995; 171:469-472.

Frieling J.T.M., Van Deuren M., Wijdenes J. Circulating interleukin-6 receptor in patients with sepsis syndrome. J Infect Dis 1995; 171:469-472.

Gaïni S., Koldkjaer O.G., Pedersen C., Pedersen S.S. Procalcitonin, lipopolysaccharide-binding protein, interleukin-6 and C-reactive protein in community-acquired infections and sepsis: a prospective study. Crit Care. 2006;10(2):R53.

Giamarellos-Bourboulis E.J. What is the pathophysiology of the septic host upon admission? Int J Antimicrob. Agents. 2010;36 (2):S2-54.

Giamarellos-Bourboulis E.J., Tsaganos T., Spyridaki E., Mouktaroudi M., Plachouras D., Vaki I., Karagianni V., Antonopoulou A., Veloni V., Giamarellou H. Early changes of CD4-positive lymphocytes and NK cells in patients with severe Gram-negative sepsis. Crit Care. 2006; 10: R166.

Giamarellos-Bourboulis EJ What is the pathophysiology of the septic host upon admission? Int J Antimicrob Agents. 2010 Dec;36 Suppl 2:S2-54;

Goris J.A., te Boekhorst T.P.A., Nuytinck J.K.S. Multiple organ failure: generalized autodestructive inflammation? Arch. Surg. 1985; 120:1109-1115.

Hammond M.E., Lapointe G.R., Feucht P.H., Hilt S., Gallegos C.A., Gordon C.A., Giedlin M.A., Mullenbach G., Tekamp-Olson P. IL-8 induces neutrophil chemotaxis predominantly via type I IL-8 receptors. J Immunol. 1995;155(3):1428-1433.

Härter L., Mica L., Stocker R., Trentz O., Keel M. Mcl-1 correlates with reduced apoptosis in neutrophils from patients with sepsis. J Am Coll Surg. 2003;197:964–973.

Hildebrand F., Pape H.C., Krettek C. The importance of cytokines in the posttraumatic inflammatory reaction Unfallchirurg. 2005;108(10):793-794, 796-803.

Holub M., Kluèkova Z., Beneda B., Hobstová J., Hužička I., Pražák J., Lobovská A. Changes in lymphocyte subpopulations and CD3+/DR+ expression in sepsis. Clin Microbiol Infect. 2000; 6: 657-660.

Jenson H.B., Pollock B.H. The role of intravenous immunoglobulin for the prevention and treatment of neonatal sepsis. Semin Perinatol. 1998;22:50-63.

Jimenez M.F., Watson W.G., Parodo J., Evans D., Foster D., Steinberg M., Rotstein O.D., Marshall J.C. Dysregulated expression of neutrophil apoptosis in the systemic inflammatory response syndrome. Arch Surg. 1997;132:1263–1270.

Keel M., Trentz O. Pathophysiology of polytrauma, Injury. 2005;36: 691–709.

Kerr A.R., Kirkham L.A.S., Kadioglu A., Andrew P.W., Garside P., Thompson H., Mitchell T.J. Identification of a detrimental role for NK cells in pneumococcal pneumonia and sepsis in immunocompromised hosts. Microbes Infect. 2005; 7:845-852.

Kulabukhov VV. Use of an endotoxin adsorber in the treatment of severe abdominal sepsis. Acta Anaesthesiol Scand. 2008 Aug;52(7):1024-5.

Kumar A.T., Sudhir U., Punith K., Kumar R., Ravi Kumar V.N., Rao M.Y. Cytokine profile in elderly patients with sepsis. Indian J Crit Care Med 2009;13:74-78.

Kumar V., Sharma A. Neutrophils: Cinderella of innate immune system. Int Immunopharmacol. 2010; 10: 1325-1334.

Kyles B.D.M., Baltimore J. Adjunctive use of plasmapheresis and intravenous immunoglobulin therapy in sepsis: a case report american journal of critical care. 2005; 14 (2): 109-112.

Laurenzi L., Natoli S., Di Filippo F., Calamaro A. Systemic and haemodynamic toxicity after isolated limb perfusion (ILP) with TNF-alpha. J Exp Clin Cancer Res. 2004;23(2): 225-231.

Lee WL, Downey GP. Neutrophil activation and acute lung injury. Curr Opin Crit Care. 2001;7:1–7

Lenz A., Franklin G.A., Cheadle W.G. Systemic inflammation after trauma Injury. 2007 Dec;38(12): 1336-1345.

Mahidhara R., Billiar T.R. Apoptosis in sepsis. Crit Care Med. 2000;28:N105–N113.

Martin C., Saux P., Mege J.L., Perrin G., Papazian L., Gouin F. Prognostic values of serum cytokines in septic shock. Intensive Care Med. 1994;20(4):272-977.

Martin C., Saux P., Mege J.L., Perrin G., Papazian L., Gouin F. Prognostic values of serum cytokines in septic shock. Intensive Care Med. 1994;20(4):272-977.

Moore F.A. The role of the gastrointestinal tract in postinjury multiple organ failure// Am. J. Surg. 1999; 178: 449–453.

Müller B., Peri G., Doni A., Perruchoud A.P., Landmann R., Pasqualini F., Mantovan A. High circulating levels of the IL-1 type II decoy receptor in critically ill patients with sepsis: association of high decoy receptor levels with glucocorticoid administration. J Leukocyte Biol. 2002;72:643-649

Murphy R., DeCoursey T. E. Charge compensation during the phagocyte respiratory burst. Bioenergetics. 2006; 1757(8): 996-1011.

Myc A., Buck J., Gonin J., Reynolds B., Hammerling U., Emanuel. The level of lipopolysaccharide-binding protein is significantly increased in plasma in patients with the systemic inflammatory response syndrome. Clin Diagn Lab Immunol. 1997; 4:113–116.

Nijhuis C. S., Vellenga E., Daenen S.J., Graaf W.T., Gietema J.A., Groen H. J., Kamps W.A., Bont E. Lipopolysaccharide-binding protein: a possible diagnostic marker for Gram-negative bacteremia in neutropenic cancer patients Intensive Care Medicine 2003; 29, 12: 2157-2161.

Oppenheim J.J., Yang D. Alarmins: chemotactic activators of immune responses. Curr Opin Immunol. 2005; 17: 359-365.

Papathanassoglou E.D.E., Moynihan J.A., McDermott M.P., Ackerman M.H. Expression of Fas (CD95) and Fas ligand on peripheral blood mononuclear cells in critical illness and association with multiorgan dysfunction severity and survival. Crit Care Med. 2001;29:709–718.

Pildal J., Gotzsche P.C. Polyclonal immunoglobulin for treatment of bacterial sepsis: a systematic review. Clin Infect Dis. 2004;39:38-46.

Pinsky M.R. Pathophysiology of sepsis and multiple organ failure:pro- versus anti-inflammatory aspects. Contrib. Nephrol. 2004; 144: 31-43.

Quinn J.V., Slotman G.J. Platelet-activating factor and arachidonic acid metabolites mediate tumor necrosis factor and eicosanoid kinetics and cardiopulmonary dysfunction during bacteremic shock. Crit Care Med. 1999;27(11):2485-2494.

Rigato O., Ujvari S., Castelo A., Salomão R. Tumor necrosis factor alpha (TNF-α) and sepsis: Evidence for a role in host defense. Infection. 1996; 24: 314–318.

Rigato O., Ujvari S., Castelo A., Salomão R. Tumor necrosis factor alpha (TNF-α) and sepsis: Evidence for a role in host defense. Infection. 1996; 24: 314–318.

Sawyer DB, Loscalzo J. Myocardial hibernation: restorative or preterminal sleep? Circulation. 2002; 105(13): 1517-1519.

Sayeed M.M. Delay of neutrophil apoptosis can exacerbate inflammation in sepsis patients: cellular mechanisms. Crit Care Med. 2004;32:1604–1606.

Segal A.W. How neutrophils kill microbe. Ann Rev Immunol 2005;23:197–223.

Segal A.W. How neutrophils kill microbe. Ann Rev Immunol 2005;23:197–223.

T. Ala-Kokko, J. Koskenkari and J. Laurila, Lipopolysaccharide adsorber in abdominal septic shock, Crit Care 13 (Suppl. 1) (2009), p. 280.

Tabata N., Azuma E., Masuda S.-I., Ido M., Sakurai M. Transient low level of IgG3 induced by sepsis Pediatrics International. 1995; 37(2): 201–202.

Takeshita S., Tsujimoto H., Kawase H., Kawamura Y., Sekine I. Increased Levels of lipopolysaccharide binding protein in plasma in children with kawasaki disease Clin Diagn Lab Immunol. 2002; 9(1): 205–206.

Thomas S., Balasubramanian K. A. Role of intestine in postsurgical complications: involvement of free radicals. Free Rad Biol Med. 2004; 36 (6): 745-756.

Vincent J.-L., Abraham E. The last 100 years of sepsis Am J Resp Crit Care Med. 2006; 173: 256-263.

Volk H.D., Reinke P., Döcke W.D. Immunological monitoring of the inflammatory process: Which variables? When to assess. Eur J Surg Suppl. 1999; 584:70-72.

Werdan K. Immunoglobulins in Sepsis: Therapeutic Use of Immunoglobulins. Sepsis. 1999; 3, 3:239-245.

Yaroustovsky M, Abramyan M, Popok Z, Nazarova E, Stupchenko O, Popov D, Plushch M, Samsonova N. Preliminary report regarding the use of selective in complex cardiac surgery patients with extensive sepsis and prolonged intensive care stay. Blood Purif. 2009;28(3):227-33.

Yegenaga I., Hoste E., Van Biesen W., Vanholder R., Benoit D., Kantarci G., Dhondt A., Colardyn F., Lameire N.: Clinical characteristics of patients developing ARF due to sepsis/systemic inflammatory response syndrome: Results of a prospective study. Am J Kidney Dis. 2004; 43 :817 –824.

Yoneda O., Imai T., Goda S., Inoue H., Yamauchi A., Okazaki T., Imai H., Yoshie O., Bloom E.T., Domae N., Umehara H. Fractalkine-mediated endothelial cell injury by NK Cells. J Immunol. 2000; 164: 4055-4062.

Zeerleder S., Hack C.E., Caliezi C., van Mierlo G., Eerenberg-Belmer A., Wolbink A., Wuillenmin W.A. Activated cytotoxic T cells and NK cells in severe sepsis and septic shock and their role in multiple organ dysfunctio. Clin Immunol. 2005;116(2): 158-165.

Zeni F., Tardy B., Vindimian M., Pain P., Gery P., Bertrand J.C. Soluble interleukin-6 receptor in patients with severe sepsis. J Infect Dis. 1995;172(2):607–608.

Zhang B., Huang Y.H., Chen Y., Yang Y., Hao Z.L., Xie S.L. Plasma tumor necrosis factor-α, its soluble receptors and interleukin-1β levels in critically burned patients. Burns. 1998;24(7):599-603.

Zhang B., Huang Y.H., Chen Y., Yang Y., Hao Z.L., Xie S.L. Plasma tumor necrosis factor-α, its soluble receptors and interleukin-1β levels in critically burned patients. Burns. 1998;24(7):599-603.

Zucker T., Kriger G. Sepsis-like syndrome caused by the Russian medication pyrogenal (Salmonella typhi endotoxin). J Exp Clin Cancer Res. 2004; Isr Med Assoc J. 2003; 5(10):750-751.

Zychlinsky A., Weinrauch Y., Weiss J. Introduction: Forum in immunology on neutrophils. Microbes and Infection. 2003; 5(14): 1289-1291.

9

Chemokine Responses to Hepatitis C Virus and Their Impact in Mediating the Treatment Responses of Antiviral Treatment

Jon Florholmen and Rasmus Goll
Research group of Gastroenterology and Nutrition,
Institute of Clinical Medicine, University of Tromsø, Tromsø
Department of Medical Gastroenterology,
University Hospital North Norway, Tromsø,
Norway

1. Introduction

The hepatitis C virus (HCV) is a global health challenge with strong regional implications (Shepard et al, 2005). Currently, about 170 million people throughout the world are chronically HCV infected and it is the most important cause of liver disease worldwide. During the last 30 years the mode of transmission in industrial countries has changed from infection by medical use of contaminated blood products to infection by shared utensils by drug abusers. The incidence of HCV infection in Europe increased during the 1990's (Rantala & van de Laar, 2008). It is unknown if this trend of increased incidence in Europe and worldwide has persisted after 2000.

Following acute HCV infection approximately 80 % of adults and between 50 to 60% of children develop chronic disease (Vogt et al, 1999). The reasons for the ineffective clearance of HCV virus is unknown, but most likely there are viral escape factors and host factors such as inappropriate immune based viral clearance. Progression of chronic HCV infection occurs in a proportion of infected subjects in a sequence via liver fibrosis to liver cirrhosis and finally death due either to liver failure or to hepatocellular carcinoma (HCC). The rate of progression is affected by various factors such as age at infection, gender, alcohol consumption, and co-infection particularly with human immunodeficiency virus (HIV), but also with hepatitis B virus (HBV) (Poynard et al, 2001). When compensated cirrhosis is established, the probability of decompensation is estimated to be 15-17 % within 2-3 years. The burden of expenses to health services due to HCV related disease has been predicted to be considerable in the future. In 2004, 23 % of all liver transplantations in Europe were related to HCV infection. Most likely the incidence of decompensated cirrhosis and HCC will increase substantially in the next few decades, due to the steady increase of HCV positive persons-at-risk (Lehman & Wilson, 2009).

Chronic HCV infection is treated with a combination of pegylated interferon (peg-IFN)-α, and the synthetic nucleoside analogue ribavirin. By this combination sustained virological response (SVR) is achieved in between 40 % and 50 % for genotype 1 and as high as approximately 85 % for genotypes 2 and 3. Due to the limited success rate of this combined therapy approach, triple therapy options have been suggested. Thus, both protease inhibitors and polymerase inhibitors has been tested as addition to PEG-interferon and ribavirin. These drugs are not approved by the authorities as standard treatment since they are still under investigation. Depending of the efficacy of triple therapy, the future need for liver transplantation may be reduced, with a considerable impact on health expenditures.

Both viral and host factors are determinants for the spontaneous elimination or persistence of HCV. The high risk for chronic infection is most likely caused by a lack of a strong and specific immune response to viral antigens. On the other hand, an overly powerful immune response may lead to acute liver failure as seen in rare cases of hepatitis A and hepatitis B. The frequent mutations of HCV are challenging to the host immune response and results in a high risk for viral escape. In the recent years HCV research has been focused on the innate and adaptive response to the virus. Special attention has been put into the role of chemokines and their receptors which are responsible for recruitment of leukocytes from blood stream to the affected tissue. It has been proposed that this is one of the most critical immunological steps for an effective clearance of the virus. We have recently reported that in the antiviral treatment, SVR is dependent on a rapid (24 hours) chemokine response (Florholmen et al, 2011). This has initiated the present review of the immunological mechanisms against the HCV with a special emphasis on the chemokine response.

2. Aims

The first part of the chapter we will review the chemokine concept and its role in the HCV pathogenesis, their role in the innate and adaptive response to HCV leading to liver inflammation and liver fibrosis. The second part will concentrate on the chemokine response during antiviral treatment using interferon, ribavirin and the new nucleoside analogues.

3. Hepatitis C virus

HCV is a positive single stranded RNA virus with regions coding for structural peptides (an envelope, 9000 bases) and regions coding for non-structural (NS) peptides (1 – 5) (Myrmel et al, 2009). Eleven genotypes have so far been described and 6 are commonly diagnosed. The Genotypes 1, 4 and 6 respond to antiviral therapy (interferon (IFN) + ribavirin) with an SVR of 50 % and 85 %, respectively. The virus has a high production of estimated 1012 virions per day, with an average half-life of 2.7 h and a turn-over rate close to 99 %. The calculated annual mutation rate is in the order of $1.5–2.0 \times 10^3$ nucleotide substitutions per site. Furthermore, the virus has no proofreading mechanisms. The naturally occurring mutations may thereby enhance resistance both to endogenous immune responses and to anti-HCV therapy. Mutations conferring resistance of hepatitis C virus to the new treatment agents, the NS3 protease inhibitors, have been described (Halfon & Locarnini, 2011). The various genotypes have not been associated to specific pathobiology. As described above, however, the pattern of genotype related resistance to therapy has been extensively documented. The molecular mechanisms of this resistance have been described to some extent. Of great interest is the interferon sensitivity-determining region (ISDR) in the non-structural NSR5 part of the virus genome. Amino acid substitutions in ISDR have been related to increased SVR of anti-HCV treatment (for review, see (Chayama & Hayes, 2011)).

4. Antiviral immune response

The immunological response to viral infection is a complex interplay between host tissue cells, the innate and adaptive immune responses. A series of mediators, systemic and paracrine, as well as cell-cell interaction will in most cases result in clearance of infection. Some viruses have developed strategies of immune evasion and can therefore establish chronic infections. In case of HCV infection, the resulting chronic inflammatory response is actually harmful to the host by driving development of fibrosis, cirrhosis, and liver failure or HCC.

Viral pathogens can enter the host in several ways, the mucosal membranes being the most frequently used. A few viruses mainly spread via direct inoculation in the bloodstream, HCV being a classic example. Each type of virus has its preferred host cell type based on specific homing mechanisms. The HCV tropism for hepatocytes and internalization process is partly characterised and involve cluster of differentiation (CD) 81 and Claudin-1 (Thorley et al, 2010).

Viral pathogens do not have metabolism and rely on modifying the host cell production apparatus to its own benefit. A range of defensive mechanisms has been developed in response to this strategy. The end result from these mechanisms is mostly death by lysis or apoptosis of the infected cell, while at the same time restricting spread of the infectious agent to neighbouring cells in the infected site. A short overview of the general immune response to viral infection with special emphasis on mechanisms related to the anti-HCV response will be given in the following.

Leukocyte trafficking is a very important feature of the immune system allowing for the immune cells to patrol the entire host organism and thereby detect any intruding microorganism, bacteria or virus. The ability to generate a rapid local response when an intruder has been detected is based on homing mechanisms which mainly are triggered by early response cytokines and chemokines. As it turns out in the case of HCV infection, chemokines may also be central in generating an effective immune response following pharmacological intervention, as a swift chemokine response early in the course of treatment can predict a sustained virological response.

4.1 Innate receptor systems

The innate immune defence consists of several specialized cell types like dendritic cells (DC's) granulocytes, natural killer (NK) cells and macrophages. A common trait for these cell types is the pattern recognition receptors (PRR's) consisting of both intracellular and transmembrane subtypes. The nucleotide oligomerization domain (NOD) receptors are intracellular and the toll like receptors (TLR's) are transmembrane receptors primarily directed towards the extracellular compartment. These innate receptors detect common motifs from pathogenic microorganisms including both bacteria and viruses. Upon triggering the receptor an intracellular pathway common to most of the TLR's involve myeloid differentiation primary response gene 88 (MyD88) and interleukin-1 receptor-associated kinase (IRAK) kinases leading to activation of NF-κ-B and transcription of pro-inflammatory cytokines.

The professional antigen presenting cell i.e. dendritic cell carry an array of pattern recognition receptors and these cells are crucial for the initiation of an adaptive response. All cell lines of the adaptive system must be stimulated by DC's in order to raise a response. The DC determines the profile of the adaptive system depending on its cytokine secretion pattern.

Most viruses have specific binding strategies for entry into host cells. This leads to a tropism of the virus rendering specific target cells its point of attack depending on the homing mechanism. Subsequently the virus particle is disassembled. At this point intracellular receptors may detect the pathogen and trigger production of early viral response cytokines – mainly type I interferons like IFN-α and -β. A possible trigger of IFN production can be double stranded RNA which has been found to stimulate type I interferons in vitro. Intracellular TLR3 is likely triggered by viral dsRNA.

4.1.1 Interferons

The family of interferons consists of three subgroups of mediators with high sequence homology. The first interferons were described by their physiological effects i.e. their ability to *interfere* with viral replication in cell cultures. The type I interferons is a group of five members: IFN -α, -β, -ω, -κ, and limitin. IFN-α and IFN-β can be secreted by practically all infected cells types following viral infection and the production of these cytokines is therefore not restricted to immune competent cells.

Type I IFN has a common receptor IFN-αβ-R which signals via the JAK-STAT pathway (JAK is short for Janus Kinase, and STAT is short for Signal Transducer and Activator of Transcription) towards the *Interferon stimulated response element* ISRE in the cell nucleus and induce transcription of several interferon inducible genes which in turn increase degradation of viral RNA and inhibit translation processes. The secreted interferon acts on both the secreting cell (autocrine stimulation) and neighbouring cells (paracrine stimulation) thus inhibiting local spread of the viral infection. Furthermore, interferons up-regulate major histocompatibility complex I (MHC-I) and thereby enhance the display of viral antigens to the adaptive effector cells (see below). Interferons also activate NK cells and thereby facilitate killing of infected cells. Thus, the entry of a virus in a cell induce production of interferons which in turn help protect neighbouring cells from infection but also facilitate killing of the infected cell by NK cells and/or antigen specific cytotoxic T cells.

4.1.2 Natural killer cells

NK cells are part of the innate immune response, and have an important role in combating viral infections in the early phase until the specific adaptive cytotoxic response is raised. The NK cell is believed to distinguish infected from normal cells via an intricate process involving both stimulatory and inhibitory signalling. A set of immunoglobulin-like receptors (Killer cell Immunoglobulin-like Receptors: KIR's) and C-type lectins are involved in activation of the NK cell. A strong inhibitory signal is presentation of MHC-I on the cell surface which may be recognized by KIR's or CD94:NKG2. As part of the microbial survival strategy many viral infections inhibit MHC-I display in order to restrain presentation of antigens to the adaptive response. This strategy removes the inhibitory signal to NK cells and the infected cells display only activation signals to the NK cells and will be eliminated. Some viruses induce conformational change of MHC-I with the same result. Thus, the NK cell may be able to detect the infected cell even if it evades the adaptive response by cytotoxic CD8+ T cells (see below).

If stimulated by IFN-α or IFN-β the NK cell increase cytotoxic activity by a factor 20-100. The activated NK cell also secretes mediators important to direct the early response patterns in the tissue. The effector action of NK cells is completed by close binding to the infected cell and may use different pathways including lysis of the cell membrane by perforins or triggering of apoptosis by interaction between Fas (CD95) and FasL (CD95L). The role of NK cells in HCV infection has been reviewed recently (Cheent & Khakoo, 2011).

4.1.3 Adaptive immune response

The adaptive immune response is antigen specific and can identify foreign antigens with great sensitivity and specificity. It consists of both humoral and cellular parts, of which especially the former can enhance the function of the innate response. Opsonising antibodies can boost the performance of innate phagocytes like neutrophil granulocytes and macrophages, and also enhance the function of an NK cell mediated cytotoxic response. The specific adaptive responses are modulated in phases: in the early response phase, activated cells undergo clonal expansion. This is followed by an effector phase where the strike against the microorganism is delivered. Finally the response is attenuated after elimination of the infectious agent – this phase is controlled by regulatory T cells (see below). In the process of down regulating the adaptive response, a small population of memory cells will remain dormant. These memory cells will be able to launch a swift and efficient adaptive response if the host should encounter the same agent at a later time.

A common feature of the adaptive immune system is that the cells are unable to generate a response without help of the innate system or other parts of the adaptive response. The T cell receptor only recognizes its epitope in the context of an MHC molecule in combination with co-stimulatory factors. Each of the adaptive cell populations are restricted by specific mechanisms. T helper (Th) cells must be stimulated by their antigen presented on MHC-II by antigen presenting cells (APC's). Cytotoxic T cells must be triggered by their epitope presented on MHC-I by the target cell. B cells bind their antigen on the B-cell receptor and internalize it for degradation and presentation on the surface by MHC-II. This allows for co-stimulation by contact with, and cytokine secretion from, Th cells with the same specificity. In this way, the B cell can also present antigens for stimulation of Th cells. The local cytokine milieu at the time of stimulation determines which effector profile the stimulated Th cell will have: IFN-γ and interleukin (IL)-12A: Th1; IL-4: Th2; transforming growth factor-β: Th3; IL-6 and TGF-β: Th17; IL-10: T regulatory-1 (Tr1).

In a viral infection, the adaptive immune response is triggered by presented antigens towards a classic Th1 profile enhancing a cytotoxic effector response. The cytotoxic CD8+ T cell is antigen specific in contrast to the NK cell, and stimulation of this cell line is primarily by Th1 cytokines like IFN-gamma and IL12A. The specificity rely on the T cell receptor recognition of the antigen as presented in the groove of a MHC-I molecule on the surface of the cell in question. Also, the cytotoxic T cell and the innate NK cell tend to mirror the Th profile in the immune response at hand, so these effector cells secrete cytokines and tend to enhance the milieu given by Th cells.

The humoral part of the adaptive response also enhances the phagocyte and cytotoxic responses by a mechanism called opsonisation. Innate immune cells like neutrophil granulocytes, macrophages and NK cells carry receptors for the stem of the antibody (the FC part). Antibodies bind their target in the binding sites, and can crosslink the target to FC receptors on the innate cell. This way a viral particle on the surface of cells can be "visualized" to innate cells. Antibodies in blood, mucosal membranes, and the extracellular space also neutralise viral particles by binding.

4.1.4 Regulatory T cells

The regulatory T cells include distinct subpopulations of which some are non-specific (CD25^{high} natural T_{reg}) and others are antigen specific (Tr1 and Th3). A common trait for regulatory T cells is the expression of forkhead family transcription factor FOXP3. The natural T_{reg}'s are generated in the thymus and characterised by a high expression of CD25 (IL-2 receptor). Natural T_{reg}'s seem to act primarily by direct cell contact similar to the actions of NK cells. In contrast, the antigen specific regulatory T cells act by secretion of cytokines like IL-10 and TGF-beta. The regulatory cytokines and direct cell contact actions keep an important brake on the immune system in general, as an uncontrolled pro-inflammatory response can lead to serious pathology and even organ destruction. Thus, the function of regulatory T cells is to balance the response of pro-inflammatory immune cells in order to keep homeostasis and avoid excessive tissue damage as well as resolving inflammation when the infection has been eliminated. The balance between pro- and anti-inflammatory stimuli is delicate. The perfect immune response is swift, efficient, and causes a minimum of damage to host cells. Of course this is a compromise and the balance may tip in either direction. In HCV infection, an overly powerful response would lead to acute liver failure and death; it has been suggested that the development of cirrhosis in longstanding HCV infection is a result of an overly aggressive chronic inflammation (Larrubia et al, 2008).

4.2 Homing and chemotaxis

All of the cell types described above must be recruited to the site of infection in order to perform their part of the anti-microbial response. Though the adaptive humoral response and antibody production in most cases takes place in the regional lymph nodes, the B cells and Th cells must still be recruited and activated. The recruitment of leukocytes to the site of infection is an intricate process controlled by homing mechanisms. Some central mechanisms of leukocyte homing will be presented in the following.

Chemotaxis is a basic behaviour seen in bacteria, primitive organisms, and several cell types in the immune system. The definition of chemotaxis is that the cell in question moves towards a higher concentration of a given chemotactic compound. As the name implies, chemokines are chemotactic compounds and a cell releasing chemokines will attract the attention of nearby immune cells.

4.2.1 Chemokines

The chemokines are a family of highly homologous small proteins with a common *Greek key* structure. These mediators have a key role in the earliest phases of infection. They can be released by many cell types in response to infectious agents and to physical damage. Chemokines can recruit cells of both innate and adaptive lines to the site of infection.

The chemokines can be divided into two main subgroups: the CC group (at least 27 members named CCL1-28) with 2 adjacent cystein residues close to the amino-terminal, and the CXC group (at least 17 members named CXCL1-17) in which the two cystein residues are spaced by a single amino-acid. This structural difference is important because each subgroup has its own set of receptors. Some receptor cross-reaction within subgroup occurs, and each chemokine may react with more than one of the receptors of the group. In addition to these main groups a few chemokines of C and CX3C group with their own receptor types have been described.

4.2.2 Chemokine receptors

The chemokine receptors have a common structure with a 7-transmembrane helix coupled to G-protein intracellular signalling. The subfamilies each have a set of chemokine receptors expressed on target cells. So far, ten CC receptors (CCR1-10) and seven CXC receptors (CXCR1-7) have been described. The system of chemokines and their receptors is quite complex and so far only partly described. However, at least theoretically, different chemokine secretion profiles combined with the receptor profiles of the target cells allow for close regulation of the homing process according to the infectious agent.

4.2.3 Chemokine effects

The chemokines trigger conformational change in the adhesion molecules (leukocyte integrins) on cell surface of leucocytes, thereby enabling a stable binding of the leukocyte to intercellular adhesion molecules (ICAM's) on the vessel wall. When the leukocyte is bound to the vessel wall it is able to squeeze between endothelial cells and enter the tissue. The cells first recruited are neutrophils, then later comes monocytes and immature dendritic cells. The chemokine activation also includes arming of the cells as effectors.

4.2.4 Homing

Upon chemokine activation endothelial cells present selectins and ICAM's on the luminal surface. Leukocytes tend to roll along the endothelial surface due to weak binding between endothelial selectin and leukocyte sialyl-Lewis^x (s-Le^x) blood group antigen. If the leukocyte integrin profile matches the ICAM a strong binding is established. This binding is enhanced further by conformational changes in the leukocyte integrin triggered by chemokine stimulation. When the cell is tightly bound, extravasation by diapedesis can be initiated. After extravasation, further movement along a chemotactic gradient to the site of infection follows.

The endothelial cells will be further activated by early response cytokines like tumor necrosis factor (TNF)-α. The chemokine activation of the neutrophil granulocyte will also stimulate the oxidative burst, which is a characteristic of the effector profile in this cell type.

4.2.5 Chemokines in the adaptive immune response

Certain chemokine receptors are expressed in certain immune profile cells. Thus a Th1 chemokine receptor set can be defined: CCR5 and CXCR3; while CCR3, CCR4 and CCR8 are linked to Th2 responses (Larrubia et al, 2008). Therefore, in a viral infection a certain subset of chemokines are especially interesting, as the Th1 response is considered the adequate and efficient response type. Ligands for the CXCR3 (Interferon gamma induced protein 10 (IP-10), Monokine induced by gamma interferon (Mig), Interferon-inducible T-cell alpha chemoattractant (I-TAC)) and CCR5 (Regulated on Activation, Normal T Expressed and Secreted (RANTES), macrophage inflammatory protein (MIP)-1-alpha, and MIP-1-beta) are theoretically crucial for the initiation of response and resolution of infection. Indeed, a frame shift mutation on the CCR5 receptor increases susceptibility to HCV infection (Woitas et al,

2002). In effect, both theoretical and experimental data support the crucial role of the chemokine response for mounting an efficient resolution of the viral infection.

4.3 Special immunobiological features of the liver

The liver is an immunotolerant organ with constitutive high expression of IL-10 and TGF-β (Crispe et al, 2006; Manigold & Racanelli, 2007). The sinusoids are inhabited by a special type of 'pit cells'; large granular lymphocytes of the NK cell trait. Data from mouse studies indicate that the NK cells of the liver tend to secrete more regulatory cytokines and less pro-inflammatory cytokines than their peripheral counterparts (Cheent & Khakoo, 2011; Lassen et al, 2010). When the HCV virus enters this environment, a proper immune response must be launched, and to this end a massive recruitment of different types of immune cells is needed. Cells of the innate immune system such as dendritic cells and NK cells are important for the initial response and stimulation of a proper adaptive Th1 response including antigen specific T helper cells, cytotoxic T cells and B cells as well as inducible regulatory T cells. All of these cell types must be recruited from the circulation and to this end an array of chemotactic signals are activated.

Chemokines have local effects on endothelium activating processes for trans-endothelial migration, and the leucocytes also have chemokine receptors activating leukocytes rolling and binding of selectins to integrin receptors. Thus chemokines have an important role in infection response allowing extravasation of leucocytes to the site of infection. As the liver has some inherent immunetolerance as mentioned above, this recruitment of external cells is especially important. Furthermore, considering the treatment of HCV with peg-IFN-α and Ribavirin the therapy may be efficient by altering the profile and composition of inflammatory cells in the liver. In this respect, the leukocyte recruitment seems have a key role in resolution of the infection.

4.3.1 Immune response to HCV infection

HCV has parenchymal liver cells as primary target utilizing CD81, claudin-1, and possibly the LDL receptor. After binding of to a target cell, the viral particle is internalized and disassembled in the cytoplasm. HCV virus has developed strategies to evade some of the basic antiviral mechanisms described above. The early IFN-β response can be blunted by cleaving adaptor proteins necessary for activating IFN transcription, and can also inhibit the JAK-STAT pathway thus inhibiting the intracellular effector events after stimulation by IFN-α.

Relatively recently a new series of λ-interferons have been described. These include the highly homologous IL-28A (IFN-λ-2), IL-28B (IFN-λ-3) and IL-29 (IFN-λ-1). Especially IL-28B has turned out to be interesting in regard to HCV infection. It seems that a firm IL-28B response is necessary for viral clearing, and that CC genotype in the rs12979860 single nucleotide polymorphism (SNP) (The Duke) in the promoter of the IL-28B gene is associated with a higher rate of spontaneous resolution of infection and also can predict response to treatment with peg-IFN-α (Langhans et al, 2011).

4.3.2 Chemokines in the context of HCV infection

Considering the immunotolerant milieu of the liver, an efficient immune response against a pathogen like HCV must be based on a considerable influx of fresh immune cells. In this respect, the chemokine response is crucial and may be one of the main factors that determine if the infection becomes chronic or is spontaneously resolved. One of the effects of peg-IFN-α therapy is to increase the pro-inflammatory response including the chemokine response allowing for fresh Th1 cells, B cells, NK cells, and dendritic cells to engage the virus. As such, the chemokine response can be seen as a common marker for a step-up in the immune response in initiation of treatment. Whether observed chemokine responses are directly triggered by the peg-IFN-α or result from a general increase in immunologic activity in the liver remains to be determined. However, as a biological marker of sustained virological response, the early rise in chemokine activity is interesting.

5. Treatment of hepatitis C

As described in the Introduction, peg-IFN-α in combination with the nucleoside analogue ribavirin is the standard treatment of HCV infection. Upcoming new drugs are albumin-INF-α, and nucleoside analogues or protease inhibitors, and nucleoside analogue/non-nucleoside analogue polymerase inhibitors. In general, these agents act via inhibitory mechanisms on the HCV gene to reduce the viral replication. These new anti HCV drugs exert their effects directly on the virus replication: protein kinase inhibitors on NS3A/B and polymerase inhibitors on NS5A/B (for review, see (Vezali et al, 2011)).

5.1 IFN-α

The mechanisms of action of peg-IFN-α are through indirect activating of the immune system and a direct antiviral mechanism at the interferon-sensitive sites of the HCV inhibiting the transcription. These mechanisms of action are rather complex and beyond the scope of this presentation. Briefly, peg-INF-α triggers a cascade of intracellular events including activations of IFN-inducible genes and increased synthesis of IFN-induced proteins (Katze et al, 2002). These proteins such as RNA-dependent protein kinase inhibit intracellular virus replication by a RNA-degrading mechanism. Peg-IFN-α also inhibits the viral replication indirectly via an immune response and most likely via activation of immune cells. These are complex mechanisms such as increased MHC-I expression and activation of immune cells with cytokine secretion. Finally, peg-IFN-α also induces an immuno-modulation in the favour of a Th1 response and an inhibition of a Th2 response (see fig 1, for review, see (Vezali et al, 2011)).

5.2 Ribavirin

The exact mode of action of ribavirin is unknown. As ribavirin alone does not inhibit the virus replication, a synergistic action together with IFN-α has been proposed. The proposed mechanisms of actions of ribavirin are: 1. an indirect host change of Th profile from a Th2 to a Th1 profile. 2. A direct inhibitory effect on the NS5B encoded RNA dependent RNA polymerase (for review, see (Lau et al, 2002)) (figure 1)

6. Chemokines in antiviral therapy

As described above, the chemokines play a pivotal role in the chemotactic immune response to HCV by acting via their specific receptors on immune active cells. The role of chemokines in the antiviral treatment is so far only incompletely understood. Of special interest for the

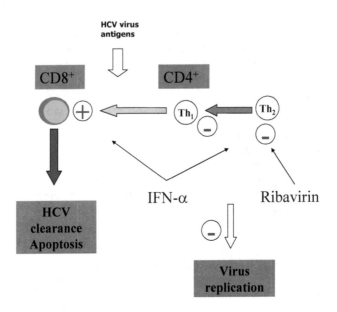

Fig. 1. Targets for antiviral therapy.

hepatic immunity is the CC chemokines macrophage inflammatory protein (MIP) -α (CCL3), MIP-1β (CCL4) and Regulated on Activation, Normal T Expressed and Secreted (RANTES) (CCL5). These chemokines are expressed by the portal vessel endothelium and recruit macrophages and lymphocytes into the liver (Ahlenstiel et al, 2004; Kusano et al, 2000). In the following we present the role of chemokines at baseline and as an early predictor of antiviral responses and clearance of the virus.

6.1 Chemokines at baseline

In one small sample sized study baseline levels before anti-HCV treatment serum levels of MIP-1β could predict a significant effect on SVR, but not eotaxin, MIP-1α, RANTES (CCL5) and IL-8 (Yoneda et al, 2011). Serum levels of MIP-3α (Yamauchi et al, 2002) have also been associated with a positive prognostic response. Moreover, increase of CXCR3 expressing CD8+ cells during treatment has been associated with achievement of viral control (Larrubia et al, 2007). Of interest was that a substitution in the ISDR was associated with response to treatment. In contrast, another study showed that baseline IL-8 level was inversely related to the response to therapy i.e. the higher IL-8 levels, the lower chance of SVR (Akbar et al, 2011). In a broad screening study of baseline CCL and CXCL chemokines, only CXCL10 was significantly associated to lack of SVR (Moura et al, 2011). In another study high CXCL10 gene expression during treatment (Sixtos-Alonso et al, 2011) and plasma level (Moura et al, 2011) were negative predictors of SVR. Finally, in two other studies baseline levels of IP10 were associated with a negative prognostic response to treatment with peg-IFN-α and ribavirin (Butera et al, 2005; Lagging et al, 2006). Interestingly, as the CCL 3-5 are produced in the portal vascular endothelium while IP-10 is produced mainly in sinusoidal endothelium and hepatocytes surrounding lobular inflammation (Zeremski et al, 2007).

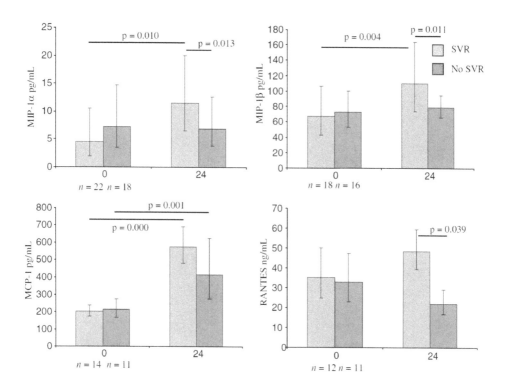

Fig. 2 Early serum chemokine responses to the treatment of chronic HCV infection. (Florholmen et al, 2011)

It is hard to interpret these apparent contradictional results of how chemokine levels can predict the response to treatment. It is of interest to note that the chemokines predicting an effective viral clearance are the CC-chemokines expressed by the portal vessel endothelium. The other chemokines predicting a lack of effect of antiviral treatment are recruited from other sources. These chemokines reflect an apparent state of viral resistance, but further studies are needed to reveal the mechanisms of action.

6.2 Early chemokine response

It is expected that an initial strong immune response is critical for a successful viral clearance in the anti HCV treatment. As far we know only one study have investigated early (24 hrs) chemokine responses during anti-HCV treatment. An early response of MIP-1α, MIP-1β, and RANTES may predict a sustained virological treatment response. MCP-1 was significantly increased but could not discriminate between SVRs and non-SVRs (Fig. 2) (Florholmen et al, 2011). However, the receiver-operator characteristic (ROC) analyses for MIP-1α, MIP-1β shows that alone, these chemokines are not suitable for clinical decisions like termination of therapy due to probable non-response (Fig. 3). Therefore, this study indicates that an early response of chemokines can be critical for an effective virus clearance during the anti-HCV treatment.

The chemokine studies mentioned above have to be interpreted with some caution both due to small sample sizes and that none of them were designed for prognostics and stratified for confounding factors.

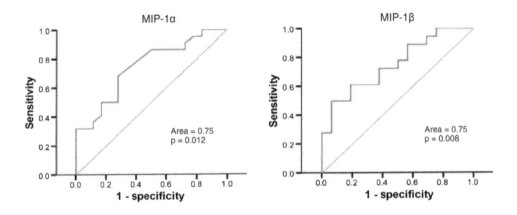

Fig. 3. ROC analysis of early chemokine response as predictor of sustained virological response (Florholmen et al, 2011).

7. New antiviral agents

The new antiviral agents based on inhibition of proteases and polymerases exert their effects on the various NS regions of the HCV genome described above. Ribavirin also has effects on an indirect mechanism of host T-cell mediation with a change from a Th2 to a Th1 profile. So far there is no evidence that the new antiviral drugs have direct suppressive effects on the HCV. Experiences from treatment of HIV show that there is a need of combination of two or more therapeutical molecules to prevent development of resistant HCV strains. So far there is an increase of SVR from 40-50 % to 75 % going from duo-therapy to triple-therapy of patients with HCV genotype 1. It would be of great interest to know if the new triple-therapy is dependent on an additional chemokine-based viral clearance for an effective treatment response. Therefore, we are waiting for further studies.

8. Concluding remarks

Chemokines seem to play a pivotal role in the immune response to HCV both to induce a spontaneous clearance during an active infection but also during the immunotherapy with peg-IFN-α and ribavirin. The mechanisms of action of chemokines are complex and still far from being fully understood. The understanding of both the successful treatment and the apparent resistance mechanisms with a virus escape from the chemokines and other immune factors is still incomplete. Most of the CC chemokines seem to play an important role in the anti virus attack. However, for other chemokines including some CXC-chemokines, increased secretions represent an apparent state of antiviral resistance to therapy. This paradox is so far poorly understood, but different compartments of chemokine production for the CC and the CXC chemokines may be a clue. It seems that the CC chemokines located in the portal vein may play a pivotal role for en effective clearance of the HCV, and the early chemokine response during antiviral treatment may be used as prognostic biomarkers. However, most of all there is a need of future studies relating viral kinetics to the chemokine responses in vivo, experimental in vitro models may contribute to a more comprehensible understanding of the role of chemokines in HCV infection.

9. References

Ahlenstiel,G.; Woitas,R.P.; Rockstroh,J., & Spengler,U. (2004). CC-chemokine receptor 5 (CCR5) in hepatitis C--at the crossroads of the antiviral immune response?, *The Journal of Antimicrobial Chemotherapy*, Vol. 53, No.6, pp. 895-898, ISSN 0305-7453.

Akbar,H.; Idrees,M.; Butt,S.; Awan,Z.; Sabar,M.F.; Rehaman,I.u.; Hussain,A., & Saleem,S. (2011). High baseline interleukine-8 level is an independent risk factor for the achievement of sustained virological response in chronic HCV patients, *Infection, Genetics and Evolution: Journal of Molecular Epidemiology and Evolutionary Genetics in Infectious Diseases*, Vol. 11, No.6, pp. 1301-1305, ISSN 1567-7257.

Butera,D.; Marukian,S.; Iwamaye,A.E.; Hembrador,E.; Chambers,T.J.; Di Bisceglie,A.M.; Charles,E.D.; Talal,A.H.; Jacobson,I.M.; Rice,C.M., & Dustin,L.B. (2005). Plasma chemokine levels correlate with the outcome of antiviral therapy in patients with hepatitis C, *Blood*, Vol. 106, No.4, pp. 1175-1182, ISSN 0006-4971.

Chayama,K. & Hayes,C.N. (2011). Hepatitis C virus: How genetic variability affects pathobiology of disease, *Journal of Gastroenterology and Hepatology*, Vol. 26 Suppl 1, pp. 83-95, ISSN 1440-1746.

Cheent,K. & Khakoo,S.I. (2011). Natural killer cells and hepatitis C: action and reaction, *Gut*, Vol. 60, No.2, pp. 268-278, ISSN 1468-3288.

Crispe,I.N.; Giannandrea,M.; Klein,I.; John,B.; Sampson,B., & Wuensch,S. (2006). Cellular and molecular mechanisms of liver tolerance, *Immunological Reviews*, Vol. 213, pp. 101-118, ISSN 0105-2896.

Florholmen,J.; Kristiansen,M.G.; Steigen,S.E.; Sørbye,S.W.; Paulssen,E.J.; Kvamme,J.M.; Konopski,Z.; Gutteberg,T., & Goll,R. (2011). A rapid chemokine response of macrophage inflammatory protein (MIP)-1-alpha, MIP-1-beta and the regulated on activation, normal T expressed and secreted chemokine is associated with a sustained virological response in the treatment of chronic hepatitis C, *Clinical Microbiology and Infection: The Official Publication of the European Society of Clinical Microbiology and Infectious Diseases*, Vol. 17, No.2, pp. 204-209, ISSN 1469-0691.

Halfon,P. & Locarnini,S. (2011). Hepatitis C virus resistance to protease inhibitors, *Journal of Hepatology*, Vol. 55, No.1, pp. 192-206, ISSN 0168-8278.

Katze,M.G.; He,Y., & Gale,M., Jr. (2002). Viruses and interferon: a fight for supremacy, *Nature Reviews.Immunology*, Vol. 2, No.9, pp. 675-687, ISSN 1474-1733.

Kusano,F.; Tanaka,Y.; Marumo,F., & Sato,C. (2000). Expression of C-C chemokines is associated with portal and periportal inflammation in the liver of patients with chronic hepatitis C, *Laboratory Investigation; a Journal of Technical Methods and Pathology*, Vol. 80, No.3, pp. 415-422, ISSN 0023-6837.

Lagging,M.; Romero,A.I.; Westin,J.; Norkrans,G.; Dhillon,A.P.; Pawlotsky,J.M.; Zeuzem,S.; von Wagner,M.; Negro,F.; Schalm,S.W.; Haagmans,B.L.; Ferrari,C.; Missale,G.; Neumann,A.U.; Verheij-Hart,E., & Hellstrand,K. (2006). IP-10 predicts viral response and therapeutic outcome in difficult-to-treat patients with HCV genotype 1 infection, *Hepatology (Baltimore, Md.)*, Vol. 44, No.6, pp. 1617-1625, ISSN 0270-9139.

Langhans,B.; Kupfer,B.; Braunschweiger,I.; Arndt,S.; Schulte,W.; Nischalke,H.D.; Nattermann,J.; Oldenburg,J.; Sauerbruch,T., & Spengler,U. (2011). Interferon-lambda serum levels in hepatitis C, *Journal of Hepatology*, Vol. 54, No.5, pp. 859-865, ISSN 0168-8278.

Larrubia,J.R.; Benito-Martinez,S.; Calvino,M.; Sanz-de-Villalobos,E., & Parra-Cid,T. (2008). Role of chemokines and their receptors in viral persistence and liver damage during chronic hepatitis C virus infection, *World Journal of Gastroenterology: WJG*, Vol. 14, No.47, pp. 7149-7159, ISSN 1007-9327.

Larrubia,J.R.; Calvino,M.; Benito,S.; Sanz-de-Villalobos,E.; Perna,C.; Perez-Hornedo,J.; Gonzalez-Mateos,F.; Garcia-Garzon,S.; Bienvenido,A., & Parra,T. (2007). The role of CCR5/CXCR3 expressing CD8+ cells in liver damage and viral control during persistent hepatitis C virus infection, *Journal of Hepatology*, Vol. 47, No.5, pp. 632-641, ISSN 0168-8278.

Lassen,M.G.; Lukens,J.R.; Dolina,J.S.; Brown,M.G., & Hahn,Y.S. (2010). Intrahepatic IL-10 maintains NKG2A+Ly49- liver NK cells in a functionally hyporesponsive state, *Journal of Immunology (Baltimore, Md.: 1950)*, Vol. 184, No.5, pp. 2693-2701, ISSN 1550-6606.

Lau,J.Y.N.; Tam,R.C.; Liang,T.J., & Hong,Z. (2002). Mechanism of action of ribavirin in the combination treatment of chronic HCV infection, *Hepatology (Baltimore, Md.)*, Vol. 35, No.5, pp. 1002-1009, ISSN 0270-9139.

Lehman,E.M. & Wilson,M.L. (2009). Epidemic hepatitis C virus infection in Egypt: estimates of past incidence and future morbidity and mortality, *Journal of Viral Hepatitis*, Vol. 16, No.9, pp. 650-658, ISSN 1365-2893.

Manigold,T. & Racanelli,V. (2007). T-cell regulation by CD4 regulatory T cells during hepatitis B and C virus infections: facts and controversies, *The Lancet Infectious Diseases*, Vol. 7, No.12, pp. 804-813, ISSN 1473-3099.

Moura,A.S.; Carmo,R.A.; Teixeira,A.L.; Teixeira,M.M., & Rocha,M.O.d.C. (2011). Soluble inflammatory markers as predictors of virological response in patients with chronic hepatitis C virus infection treated with interferon-alpha plus ribavirin, *Memórias Do Instituto Oswaldo Cruz*, Vol. 106, No.1, pp. 38-43, ISSN 1678-8060.

Myrmel,H.; Ulvestad,E., & Asjø,B. (2009). The hepatitis C virus enigma, *APMIS: Acta Pathologica, Microbiologica, Et Immunologica Scandinavica*, Vol. 117, No.5-6, pp. 427-439, ISSN 1600-0463.

Poynard,T.; Ratziu,V.; Charlotte,F.; Goodman,Z.; McHutchison,J., & Albrecht,J. (2001). Rates and risk factors of liver fibrosis progression in patients with chronic hepatitis c, *Journal of Hepatology*, Vol. 34, No.5, pp. 730-739, ISSN 0168-8278.

Rantala,M. & van de Laar,M.J.W. (2008). Surveillance and epidemiology of hepatitis B and C in Europe - a review, *Euro Surveillance: Bulletin Européen Sur Les Maladies Transmissibles = European Communicable Disease Bulletin*, Vol. 13, No.21, 1560-7917.

Shepard,C.W.; Finelli,L., & Alter,M.J. (2005). Global epidemiology of hepatitis C virus infection, *The Lancet Infectious Diseases*, Vol. 5, No.9, pp. 558-567, ISSN 1473-3099.

Sixtos-Alonso,M.S.; Sanchez-Munoz,F.; Sanchez-Avila,J.F.; Martinez,R.A.; Dominguez Lopez,A.; Vargas Vorackova,F., & Uribe,M. (2011). IFN-stimulated gene expression is a useful potential molecular marker of response to antiviral treatment with Peg-IFN-alpha 2b and ribavirin in patients with hepatitis C virus genotype 1, *Archives of Medical Research*, Vol. 42, No.1, pp. 28-33, ISSN 1873-5487.

Thorley,J.A.; McKeating,J.A., & Rappoport,J.Z. (2010). Mechanisms of viral entry: sneaking in the front door, *Protoplasma*, Vol. 244, No.1-4, pp. 15-24, ISSN 1615-6102.

Vezali,E.; Aghemo,A., & Colombo,M. (2011). Interferon in the treatment of chronic hepatitis C: a drug caught between past and future, *Expert Opinion on Biological Therapy*, Vol. 11, No.3, pp. 301-313, ISSN 1744-7682.

Vogt,M.; Lang,T.; Frösner,G.; Klingler,C.; Sendl,A.F.; Zeller,A.; Wiebecke,B.; Langer,B.; Meisner,H., & Hess,J. (1999). Prevalence and clinical outcome of hepatitis C infection in children who underwent cardiac surgery before the implementation of blood-donor screening, *The New England Journal of Medicine*, Vol. 341, No.12, pp. 866-870, ISSN 0028-4793.

Woitas,R.P.; Ahlenstiel,G.; Iwan,A.; Rockstroh,J.K.; Brackmann,H.H.; Kupfer,B.; Matz,B.; Offergeld,R.; Sauerbruch,T., & Spengler,U. (2002). Frequency of the HIV-protective CC chemokine receptor 5-Delta32/Delta32 genotype is increased in hepatitis C, *Gastroenterology*, Vol. 122, No.7, pp. 1721-1728, ISSN 0016-5085.

Yamauchi,K.; Akbar,S.M.F.; Horiike,N.; Michitaka,K., & Onji,M. (2002). Increased serum levels of macrophage inflammatory protein-3alpha in chronic viral hepatitis:

prognostic importance of macrophage inflammatory protein-3alpha during interferon therapy in chronic hepatitis C, *Journal of Viral Hepatitis*, Vol. 9, No.3, pp. 213-220, ISSN 1352-0504.

Yoneda,S.; Umemura,T.; Joshita,S.; Ichijo,T.; Matsumoto,A.; Yoshizawa,K.; Katsuyama,Y.; Ota,M., & Tanaka,E. (2011). Serum chemokine levels are associated with the outcome of pegylated interferon and ribavirin therapy in patients with chronic hepatitis C, *Hepatology Research: The Official Journal of the Japan Society of Hepatology*, Vol. 41, No.6, pp. 587-593, ISSN 1386-6346.

Zeremski,M.; Petrovic,L.M., & Talal,A.H. (2007). The role of chemokines as inflammatory mediators in chronic hepatitis C virus infection, *J Viral Hepat.*, Vol. 14, No.10, pp. 675-687, ISSN

10

Synthetic Peptide Vaccines

Alexandr A. Moisa and Ekaterina F. Kolesanova
Institute of Biomedical Chemistry, Russian Academy of Medical Sciences
Moscow,
Russia

1. Introduction

Vaccination was discovered more than 200 years ago and quickly distributed around the whole Europe despite of the fact that mechanisms of protective effects of vaccines remained unclear for a long time. New vaccines appeared only at the end of XIX century and mainly during the last century after detailed studies of infectious processes, microorganisms inducing these infections, and mechanisms of immune defense. During this period many effective vaccines were developed; they controlled and even totally eliminated some dangerous infectious diseases (Makela, 2000). Now about 40 human diseases are controlled by vaccination (Uchaikin & Shamsheva, 2001). However, for some infections vaccine prophylaxis and vaccine therapy have not been developed yet. These include AIDS and hepatitis C (Barrett & Stanberry, 2009). Situation with these infections is complicated by lack of effective therapeutics, causing full elimination of the human immunodeficiency virus causing AIDS and therapeutics, which would be effective in all patients infected with hepatitis C virus (HCV) (Barrett & Stanberry, 2009). It results in the high chronization degree of these infections (almost 100% in the case of HIV infection and 70−80% in the case of HCV), which basically become lethal ones (Barrett & Stanberry, 2009). Numerous efforts to develop vaccines against these diseases still remain unsuccessful; however, problems associated with the development of such vaccines stimulated large-scale studies of the interaction of infectious agents with the immune system, mechanisms of the immune response, structural basis of immunogenicity and antigenicity, methodology and technology for the development of new generation vaccines.

Traditional vaccines are subdivided into alive (attenuated microorganisms or viral cultures), dead, or corpuscular (inactivated infectious agents) and subunit, or chemical vaccines (individual immunogenic components of infective agents) (Uchaikin & Shamsheva, 2001). The latter vaccines are free from side effects that appear after inoculation of the whole pathogenic agents. Traditional technology has been employed for the development of effective vaccines against many infections (Uchaikin & Shamsheva, 2001); however, now this technology tends to be avoided in many cases because the preparation and use of such vaccines is associated with some problems (Liljeqvist & Stahl, 1999), including:

- expensive cultivation of pathogenic bacteria, viruses or protozoa for industrial production of vaccines or immunogenic components;
- risk of infectious agent leaks;

-   side effects during administration; first of all, increased reactogenicity, which cannot be excluded even in the case of subunit vaccines;
-   expensive purification and detoxification of vaccine products;
-   high genetic variability of an infectious agent; this complicates the detection of chemical components, which can induce an immune response against all its strains;
-   significant structural changes of an infectious agent during its life cycle in the host organism that lead to the changes of its antigenic properties.

Solution of these problems requires elaboration of novel approaches to vaccine development based on knowledge of an antigenic structure of a pathogen, immune response of the host organism to the pathogen or its components, and mechanisms responsible for the modification of strength and direction of this response. Such combined approach that includes the arsenal of methods of bioinformatics, molecular biology, organic chemistry, experimental and clinical immunology is known as "reverse vaccinology". It is aimed at the identification, study of antigenic and immunogenic properties, construction and production of highly purified preparations of novel recombinant and synthetic immunogens and their use for the development of new generation vaccines (Rappuoli, 2001). Synthetic peptide vaccines considered in this review belong to vaccines developed by this approach. Here we do not discuss problems of the development of anticancer vaccines, because of special approaches required for that. One can address available papers, including reviews (Palena et al, 2006, Machiels et al, 2002, Garg et al., 2010) that describe this question.

2. What are peptide vaccines and what are their advantages?

Synthetic peptide vaccines represent fragments of protein antigen sequences, which are synthesized from amino acids and assembled into a single molecule or a supramolecular complex or just mechanically mixed; they are recognized by the immune system and induce the immune response (Sesardic, 1993). This immune response may involve either cytotoxic T-cells or B-cells (i.e. directed to elaboration of specific antibodies) or combine both possible pathways (Bijker et al., 2007). Fragments of protein molecules exhibiting B- and/or T-epitope activity are the main components of peptide vaccines, which determine the direction and specificity of the immune response. Such vaccines may also contain some individual compounds or supramolecular complexes (e.g. micelles, liposomes, polymer particles, etc.), which can nonspecifically or specifically activate certain stages of the immune response to peptides and therefore potentiate this response (Vogel & Alving, 2002). Increase in chemical stability of peptides is achieved by their attachment to carriers, which simultaneously act as activators of the immune response (Aguilar & Rodriguez, 2007).

Peptide vaccines are characterized by the following advantages over traditional vaccines based on dead pathogens, and also subunit and recombinant vaccines (Ben-Yedidia & Arnon, 1997; van der Burg et al., 2006):

-   Relatively inexpensive and safe production technologies.
-   Ability to induce the immune response to those structural elements of a protein antigen, which exhibit weak immunogenicity within the whole antigen molecule.
-   High standardization.
-   Lack of components possessing high reactogenicity (lipopolysaccharides, toxins).

- Possibility of removal of antigen fragments exhibiting allergenicity and cross-reactivity to own molecules of the vaccinated organism.
- Possibility of conjugation of various peptides from different antigens to the same carrier.

3. Steps for the synthetic peptide vaccine development

The development of a candidate synthetic peptide vaccine includes the following steps (Rappuoli, 2001, Sobolev et al., 2005):

1. Selection of immunoactive peptide fragments of protein antigen(s) of an infectious agent and construction of a peptide antigen (or several antigens).
2. Chemical synthesis of peptide antigens and their conjugation (if necessary) to a carrier.
3. Immunogenicity testing of resultant constructs on laboratory animals, determination of specificity of antibodies (elaborated to these constructs) and their protective properties.
4. Preclinical trials of selected antigens.
5. The development of the candidate vaccine and laboratory technology for its production and elaboration of samples for testing.
6. Preclinical and clinical trials of the candidate vaccine samples.

Steps 4−6 are usually determined by sanitary rules and methodical instructions approved by the corresponding governmental control services (in Russian Federation: State Sanitary and Epidemiologic Inspection (Sanitary Rules, 1995, 1998; Methodical Recommendations, 1998); in the USA: Food and Drug Administration (FDA)). Steps 1−3 are discussed in this review.

3.1 Selection of antigenic determinants for immunogenic constructs

First of all, one should take into account the type of the immune response directed to the pathogen neutralization and providing vaccine therapy and/or vaccine prophylaxis: cytotoxic response realized by specific cytotoxic T-lymphocytes, or specific humoral response, which involves the conversion of B-lymphocytes activated by a particular antigen into plasma cells that generate specific neutralizing antibodies (Sobolev et al., 2005). General features of mechanisms responsible for the formation of the specific immune response to various foreign antigens are comprehensively considered in textbooks (Male et al., 2006, Abbas & Lichtman, 2011). Taking into account these common mechanisms, vaccines directed to the generation of cytotoxic immune response should contain cytotoxic T-epitopes as obligatory components, which are often supplemented by class 1 T-helper epitopes (van der Burg et al., 2006). Vaccines that induce antibody formation should contain B-epitopes and T-helper epitopes as obligatory components (van der Burg et al., 2006). It is essential that the B-epitope components of such vaccines should originate from antigens from virulent strains and the generated antibodies should suppress virulence (Sesardic, 1993).

If antigens and virulence factors of an infectious agent remain unknown, it is possible to predict them by means of the "reverse vaccinology", which employs computer analysis of biopolymer structures (first of all their nucleotide and amino acid sequences of genome and proteome, respectively). The technology of this process has been highlighted in the reviews (Rappuoli, 2001, Sobolev et al., 2005, Barocchi et al., 2007). In order to prove the antigenicity and virulence of predicted protein molecules they are expressed and tested for the interaction with antibodies obtained from patients with corresponding infections and for their ability to cause pathological reactions in animals (Rappuoli, 2001). Now, high-throughput screening methods for antigen detection in microorganism proteomes have appeared. These include SERPA technology (SERological Proteome Analysis) and antigenome analysis (Klade, 2002; Ling et al., 2004; Tedeschi et al., 2009,Vytvytska et al., 2002, Målen et al., 2008; Glowalla et al., 2009; Meinke et al., 2005; Felgner et al., 2009; Fritzer et al., 2010). The first method consists in the separation of protein components of the cultivated infectious agent by two-dimensional electrophoresis followed by subsequent visualization of antigenically active proteins by immunoblotting with antibodies from sera of patients with corresponding diseases (Målen et al., 2008; Glowalla et al., 2009; Meinke et al., 2005; Felgner et al., 2009; Fritzer et al., 2010). The second approach includes preparation (by means of heterologous expression) of a library of proteins and their fragments encoded by the library of genome fragments of the infectious agent followed by subsequent testing of expressed proteins for antigenicity (evaluated by interaction with antibodies from sera of infected patients) and then for immunogenicity in experiments by immunizing laboratory animals (Felgner et al., 2009; Fritzer et al., 2010; Meinke et al., 2005). Antigenomic analysis excludes the cultivation of a pathogenic organism of interest; it is applicable in the case of microorganisms with small and completely sequenced genomes. To the contrary, SERPA technology is suitable for the determination and characterization of primary structures of the most diagnostically and therapeutically important antigens of infectious agents with incompletely sequenced genomes.

The next task consists in the identification of peptides corresponding to B- and T-epitopes. If tertiary structure of the peptide antigen and/or its sites involved in the binding with antibodies neutralizing its virulent properties are known, the task implies the selection and design of a peptide (or peptides) that is the best model of the already known B-epitope (Rodriguez et al., 2007, Haro et al., 2003). However, tertiary structures of antigens may be unknown; and also, this approach detects only B-epitopes, but not T-epitopes, recognized as linear peptides. Frequently, most probable B- and T-epitope selection is performed via the antigen amino acid sequence analysis with the help of bioinformatics approaches. The principal technology of this process has been well described in many reviews (Sobolev et al., 2005, Sobolev et al., 2003, He et al., 2010). It should be noted that computer-based epitope prediction capabilities are constantly extended: appearance of new information on mapped B- and T-epitopes results in the more exact specification of corresponding patterns and, consequently, in increased effectiveness of corresponding program products. New, more convenient interfaces are developed for servers containing epitope databases and prediction tools; the development of integrated servers allows to search for possible B- and T-epitopes and combine them into putative immunogenic constructions at one place (Sieker et al., 2009; Wiwanitkit, 2009; MacNamara et al., 2009; Lin et al., 2008; Perry et al., 2008; Roggen, 2006; Tian et al., 2009; Schuler et al., 2007).

However, accuracy of prediction of B- and T-helper epitopes from antigen amino acid sequences remains rather low, and many researchers prefer experimental identification of these epitopes (especially taking into account existing methods of high-throughput screening). Peptide scanning by means of partially overlapping fragments of protein antigen amino acid sequences obtained by multiple parallel synthesis allows to map both linear B-epitopes and also helper and cytotoxic T-epitopes (Castric & Cassels, 1997; Tribbick, 2002). B-epitopes are detected by testing peptides for their interaction with antisera obtained against the whole protein antigen and also sera of infected patients (there are many examples of such studies, for example, antigenic mapping of HCV envelope proteins (Kuzmina et al., 2009; Olenina et al., 2002)). Besides chemical synthesis, fragments of antigen amino acid sequences for B-epitope mapping are also obtained by genetic engineering approach: by means of construction of expression libraries of fragments as chimeras with easily expressed and purified proteins (Bongartz et al., 2009). Peptides of various lengths (from 6 to 20 and even more residues) are used for antigen scanning for B-epitopes; however, it should be noted that peptides longer than 10 residues may contain more than one linear B-epitope (Olenina et al., 2002). Besides the determination of linear B-epitopes attempts are undertaken to map and model conformational epitopes by synthetic and also phage display combinatorial peptide libraries that cover a large number of amino acid sequences from 6 to 15 residues (Pereboeva et al., 2000). In addition, B-epitopes may be determined by means of mass-spectrometry analysis of antigen-antibody complexes via the determination of an antigen site protected against proteolysis or modification by an antibody paratope (Castric & Cassels, 1997; Lu et al., 2009). Fragments of antigen molecules exhibiting T-epitope activity are detected by their ability to induce proliferation of T-lymphocytes in culture (Ahmed & Maeurer, 2009). Cytotoxic T-epitopes have a limited length (8−11 residues) and must have free N-terminal amino and C-terminal carboxyl groups; it is determined by the structure of the MHC I binding pocket. In the case of helper T-epitope determination, longer peptides, often with amidated C-terminal carboxyl groups, are used (Tribbick, 2002). The type of helper epitope activity (Th1 or Th2) is determined by ELISPOT technology. This technology allows large-scale screening of peptides, putative T-helper epitopes, via the determination of the cytokine profile (gamma-interferon, interleukins 2, 4, 10, etc) secreted by T-lymphocytes stimulated by corresponding peptides (Kalyuzhny, 2005; Wulf et al., 2009). Peptide vaccines usually contain such T-helper epitope, which exhibits affinity towards several most widespread (in a given population) Human Leukocyte Antigen (HLA) alleles (so-called universal, or promiscuous T-epitope), or an antigen fragment containing several overlapping T-epitopes of different specificity towards HLA (Sobolev et al., 2005, Panina-Bordignon et al., 1989; Jackson et al., 2002). Several cytotoxic T-epitopes with different specificity towards HLA are included into candidate peptide vaccines for induction of cytotoxic response (Bermúdes et al., 2007; Lauer et al., 2004).

3.2 Construction of peptide immunogen

Formation of a single immunogenic construction from predicted or experimentally determined B- and T-epitopes provides optimal recognition of all the components of this construction by the immune system. For example, the integration of a linear B-epitope and a helper T-epitope in a single molecule results in their penetration into the same B-lymphocyte, which will be converted into a plasma cell producing antibodies of a desired specificity (Moss et al., 2007). B- and T-epitopes may be located far away from each other in a parent protein antigen molecule; moreover, they may originate even from different proteins of the infectious agent and even from different microorganisms. For example, the universal human T-helper epitope of tetanus toxin, QYIKANSKFIGITE, is frequently used in immunogenic constructions in combinations with various peptide B-epitopes for high population coverage of a candidate vaccine (Panina-Bordignon et al., 1989). Combination of a fragment, which is supposed to induce a specific antibody, but is characterized by weak (if any) immunogenicity within the whole protein antigen, with the universal T-helper epitope allows the induction of such specific humoral response in the vaccinated organism that could not be achieved by the immunization with the whole antigen. It is one of advantages of peptide vaccines. Insertion of a short flexible linker between B- and T-epitopes provides a free rotation of the B- and T-helper parts versus each other and therefore promotes independent recognition by corresponding receptors of immunocompetent cells (Moss et al., 2007). In some cases overlapping B- and T-helper epitopes are used as they are located in the protein antigen molecule (e.g. synthetic peptide immunogens from protein VP1 of foot-and-mouth disease virus (Kupriianova et al., 2000)).

Synthetic immunogenic constructs can be represented by both linear oligopeptides and more complex structures such as branched dendrimers (so-called lysine "trees") (Tam, 1988; Van Regenmortel & Muller, 1999), cyclic or linear unbranched oligomers conjugated (via their side chain functional groups) with either individual B- and T-epitopes or such constructs as T-epitope−linker−B-epitope/B-epitope−linker-T-epitope (Jackson et al., 2002). Complex structures are less sensitive to proteolysis and therefore they have higher stability during administration to the body and form higher local concentrations of the immunogen (Sobolev et al., 2005). However, such structures are more difficult to obtain; in addition, their complex surface structure can interfere with the recognition of individual linear B-epitopes included into these constructs (Van Regenmortel & Muller, 1999). Optimal co-location of B- and T-epitopes is selected experimentally by comparing the immugenicity of constructs with different structures (Van Regenmortel & Muller, 1999). A general principle of the effective immune response to B-epitope consists in its close proximity to T-helper epitope(s). Binding of the B-epitope to a B-lymphocyte receptor seems to protect the neighboring T-helper epitope against endosomal cleavage (Moss et al., 2007).

Synthetic peptide vaccines based on cytotoxic and Th1-epitopes represent mechanical mixtures of peptides corresponding to various T-epitopes from one or several antigens of an infectious agent (Jackson et al., 2002). The design of monomolecular constructs is not required because in contrast to the B-T-epitope construction these T-epitopes can independently bind to various cells of the immune system.

The monomolecular immunogenic constructions can also include components with adjuvant functions (see below).

3.3 Immunogen synthesis

Peptide components for synthetic vaccines are obtained by means of solid phase peptide synthesis and peptide synthesis in solution (Sobolev et al., 2005, Sieker et al., 2009; Jackson et al., 2002, Tam, 1988; Van Regenmortel & Muller, 1999). In the case of constructs that include B- and T-helper epitopes representing rather long peptides (exceeding 20 residues) an automated solid phase synthesis or a combination of solid phase synthesis of separate immunogen fragments followed by their condensation into a single peptide in solution are preferable (Lloyd-Williams et al., 1997; Bruckdorfer et al., 2004; Mitsuaki et al., 1987; Rinnova et al., 1999). Solid phase peptide synthesis developed by Merrifield in the beginning of 1960th, now represents rather routine procedure due to numerous studies and automation of this process (Lloyd-Williams et al., 1997). The major advantage of solid phase synthesis over synthesis in solution consists in that there is no need in the purification of a resultant product after each round of peptide chain elongation. The product remains covalently bound to a polymer support up to the end of synthetic procedure, and unreacted components, activators and improper products are washed away by a solvent flow. It significantly accelerates the solid phase protein synthesis compared to the synthesis in solution (Bruckdorfer et al., 2004). Use of microwave irradiation significantly accelerates the solid phase synthesis process and increases its efficiency: synthesis of peptides of 40 residues long takes less than one day and results in good yields. It is especially useful for the synthesis of peptides, which tend to aggregate on the support (Sabatino & Papini, 2008). Of course, synthesis of each peptide requires experimental selection of the most effective protocol and initial amino acid derivatives, which allow to obtain the final product with a maximal yield (Lloyd-Williams et al., 1997). Now the most popular peptide synthesis employs amino acid derivatives protected at alpha-amino group with 9-fluorenyl(methoxycarbonyl) (FMOC). In contrast to synthesis using *tert*-butyl(oxycarbonyl)(BOC)-amino acid derivatives it does not require the use of such strong acid as HF to cleave the synthesized peptide from the support at the end of the process. FMOC-amino acids are preferably used in large-scale peptide synthesis that may yield tens and even hundred kilograms of peptides (Bruckdorfer et al., 2004). Since it is difficult to obtain long peptides (exceeding 30 residues) with good yield and separate them from contaminants differing by $1-2$ residues, such peptides are synthesized as $2-3$ fragments with protected side chain functional groups and then these fragments are linked together (in solution) into a single molecule (Mitsuaki et al., 1987; Rinnova et al., 1999). The same approach is used for conjugation of B-T-epitope constructions or individual epitopes with lysine dendrimers, cyclic or linear oligomer matrix structures. Methods of chemoselective cross-links used for conjugation of peptides with oligomer carriers are discussed elsewhere (Jackson et al., 2002). Non-disturbance of epitope structures during cross-linking is achieved via the introduction of additional modifiable groups or amino acid residues into synthesized peptides. Most frequently, conjugation is performed by thioalkylation (in this case cysteine residue is included into one component of the construct, whereas monochloroacetyl or maleimide group is included into another component), hydrazone or oxime formation (serine residue is included into one component, in which the CH_2OH group is oxidized to CHO by periodic acid, while monohydrazide of succinic or benzoic acid or aminooxyacetic acid residue is included into another component), and formation of thiazolidine or oxazolidine cycle (in this case the CH_2OH group of serine residue included into one component is oxidized to CHO and additional serine or cysteine residue is included into another component). In addition, some companies (e.g. Novabiochem and Bachem, both from Switzerland) produce supports for solid phase peptide synthesis with preformed lysine dendrimers, on which peptide synthesis can be performed.

3.4 Adjuvants for peptide vaccines

Formation of strong and long-term specific immune response to antigens is an important task for creation of any vaccine. It is achieved by an additional nonspecific stimulation of the immune system cells, specific targeted antigen delivery to the immunocompetent cells and their constant activation by the antigen due to its depositing and protection against protease cleavage. These functions are attributed to adjuvants (from Latin *adjuvans, adjuvantis*: aiding, helping), which are included into vaccine preparations (Aguilar & Rodriguez, 2007). In vaccines prepared from attenuated and killed infectious agents structural elements of the microorganisms such as cell walls, membranes and their components (polysaccharides, lipopolysaccharides, phospholipids, etc.) play the adjuvant role (Uchaikin & Shamsheva, 2001, Aguilar & Rodriguez, 2007). Subunit vaccines contain added adjuvants, which promote the depositing of antigens (via their adsorption) and nonspecific stimulation of the immune response (lymphocyte and macrophage attraction to the injection site due to the inflammatory reaction development); usually aluminium salts or hydroxide are used for this purpose (Aguilar & Rodriguez, 2007; Uchaikin & Shamsheva, 2001). Adjuvant selection becomes especially important during development of synthetic peptide vaccines, because peptides are usually well soluble in aqueous media, readily subjected to proteolysis and are not deposited at the administration site. Peptide constructs are targeted to the activation of immune response of a narrow specificity, and they do not provide attraction and activation of cells participating in the nonspecific immune response, which potentiate and direct the specific response. Aluminum hydroxide and salts poorly adsorb peptides, weakly activate immunocompetent cells and do not potentiate the immune response to peptide antigens (Jackson et al., 2002). Search for new adjuvants for peptide vaccines against human infectious diseases includes adjuvants approved to animal use and also immunomodulators (Aguilar & Rodriguez, 2007, Jackson et al., 2002).

Oil-based adjuvants, for example, Freund's complete adjuvant (which contains a suspension of killed *Mycobacterium tuberculosis* cells or their lipopolysaccharides in a mineral oil with lanolin) are used in laboratory studies of immunogenicity on animals for a long time. However, Freund's adjuvant is rather toxic, exhibits high reactogenicity and can induce formation of necrotic ulcers at the injection site (Allison & Byars, 1991). Now less toxic and reactogenic oil-based adjuvants (Montanide series) have been developed; they are used in some peptide vaccines that are under clinical trials (Ahmed & Maeurer, 2009; Roestenberg et al., 2008).

Saponins (e.g., QuilA, an extract from *Quillaja saponaria*, in which 23 different saponins have been identified), plant glycosides with surfactant properties, which form micelles in solution, are also used as adjuvants. QuilA is too toxic for use in humans, but its fraction QS-21, which is less toxic and induces an effective T-cell response against antigens, is considered as a prospective adjuvant for peptide vaccines (Allison & Byars, 1991; Kensil, 1996; Takahashi et al., 1990). Saponins are used as adjuvants in the immunostimulating complexes (abbreviated as ISCOMs), which represent mixed micelles of saponin and cholesterol of 40 nm in diameter where hydrophobic and amphipathic antigens are inserted. ISCOMs represent a convenient system for antigen delivery to antigen presenting cells; these particles can penetrate into such antigen-presenting cells as dendritic cells and macrophages, and hence increase the efficiency of antigen presentation (Allison & Byars, 1991; Singh et al., 2006).

Improvement in peptide antigen transport to antigen presenting cells also occurs using the polycations poly-L-lysine, poly-L-arginine and chitosan as adjuvants (Schlaphoff et al., 2007; Svirshchevskaya et al., 2009). Effectiveness of the polymeric polycation polyoxidonium (which has been shown to nonspecifically activate cell immune response (Khaitov & Pinegin, 2005)) as the adjuvant for synthetic peptide vaccines is still questionable (Olenina et al., 2003).

Currently adjuvants synthesized on the basis of pathogen-associated unique highly conserved molecular structures are widely used; they do not have analogues in macroorganisms and trigger nonspecific immune response via pattern-recognizing receptors (e.g. Toll like receptors) [Düesberg et al., 2002; Chua et al., 2007; Jackson et al., 2004]. Dipalmitoyl glyceryl-S-cysteine (Pam$_2$Cys) (Düesberg et al., 2002; Chua et al., 2007; Jackson et al., 2004; Deliyannis et al., 2006), a synthetic analogue of the lipid fragment of macrophage activating lipopeptide-2 isolated from *Mycoplasma fermentans* membranes (Zeng et al., 2002) is one of such structures. Pam$_2$Cys has been used in some candidate synthetic peptide vaccines against hepatitis C virus; these vaccines consist of cytotoxic HLA-A2-specific T-epitope of the HCV NS5B protein or of highly immunogenic hypervariable region 1 of HCV E2 envelope protein and a foreign CD4+ T-helper epitope (Engler et al., 2004; Torresi et al., 2007; Chua et al., 2008). Synthetic peptide constructs also contain the other lipid group, Pam$_3$Cys, which represents an N-terminal fragment of *E. coli* lipoprotein (Zeng et al., 2000; Müller et al., 2002). The immunogenic constructs based on the peptide covalently linked to Pam$_3$Cys induce an effective immune response after both parenteral and intranasal administration; the raised protective antibodies belong to immunoglobulin A type (Müller et al., 2002), which are important components of the mucosal immune response.

Frequently, peptide constructs containing fatty acid residues and also hydrophobic peptides are included into liposomes. Liposome-associated antigens are protected against proteolysis, they arrive directly to the antigen-presenting cells and this potentiates the immune response (Engler et al., 2004; Kaplun et al., 1999; Scheerlinck & Greenwood, 2006, 2008). Besides antigens, liposomes also contain proteins promoting liposome fusion with cell membranes, such as influenza virus hemagglutinin; such particles are known as virosomes (Kaplun et al., 1999; Scheerlinck & Greenwood, 2008). Virosomes use routes that are natural for viral particles and the antigen fragment is exposed on the surface of the antigen-presenting cells in the complex with MHC II (i.e. in the form recognized by T-helpers). Antigen incorporation into nanoparticles of 20−40 nm in size (virosomes, liposomes, ISCOMs) improves its presentation because such particles are readily absorbed by antigen-presenting dendritic cells (Jackson et al., 2004; Scheerlinck & Greenwood, 2006, 2008).

Besides liposomes and ISCOMs antigens may be also incorporated into biodegradable polymeric microspheres for storage and protection against proteolysis. Such microcapsules (size less than 10 (mu)m) that consist of polylactide, polyglycolide or their copolymer may be used for peroral antigen administration because they are insoluble in gastric juice and may provide gradual antigen release (Eldridge et al., 1991; Cox et al., 2006; Scheerlinck & Greenwood, 2006).

3.5 Evaluation of efficiency and protectivity of the immune response to synthetic peptide immunogens

Studies of peptide constructs begin with the determination of their immunogenicity (i.e. their ability to induce the immune response programmed during the design of these constructs) (Sobolev et al., 2005, Sobolev et al., 2003, Jackson et al., 2002). If a peptide immunogen includes B- and T-helper epitopes, it should induce production of antibodies against its B-epitope and also against the protein, which "borrowed" the fragment corresponding to this B-epitope; usually such experiments are performed on laboratory animals. The higher the proportion of animals developed such immune response (among total number of immunized animals) the more universal T-helper epitope included into the construct is. Immunogenicity of a mixture of peptides corresponding to cytotoxic T-epitopes is initially elucidated by appearance of cytotoxic T-lymphopcytes of a certain specificity in immunized animals (Kalyuzhny, 2005; Wulf et al., 2009). Subsequently, effectiveness of the cytotoxic immune response is evaluated in a mixed cell culture by the degree of infected cell killing by cytotoxic T-lymphocytes obtained from immunized animals or cell cultures stimulated by the investigated peptide immunogens (Lauer et al., 2004; Schlaphoff et al., 2007; Takahashi et al., 1990). Protectivity of the specific humoral response induced by peptide immunogen administration is determined by the neutralizing effect of antibodies on the penetration of an infectious agent to the target cell or by inactivation of a toxin produced by the infectious agent (Sobolev et al., 2005, Sobolev et al., 2003; Law et al., 2008). If animals are also susceptible to this disease an investigation of the protective effect of the immunization by the peptide antigen is performed on animals. Strains of small rodents are the most convenient animal models from the viewpoint of maintenance. However, there are situations when no laboratory animal is susceptible to a certain disease. In such cases severe combined immunodeficiency (SCID) mice with xenotransplanted human cells or tissues are used: in the case of malaria these are SCID mice with transplanted human erythrocytes (Badell et al., 2000), in the case of hepatitis C these are SCID mice with transplanted human hepatic tissue (Guévin et al., 2009; Zhu et al., 2006). Alternatively, researchers limit their experiments by testing protectivity of the immune response in cell cultures. For example, testing of virus neutralizing activity of antibodies produced in response to hepatitis C virus (HCV) antigens is performed in experiments by blockade of the entry of the virus or virus-like particles carrying HCV envelope proteins on their surfaces into primary hepatocytes or into hepatoma cell culture (Law et al., 2008).

It should be noted that not only the strength of the protective immune response but also its duration after the last immunogen administration is crucial. If an infectious agent exhibits high genetic variability, it is important to elucidate whether the immune response to a particular peptide immunogen is strain or isolate-specific. Only after this step of studies the synthetic peptide immunogenic construction may be submitted to preclinical and clinical trials (Rappuoli, 2001, Sobolev et al., 2005, Sobolev et al., 2003).

4. Examples of synthetic vaccines reaching stages of clinical trials

4.1 Peptide vaccines against malaria

Development of peptide vaccines against malaria started in 1970th and in spite of first unsuccessful attempts it is still considered as a perspective direction (Epstein et al., 2007). Malaria is caused by *Plasmodium* parasites, which undergo several developmental stages in the human body and each stage of its development is characterized by different protein and therefore antigenic structures. Forty perspective protective *Plasmodium* antigens have been identified and they are used for the development of various types of anti-malaria vaccines targeted to various stages of the parasite life cycle. Interest in the development of peptide vaccines is determined by genetic and therefore antigenic differences in local populations of *Plasmodium*; this does not allow to form the isolate-nonspecific protective immune response during administration of the whole infectious agent or its protein antigens than belong to one of many strains (Takala & Plowe, 2009). In addition, it is easier to develop a multiantigenic vaccine based on synthetic peptides, which would induce formation of the immune response against various stages of the parasite development (with minimal reactogenicity).

In 1980, clinical trials of the first synthetic anti-malaria vaccine Spf66 against *Pl. falciparum* in the asexual stage of development started (Urdaneta et al., 1998). This vaccine consisted of three fragments of three various surface antigens of the merozoite with the repeated PNAN fragment of sporozoite CS protein between them. However, efficiency of Spf66 in clinical trials significantly varied in dependence of geographical regions and subsequent trials were interrupted (Graves & Gelband, 2007).

Now three candidate vaccines against malaria are under various phases of clinical trials. Two of them contain long (> 70 amino acid residues) synthetic peptide immunogens inducing antibody production to two surface *Plasmodium* proteins at the shizont stage: merozoite surface protein 3 (MSP3) and glutamate rich protein (GLURP). These immunogens are MSP-3-LSP (Long synthetic protein) that represents the MSP-3 fragment including the residues 186-276 [Bouharoun-Tayoun, 1995] and GLURP-LPS that represents the GLURP fragment including the residues 85-213 (Dodoo et al., 2000; Theisen et al., 2000, 2001). These peptide immunogens were highly conservative for all plasmodium isolates; they induced formation of cytophilic antibodies of IgG1 and IgG3 subclasses; via opsonizing shizonts they attracted monocytes that caused shizont lysis (Theisen et al., 2001; Soe et al., 2004). Phase I clinical trials (Druilhe et al., 2005; Sirima et al., 2009) demonstrated formation of long (at least 1 year) immune response to these vaccines. At the moment Phase IIb clinical trial of the MSP3-LSP vaccine continues (http://www.amanet-trust.org/ext/reports /newsletters/issue23June08.pdf).

Preparations of the virosomal peptide vaccines PEV302 and PEV301 jointly developed by Swiss Tropical Institute and Pevion Biotech Ltd on the basis of fragments of the sporozoite CS protein and apical membrane antigen 1 (AMA-1) are under Phase I clinical trials (AMANET). PEV302 is a 39-mer cyclic peptide containing five highly conservative NPNA repeats of the CS protein; the peptide is conjugated with phosphatidylethanolamine and included into a phosphorlipid particle together with influenza virus hemagglutinin (Okitsu et al., 2007). PEV301 is a similar virosomal preparation that contains another (49-mer) peptide including rather conservative loop I of AMA-1 domain III, also conjugated with phosphatidylethanolamine. It was demonstrated that both peptide containing virosomal preparations induced production of antibodies inhibiting sporozoite invasion of liver cells and erythrocytes (Okitsu et al., 2007; Thompson et al., 2008).

4.2 Synthetic peptide vaccines against HCV

Hepatitis C virus (HCV) exhibits extremely high genetic variability and therefore employment of the traditional approach for vaccine development based on attenuated or inactivated virus strain is ineffective in the case of HCV (Barrett & Stanberry, 2009). This determines the need of nontraditional approaches for the development of anti-HCV vaccines, particularly, synthetic vaccines. HCV envelope proteins are characterized by high variability of their amino acid sequences and the presence of a large number of glycosyl residues similar to those present in host glycoproteins; this complicates the development of effective isolate-nonspecific neutralizing antibody production. At the same time the importance of the cytotoxic immune response in HCV eliminations in patients with spontaneous reconvalescence has been demonstrated (Freeman et al., 2003; Tester et al., 2005). It determined the interest in the development of therapeutic peptide vaccines stimulating the cytotoxic response to the virus. These candidate peptide anti-

HCV vaccines represent either a mixture of several peptides or a single multiepitope polypeptide.

4.2.1 Synthetic peptide vaccines based on CTL epitopes

IC41 is a therapeutic candidate vaccine developed by Intercell AG (Austria); it contains 5 synthetic peptides (2 fragments of the core protein, residues 23−44 and 132−140; 2 fragments of the nonstructural protein NS3, residues 1073−1081 and 1248-1261; one fragment of the NS4 protein, residues 1764−1786; all fragments are taken from HCV genotype I and numeration of amino acid residues is shown by the sequence of HCV polyprotein) and poly-L-arginine as the adjuvant stimulating penetration of the peptide antigens into cells. these peptides contain 3 T-helper epitopes (core protein, residues 23−44; NS3, residues 1248−1261; NS4, residues 1767−1786) and five HLA-A2-specific cytotoxic T-epitopes (core protein, residues 35-44 and 132−140; NS3 1073−1081; NS4, residues 1764−1772) (Schlaphoff et al., 2007). The fragments 23−44, 132−140, 1248−1261, 1764−1772 are conservative in various HCV genotypes (the identify of their sequences in the subtypes 1a, 1b, and 2 is not less than 87%) (Lauer et al., 2004). The NS3 fragment 1073−1081 differs in various HCV genotypes (the identity did not exceed 15%); however, vaccine developers used this peptide as one of effective T-epitopes typical for the HCV genotype 1a frequently detected in Europe (Firbas et al., 2006). Phase I clinical trials have shown that the IC41 vaccine induces formation of HCV-specific CD8+ T-lymphocytes in healthy patients and is well-tolerated in patients (Klade et al., 2008). In Phase II clinical trials HLA-A2 positive patients with chronic hepatitis C received 6 doses of the vaccine with a 4-week interval between doses; although the content of circulating HCV RNA was not decreased, the increase in HCV specific CD8+ specific lymphocytes was observed in 25% of patients (Lauer et al., 2004). In the other study 66% of patients with chronic hepatitis C (genotype 1) resistant to the standard therapy demonstrated a small but statistically significant decrease in HCV RNA observed 6 months after vaccination with IC41 (Klade et al., 2008).

Another CTL T-epitope-based vaccine was developed in Japan. It included a HLA-A2-restricted HCV core protein-derived 35-44 fragment as CTL T-epitope injected in an emulsion with incomplete Freund's adjuvant during Phase I clinical trial. About 25% patients (non-responders for the previous interferon plus ribavirin treatment) positively responded to vaccinations: alanine aminotransferase activity was lowered, and some patients showed the decline of viral load. However, all patients received more than 10 vaccinations, and some received even more than 50 injections of the peptide formulation (Yutani et al., 2009).

4.2.2 Virosome-based peptide vaccine

This vaccine developed by Pevion Biotech Ltd is under Phase I clinical trials. The virosome envelope consists of phospholipids with included influenza virus hemagglutinin and neuraminidase. The virosome contains a synthetic fragment of HCV core protein of 132 residues in length, which induced formation of virus specific cytotoxic T-cells producing [gamma]-interferon in HLA-A2.1 transgenic mice (Amacker et al., 2005).

4.3 Synthetic peptide vaccine against human papillloma virus, strain 16

This vaccine has been developed in the Center for Genetic Engineering and Biotechnology, Havana, Cuba, and undergoes Phase II clinical trial now. It consists of HLA-A2-restricted human papilloma virus strain 16 (HPV16) E7 T-epitope incorporated into very small size proteoliposomes. Four vaccinations with this vaccine resulted in the clearance from HPV16 in 3 out of 7 immunized patients and in complete or at least partial regression of cervical lesions caused by HPV infection (Solares et al., 2011).

4.4 Synthetic vaccine against foot-and-mouth disease

Although inactivated vaccine against foot-and-mouth disease (FMD) may effectively protect animals it has some serious drawbacks such as: a) slow formation of the immune response and existing risk of viral infection of vaccinated animals before the development of the adaptive immune response; b) appearance of virus carriers even after successful vaccination; c) difficulties with discrimination of vaccinated animals from convalescence and infected animals (Barrett & Stanberry, 2009).

During many years researchers try to develop alternative vaccines against FMD virus. Synthetic peptide vaccines based on the VP1 peptide fragments 135−160 and 200-213 containing virus neutralizing B-epitopes (Strohmaier et al., 1982) and the fragments of the same protein 20−41 and 170−189 containing T-helper epitopes (Collen et al., 1991; Volpina et al., 1993) are considered as possible variants. A synthetic vaccine based on the VP1 protein fragment 135−159 (FMD virus, strain 22) has been developed in M. M. Shemyakin and Yu. A. Ovchinnikov Institute of Biooeganic Chemistry (Russian Academy of Sciences); this vaccine provided antiviral protection within one year after a single immunization (Volpina et al., 1993, 1999). It is the only synthetic peptide vaccine approved in Russia for the use in veterinary (Volpina et al., 1999).

4.5 Dendrimeric peptide vaccine against swine fever virus

Three dendrimeric peptide constructs were prepared from three different fragments of the classical swine fever virus (CSFV) envelope protein E2 (as B-epitopes) and T helper epitope from the NS3 protein of the same virus (Tarradas et al., 2011). Each dendrimer contained four copies of one of the putative B-epitopes linked to the T-epitope. Intramuscular injections with these dendrimers significally reduced the pig lethality after the challenge with the lethal dose of CSFV though no netralizing antibodies were detected in animal blood.

5. Examples of peptide immunogens under current successful development

5.1 Peptide immunogens for universal anti-flu vaccines

Current influenza vaccines protect mostly against homologous virus strains. However, while facing the danger of new pandemics expected from the transmittance of mutated bird and swine flu viruses to humans, the development of a broadly protective anti-flu vaccine is of great importance. Several groups succeeded in preparing conserved synthetic peptide immunogens derived from hemagglutinin and matrix M2 protein of the influenza virus. These fragments were shown to be conserved in various virus strains. Corresponding synthetic peptides conjugated with carrier protein keyhole limpet hemocyanin were able to elicit broadly specific immune response in mice and protect them from the influenza infection caused by different virus strains (Stanekova et al., 2011; Wang et al., 2010).

5.2 Peptide immunogens for anti-HCV vaccines under development

Antibodies protective against HCV infection should attack HCV envelope proteins, since these proteins are responsible for targeting the virus into the host cells, where its replication occurs (Gal-Tanamy et al., 2009; Voisset & Dubuisson, 2004). However, HCV envelope proteins demonstrate the highest sequence variability, with regard to HCV genetic variants, among all viral proteins (Sobolev et al., 2000). Though the immunization with the full-size HCV envelope proteins can elicit virus-neutralizing antibodies, these antibodies are specific to certain HCV genetic variants, relative to the one, from which the envelope proteins used for immunization, are taken (Elmowalid et al., 2007; Alvarez-Lajonchere et al., 2009). Several highly conserved sites were determined in HCV envelope proteins E1 and E2 (Sobolev et al, 2000); however, most these sites did not elicit specific antibodies because of insufficient T-lymphocyte help resulting from the absence of T-helper epitopes in the vicinity. Conjugation of putative B-epitopes, derived from HCV envelope proteins, to promiscuous T-helper epitopes from other sources (Torresi et al., 2007) or to the carrier protein, keyhole limpet hemocyanin (El Awady et al., 2010; El Abd et al., 2011), resulted in the formation of immunogens capable of producing antibodies specific for the whole HCV envelope proteins and viral particles. However, the use of foreign T-epitopes and carrier proteins leads to the formation of T helper memory cells that are non-specific for HCV and hence, will not be activated upon HCV infection.

We performed a search for putative T-helper epitope motifs in HCV envelope proteins with the help of SYFPEITHI Database and detected several conserved fragments that contain a number of such motifs of different specificity with regard to HLA allele products. Hence these fragments can be considered as broadly specific T helper epitopes. Several artificial peptide constructs were made on the basis of one such E2 protein fragment (CR2; fragment designation here and in the table 1 in accordance with Sobolev et al., 2000) and three fragments from the same protein, shown to be responsible for the interaction of HCV with heparan-sulphates (Olenina et al., 2005). These artificial constructs were synthesized and tested for their immunogenicity on rats (table 1). The constructs were shown to be highly immunogenic in the absence of any carrier besides Freund's adjuvant and able to elicit antibodies that interacted with full-size envelope proteins. The mixture of all six constructs showed the comparable immunogenicity and enhanced ability in eliciting anti-E2 antibodies. Five out of six constructs as well as the mixture of constructs elicited antibodies capable of binding HCV from patient plasma(fig. 1) (Kolesanova et al., 2011).

5.3 Other important examples of peptide immunogens

An interesting example of the peptide immunogen has been developed for the candidate anti-anthrax vaccine. The current vaccines for anthrax though being efficient, require extensive immunization protocols, and one of the reasons for it is the absence of antibodies against the linear determinant in domain 2 of *Bacillus anthracis* protective antigen. Two multiple antigenic peptides composed of the fragment 304-319 (loop-neutralizing determinant) of *B. anthracis* protective antigen and a promiscuous T-helper epiope from *Pl.*

Peptide	Antibody titer*		
	Against peptide	Against E2 protein	Against E1E2 heterodimer
CR2-linker-CR3	1:32000	1:50-1:100 (3)	1:50-1:100 (3)
CR3-linker-CR2	1:8100	1:50-1:100 (3)	1:50-1:100 (3)
PRR1-linker-CR2	1:900	1:50 (1)	1:50 (1)
CR2-linker-PRR1	1:9200	1:50(2)	1:50(2)
CHR-linker-CR2	1:5600	1:50 (2)	1:50 (2)
CR2-linker CHR	1:2700	1:50 (1)	1:50 (1)
Mixture of 6	1:2000-1:24000 depending on peptide	1:150 (3)	1:100 (3)

* Numbers in brackets show the number of animal antisera samples containing corresponding antibodies. Number of rats in experimental groups – 5; the group immunized with mixture of the constructs consisted of 4 species.

Table 1. Artificial peptide constructs made from E2 HCV protein fragments and their immunogenicity testing results.

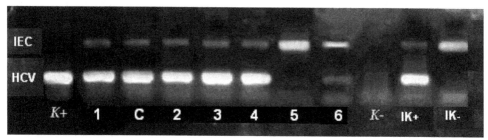

Fig. 1. HCV binding to antibodies elicited by artificial peptide constructs made from envelope protein E2 conserved fragments – PCR detection. Numbers in the line below designate the number of the construct used for the immunization (see table 1), C – mixture of all 6 constructs. K+ and K- - positive and negative control probes; IK+ and IK- - positive and negative internal controls; IEC – internal experiment control PCR product; HCV – HCV-derived PCR product.

falciparum were prepared with the B-T or T-B order of epitope determinants. Rabbits immunized with both constructs were efficiently protected from the lethal infection caused by aerosolized spores of B. anthracis. (Oscherwitz et al., 2010).

Peptide immunogens are also of interest as immunogens for anti-allergic vaccines. Since the aim of these vaccine preparation is to elicit antibodies that bind and clear off allergens from blood for preventing an allergic reaction, full-size allergen molecules can hardly be applied as immunogens. Allergen-derived epitope structures devoid of determinants responsible for causing allergic reactions are used instead. The development of the peptide immunotherapy peptide-based vaccine for cat allergy can be considered as one of such examples (Worm et al., 2011). Several peptides derived form the cat allergen Fel d1 that were identified as T-helper lymphocyte-stimulating molecules and synthesized, were safe and well tolerated in human volunteers. This vaccine was efficient in very small doses (3 nmols) and did not cause any allergic reactions that are caused by the full-size allergen molecule. Hence these peptide immunogens and the methodological basis for their development can be further used for the preparation of anti-allergic vaccines of other kinds.

6. Conclusions

Now there is a good background for the selection of immunogens targeted to those immune processes, which should be triggered by future vaccines. However, at the moment all known synthetic peptide vaccines against agents causing infectious diseases in man are at various stages of clinical trials (http://clinicaltrials.gov/ct2/results?term=vaccine). This situation is associated with the following circumstances: difficulties in reproduction of native conformation of protein antigenic sites, some B-cell epitopes recognized by neutralizing antibodies are discontinuous rather than linear ones; peptides are easily subjected to proteolysis. Peptides themselves are weakly immunogenic and such vaccine requires careful selection of an adjuvant. In the case of peptide vaccines salts and aluminum hydroxide, the adjuvants approved in all countries, are ineffective, whereas more effective adjuvants (for peptides) are not approved for clinical application in humans in most countries (e.g. they are forbidden for human use in the USA (Common Ingredients in U.S. Licensed Vaccines)). Nevertheless, deeper knowledge on structures of antigens of infectious agents, mechanisms of immune response formation, development of technologies for large-scale synthesis of long peptides, preparation of stabilized nanoparticles and the development of effective and safe adjuvants give hope that the effective peptide vaccines will be developed in the future.

7. Acknowledgements

The work on this chapter was supported with RFBR grant No. 09-04-12117 and the Federal program "Research and development on priority directions in scientific and technological complex of Russia in 2007-2012" contract No. 16.512.11.2069   (theme No. 2011-1.2-512-017-031).

8. References

Abbas, A.K. & Lichtman, A.H. (2011). *Basic Immunology: Functions and Disorders of the Immune System*. Saunders/Elsevier, ISBN 978-1-4160-5569-3, Philadelphia, PA, USA.

Aguilar, J.C. & Rodriguez, E.G. (2007) Vaccine Adjuvants Revisited. *Vaccine*, Vol. 25, No.19 (May 10, 2007), pp. 3752-3762, ISSN 0264-410X.

Ahmed, R.K. & Maeurer, M.J., (2009). T-Cell Epitope Mapping. In: *Methods Mol. Biol.*, Vol. 524, No. 4. *Epitope Mapping Protocols*, M. Schutkowski & Reineke, U. (Eds.), pp. 427-438, Humana Press, ISBN 978-1-59745-450-6_32.

Allison, A.C. & Byars, N.E. (1991) Immunological Adjuvants: Desirable Properties and Side-Effects. *Mol. Immunol.*, Vol. 28, No.3 (March 1991), pp. 279-284, ISSN 0161-5890.

Alvarez-Lajonchere, L., Shoukry, N. H., Gra, B., Amador-Canizares, Y., Helle, F., Bedard, N., Guerra, I., Drouin, C., Dubuisson, J., Gonzalez-Horta, E. E., Martınez, G., Marante, J., Cinza, Z., Castellanos, M. & Duenas-Carrera, S. (2009). Immunogenicity of CIGB-230, a Therapeutic DNA Vaccine Preparation, in HCV-Chronically Infected Individuals in a Phase I Clinical Trial. *J. Viral Hepat.*, 16, No. 2, (March 2009), pp.156-167, ISSN 1352-0504.

Amacker, M., Engler, O., Kammer, A.R., Vadrucci, S., Oberholzer, D., Cerny, A., & Zurbriggen, R., (2005) Peptide-Loaded Chimeric Influenza Virosomes for Efficient In Vivo Induction of Cytotoxic T Cells. *Int. Immunol.*, Vol. 17, No. 6, (June 2005), pp. 695-704, ISSN 0953-8178.

AMANET Launches Large-Scale Testing of Candidate Malaria Vaccine MSP3-LSP in Mali. Available at:
http://www.amanet-trust.org/ext/reports/newsletters/issue23June08.pdf

Badell, E., Oeuvray, C., Moreno, A., Soe, S., van Rooijen, N., & Bouzidi, A. (2000). Human Malaria in Immunocompromized Mice. An in Vivo Model to Study Defense Mechanisms against *Plasmodium falciparum*. *J. Exp. Med.*, Vol. 192, No. 11, (December 4, 2000), pp. 1653-1660, ISSN 0022-1007.

Barocchi, M.A., Censini, S., & Rappuoli, R. (2007) Vaccines in the Era of Genomics: the Pneumococcal Challenge. *Vaccine*, Vol. 25, No. 16 (April 20, 2007), pp. 2963-2973, ISSN: 0264-410X.

Barrett, A.D.T. & Stanberry, L.R. (Eds.). (2009). *Vaccines for Biodefense and Emerging and Neglected Diseases*, Elsevier Inc., ISBN 978-0-3-69408-9.

Ben-Yedidia, T. and Arnon, R., (1997) Design of Peptide and Polypeptide Vaccines. *Curr. Opin. Biotechnol.*, Vol. 8, No.4 (August, 1997), pp. 442-448, ISSN 0958-1669.

Bermúdes, A., Reyes, C., Guzmán, F., Vanegas, M., Rosas, J., Amador, R., Rodríguez, R., Patarroyo, M.A., & Patarroyo, M.E. (2007). Synthetic Vaccine Update: Applying Lessons Learned from Recent SPf66 Malarial Vaccine Physicochemical, Structural and Immunological Characterization. *Vaccine*, Vol. 25, No. 22 (May 30, 2007), pp. 4487-4501, ISSN: 0264-410X.

Bijker, M.S., Melief, C.J., Offringa, R., and van der Burg, S.H., (2007) Design and Development of Synthetic Peptide Vaccines: Past, Present and Future. *Expert Rev. Vaccines*, Vol. 6, No.4 (August, 2007), pp. 591-603, ISSN 1476-0584.

Bongartz, J., Bruni, N., & Or-Guil, M. (2009). Epitope Mapping Using Randomly Generated Peptide Libraries. In: *Methods Mol. Biol.*, Vol. 524, No. 4. *Epitope Mapping Protocols*, M. Schutkowski & Reineke, U. (Eds.), pp. 237-246, Humana Press, ISBN 978-1-59745-450-6_32.

Bouharoun-Tayoun, H., Oeuvray, C., Lunel, F., & Druilhe, P. (1995). Mechanisms Underlying the Monocyte-Mediated Antibody-Dependent Killing of *Plasmodium falciparum* Asexual Blood Stages. *J. Exp. Med.*, Vol. 182, No. 2, (August 1, 1995), pp. 409-418, ISSN 0022-1007.

Bruckdorfer, T, Marder, O., & Albericio, F. (2004). From Production of Peptides in Milligram Amounts for Research to Multi-tons Quantities for Drugs of the Future. *Curr. Pharm. Biotechnol.*, Vol. 5, No. 1, (February 2004), pp. 29-43.

van der Burg, S.H., Bijker, M.S., Welters, M.J., Offringa, R., & Melief, C.J. (2006) Improved Peptide Vaccine Strategies, Creating Synthetic Artificial Infections to Maximize Immune Efficacy. *Adv. Drug. Deliv. Rev.*, Vol. 58, No.8, (October 1, 2006), pp. 916-930, ISSN 0169-409X.

Castric, P.A. & Cassels, F.J. (1997) Peptide Epitope Mapping in Vaccines. *J. Ind. Microbiol. Biotechnol.*, Vol. 19, No.1 (July 1997), pp. 56-57.

Chua, B.Y., Eriksson, E.M., Brown, L.E., Zeng, W., Gowans, E.J., Torresi, J., & Jackson, D.C. (2008). A Self-Adjuvanting Lipopeptide-Based Vaccine Candidate for the Treatment of Hepatitis C Virus Infection. *Vaccine*, Vol. 26, No.31, (September 2, 2008), pp. 4866-4875, ISSN 0264-410X.

Chua, B.Y., Zeng, W., Lau, Y.F., & Jackson, D.C. (2007) Comparison of Lipopeptide-Based Immunocontraceptive Vaccines Containing Different Lipid Groups. *Vaccine*, Vol. 25, No. 1 (January 2, 2007), pp. 92-101, ISSN 0264-410X.

Collen, T., Dimarchi, D., & Doel, T.R. (1991) A T Cell Epitope in VP1 of Foot-and-Mouth Disease Virus is Immunodominant for Vaccinated Cattle. *J. Immunol.*, Vol. 146, No. 2 (January 15, 1991), pp. 749-755, ISSN 0022-1767.

Common Ingredients in U.S. Licensed Vaccines. (July, 2011). In: Vaccine Safety & Availability,   7.07.2011,   Available   from http://www.fda.gov/BiologicsBloodVaccines/SafetyAvailability/VaccineSafety/ucm187810.htm.

Cox, E., Verdonck, F., Vanrompay, D., & Goddeeris, B. (2006). Adjuvants Modulating Mucosal Immune Responses or Directing Systemic Responses towards the Mucosa. *Vet. Res.*, Vol. 37, No. 3, (May-June 2006), pp. 511-539, ISSN 0928-4249.

Deliyannis, G., Kedzierska, K., Lau, Y.F., Zeng, W., Turner, S.J., & Jackson, D.C. (2006) Intranasal Lipopeptide Primes Lung-Resident Memory CD8+ T Cells for Long-Term Pulmonary Protection against Influenza. *Eur. J. Immunol.*, Vol. 36, No. 3 (March, 2006), pp. 770-778, ISSN 0014-2980.

Dodoo, D., Theisen, M., Kurtzhals, J.A., Akanmori, B.D., Koram, K.A., Jepsen, S., Nkrumah, F.K., Theander, T.G. & Hviid, L. (2000). Naturally Acquired Antibodies to the Glutamate-Rich Protein are Associated with Protection against *Plasmodium falciparum* Malaria. *J. Infect. Dis.*,@ 2000, vol. 181, pp. 1202-1205, ISSN 0022-1899.

Druilhe, P., Spertini, F., Soesoe, D., Corradin, G., Mejia, P., Singh, S., Audran, R., Bouzidi, A., Oeuvray, C., & Roussilhon, C. (2005). A Malaria Vaccine that Elicits in Humans Antibodies Able to Kill *Plasmodium falciparum*. *PLoS Med.*, Vol. 2, No. 11, e344 . Available at http://www.plosmedicine.org/article/info%3Adoi%2F10.1371%2Fjournal.pmed.0020344.

Düesberg, U., von dem Bussche, A., Kirschning, C., Miyake, K., Sauerbruch, T., & Spengler, U. (2002). Cell Activation by Synthetic Lipopeptides of the Hepatitis C Virus (HCV)–Core Protein Is Mediated by Toll Like Receptors (TLRs). *Immunol. Lett.*, Vol. 84, No.2 (December 1, 2002), pp. 89-95, ISSN 0165-2478.

El Abd, Y.S., Tabll, A.A., Bader El Din, N.G., Hosny, A.E., Moustafa, R.I., El-Shenawy, R., Atef, K. & El-Awady, M.K. (2011). Neutralizing Activities of Caprine Antibodies towards Conserved Regions of the HCV Envelope Glycoprotein E2. *Virol. J.*, Vol. 8, No. 1, (August 5, 2011), p.391, ISSN 1743-422X.

El-Awady, M.K., Tabll, A.A., Yousif, H., El-Abd, Y., Reda, M., Khalil, S.B., El-Zayadi, A.R., Shaker, M.H. & Bader El Din, N.G. (2010). Murine Neutralizing Antibody Response and Toxicity to Synthetic Peptides Derived from E1 and E2 Proteins of Hepatitis C Virus. *Vacc ine*, Vol. 28, No. 52 (December, 6, 2010), pp. 8338-8344, ISSN 0264-410X.

Eldridge, J.H., Staas, J.K., Meulbroek, J.A., Tice, T.R., & Gilley, R.M. (1991). Biodegradable and Biocompatible Poly(DL-Lactide-co-Glycolide) Aicrospheres as an Adjuvant for Staphylococcal Enterotoxin B Toxoid which Enhances the Level of Toxin-Neutralizing Antibodies. *Infect. Immun.*, Vol. 59, No. 9, (September 1991), pp. 2978-2983, ISSN 0019-9567.

Elmowalid, G.A., Qiao, M., Jeong, S.H., Borg, B.B., Baumert, T.F., Sapp, R.K., Hu, Z., Murthy, K., Liang, T.J. (2007). Immunization with Hepatitis C Virus-Like Particles Results in Control of Hepatitis C Virus Infection in Chimpanzees. Proc. Natl. Acad. Sci. USA, Vol. 104, No. 20, (May 15, 2007), pp.8427-8432, ISSN 0027-8424.

Engler, O.B., Schwendener, R.A., Dai, W.J., W@lk, B., Pichler, W., Moradpour, D., Brunner, T., & Cerny, A. (2004). A Liposomal Peptide Vaccine Inducing CD8+ Cells in HLA-A2.1 Transgenic Mice, which Recognise Human Cells Encoding hepatitis C Virus (HCV) Proteins. *Vaccine,* Vol. 23, No. 1, (November 15, 2004), pp. 58-68, ISSN 0264-410X.

Epstein, J.E., Giersing, B., Mullen, G., Moorthy, V., & Richie, T.L.,(2007) Malaria Vaccines: Are We Getting Closer? *Curr. Opin. Mol. Ther.*, Vol. 9, No. 1, (February 2007), pp. 12-24, ISSN 1464-8431.

Firbas, C., Jilma, B., Tauber, E., Buerger, V., Jelovcan, S., & Lingnau, K., Buschle, M., Frisch, J., Klade, C.S. (2006) Immunogenicity and Safety of a Novel Therapeutic Hepatitis C Virus (HCV) Peptide Vaccine: a Randomized, Placebo Controlled Trial for Dose Optimization in 128 Healthy Subjects. *Vaccine,* Vol. 24, No. 20, (May 15, 2006), pp. 4343-4353, ISSN 0264-410X.

Felgner, P.L., Kayala, M.A., Vigil, A., Burk, C., Nakajima-Sasaki, R., Pablo, J., Molina, D.M., Hirst, S., Chew ,J.S.W., Wang, D., Tan, G., Duffield, M., Yang, R., Neel, J., Chantratita, N., Bancroft, G., Lertmemongkolchai, G., Davies, D.H., Baldi, P., Peacock, S., & Titball, R.W. (2009) A *Burkholderia pseudomallei* Protein Microarray Reveals Serodiagnostic and Cross-Reactive Antigens. *Proc. Natl. Acad. Sci. USA*, Vol. 106, No.32, (August 11, 2009), pp. 13499-13504, ISSN 0027-8424.

Freeman, A.J., Pan, Y., Harvey, C.E., Post, J.J., Law, M.G., White, P.A., Rawlinson, W.D., Lloyd, A.R., Marinos, G. & French, R.A. (2003). The Presence of an Intrahepatic Cytotoxic T Lymphocyte Response is Associated with Low Viral Load in Patients with Chronic Hepatitis C Virus Infection.*J. Hepatol.*, Vol. 38, No. 3, (March 2003), pp.349-356, ISSN 0168-8278.

Fritzer, A., Senn, B.M., Minh, D.B., Hanner, M., Gelbmann, D., Noiges, B., Henics, T., Schulze, K., Guzman, C.A., Goodacre, J., von Gabain, A., Nagy, E. & Meinke, A.L. (2010) Novel Conserved Group A Streptococcal Proteins Identified by the

Antigenome Technology as Vaccine Candidates for a non-M Protein-Based Vaccine. *Infect Immun.*, Vol.78, No.9, (September, 2010), pp. 4051-4067, ISSN 1098-5522.

Gal-Tanamy M., Walker C., Foung S., Lemon S.M. (2009). Hepatitis C. In: *Vaccines for Biodefence and Emerging and Neglected Diseases*, A.T. Barrett and L.R. Stanberry (Eds.). Academic Press, London-Amsterdam-Burlington-San Diego, pp. 413-440, ISBN 978-0-3-69408-9.

Garg, A.D, Nowis, D., Golab, J., Vandenabeele, P., Krysko, D.V., & Agostinis, P. (2010) Immunogenic cell death, DAMPs and anticancer therapeutics: an emerging amalgamation. *Biochim Biophys Acta,* Vol.1805, No.1 (January, 2010), pp.53-71, ISSN 0304-419X.

Glowalla, E., Tosetti, B., Krönke, M., & Krut, O. (2009) Proteomics-Based Identification of Anchorless Cell Wall Proteins as Vaccine Candidates against *Staphyllococcus aureus*. *Infect. Immun.*, Vol. 77, No. 7, (July, 2009), pp. 2719-2729, ISSN 1098-5522.

Graves, P. & Gelband, H. (2007). Vaccines for Preventing Malaria. *Cochrane Database Sys. Rev.*, No. 4, July 18, 2007. Available at http://onlinelibrary.wiley.com/doi/10.1002/14651858.CD000129.pub2/pdf.

Guévin, C., Lamarre, A., & Labonté, P. (2009). Novel HCV Replication Mouse Model Using Human Hepatocellular Carcinoma Xenografts.*Antiviral Res.*, Vol. 84, No. 1, (October 2009), @ 2009, pp. 14-22, ISSN 0166-3542.

Haro, I., Pérez, S., García, M., Chan, W.C., Ercilla, G. (2003). Liposome Entrapment and Immunogenic Studies of a Synthetic Lipophilic Multiple Antigenic Peptide Bearing VP1 and VP3 Domains of the Hepatitis A Virus: a Robust Method for Vaccine Design. *FEBS Lett.*, Vol. 540, No. 1-3, (April 10, 2003), pp. 133-140, ISSN .

He, Y., Rappuoli, R., De Groot, A.S. & Chen, R.T. (2010). Emerging Vaccine Informatics. *J. Biomed. Biotechnol.*, 2010; 2010: 218590 (June 15, 2011), ISSN 1110-7251.

Jackson, D.C., Lau, Y.F., Le, T., Suhrbier, A., Deliyannis, G., & Cheers, C. (2004). A Totally Synthetic Vaccine of Generic Structure that Targets Toll-Like Receptor 2 on Dendritic Cells and Promotes Antibody or Cytotoxic T Cell Responses. *Proc. Natl. Acad. Sci. USA*, Vol. 101, No. 43 (October 26, 2004), pp. 15440-15445, ISSN 0027-8424.

Jackson, D.C., Purcell, A.W., Fitzmaurice, C.J., Zeng, W., & Hart, D.N. (2002) The Central Role Played by Peptides in the Immune Response and the Design of Peptide-Based Vaccines against Infectious Diseases and Cancer. *Curr. Drug Targets*, Vol. 3, No.2, (April 2002), pp. 175-196, ISSN 1389-4501.

Kalyuzhny, A.E., (Ed.). (2005) *Handbook of ELISPOT. Methods and Protocols*, Humana Press, ISBN 978-1-58829-469-2.

Kaplun, A.P., Le Bang Shon, Krasnopolskii, Yu.M., & Shvets, V.I. (1999). Liposomes and Other Nanoparticles as Drug Delivery Means. *Vopr. Med. Khim.*, Vol. 45, No. 1, pp. 3-12, ISSN 0042-8809.

Khaitov, R.M. & Pinegin, B.V. (2005). Modern Views on the Polyoxidonium Mechanism of Action. *Immunologiya*, No. 4, (April 2005), pp. 197-205.

Kensil, C.R. (1996). Saponins as Vaccine Adjuvants. *Crit. Rev. Ther. Drug. Carrier. Syst.*, Vol. 13, No. 1-2, pp. 1-55, ISSN 0743-4863.

Klade, C.S. (2002) Proteomics Approaches towards Antigen Discovery and Vaccine Development. *Curr. Opin. Mol. Ther.*, Vol. 4, No. 3, (June, 2002), pp. 216-223, ISSN 1464-8431.

Klade, C.S., Wedemeyer, H., Berg, T., Hinrichsen, H., Cholewinska, G., Zeuzem, S., Blum, H., Buschle, M., Jelovcan, .S, Buerger, V., Tauber, E., Frisch, J., Manns, M.P. (2008) Therapeutic Vaccination of Chronic Hepatitis C Nonresponder Patients with the Peptide Vaccine IC41. *Gastroenterology*, Vol. 134, No. 5, (May 2008), pp. 1385-1395, ISSN 0016-5085.

Kolesanova, E.F., Farafonova, T.E., Moisa, A.A., Aleshina, E.Yu., Pyndyk, N.V., Sobolev, B.N. & Archakov, A.I. (2011). Development of Peptide Immunogens for Anti-HCV Vaccine. In: *Peptide Science 2010*, N. Fujii & Y. Kiso (Eds.), p.33, The Japanese Peptide Society, Osaka, ISBN 978-4-931541-11-5.

Kupriianova, M.A., Zhmak, M.N., Koroev, D.O., Chepurkin, A.V., Volpina, O.M., & Ivanov, V.T. (2000). Synthetic Peptide Designs Based on Immunoactive Fragments of the VP1 Protein of the Foot-and-Mouth Disease Virus Strain A22. *Bioorgan. Khim. (Russ.)*, Vol. 26, No.12 (December 2000), pp. 926-933.

Kuzmina, T.I., Olenina L.V., Sanzhakov, M.A., Farafonova, T.E., Abramikhina, T.V., Dubuisson, J., Sobolev, B.N., & Kolesanova, E.F. (2009). Antigenicity and B-Epitope Mapping of hepatitis C Virus Envelope Protein E2. *Biochemistry (Moscow) Supplement Series B: Biomedical Chemistry*, Vol. 3, No. 2, pp. 177–182, ISSN 1990-7508.

Lauer, G.M., Barnes, E., Lucas, M., Timm, J., Ouchi, K., Kim, A.Y., Day, C.L., Robbins, G.K., Casson, D.R., Reiser, M., Dusheiko, G., Allen, T.M., Chung, R.T., Walker, B.D., & Klenerman, P., (2004). High Resolution Analysis of Cellular Immune Responses in Resolved and Persistent Hepatitis C Virus Infection. *Gastroenterology*, Vol. 27, No. 3 (September, 2004), pp. 924-936, ISSN 0016-5085.

Law, M., Maruyama, T., Lewis, J., Giang, E., Tarr, A.W., Stamataki, Z., Gastaminza, P., Chisari, F.V., Jones, I.M., Fox, R.I., Ball, J.K., McKeating, J.A., Knellerman, N.M. & Burton, D.R. (2008). Broadly Neutralizing Antibodies Protect against Hepatitis C Virus Quasispecies Challenge. *Nat Med.*, Vol. 14, No. 1, (January 14, 2008), pp. 25-27, ISSN 1078-8956.

Liljeqvist, S. & Stahl, S.J. (1999).Recombinant Subunit Vaccines: Protein Immunogens, Live Delivery Systems or Nucleic Acid Vaccines. *J. Biotechnol.*, Vol.73, No.1, pp.1-33, ISSN 0168-1656.

Lin, H.H., Zhang, G.L., Tongchusak, S., Reinherz, E.L., & Brusic, V. (2008) Evaluation of MHC-II Peptide Binding Prediction Servers: Applications for Vaccine Research. *BMC Immunol.*, Vol. 9, No.8, (March 16, 2008), ISSN 1471-2172. Available at: http://www.biomedcentral.com/1471-2172/9/8.

Ling, E., Feldman, G., Portnoi, M., Dagan, R., Overweg, K., Mulholland, F., Chalifa-Caspi, V., Wells, J., & Mizrachi-Nebenzahl, Y. (2004). Glycolytic Enzymes Associated with the Cell Surface of *Streptococcus pneumoniae* are Antigenic in Humans and Elicit Protective Immune Responses in the Mouse. *Clin. Exp. Immunol.*, Vol. 138, No. 2, (November, 2004), pp. 290-298, ISSN 0009-9104.

Lloyd-Williams, P., Albericio, F., & Giralt, E. (1997). *Chemical Approaches to the Synthesis of Peptides and Proteins*, CRC Press LLC, New York, ISBN 978-0-84939-142-2.

Lu, X., DeFelippis, M.R., & Huang, L. (2009). Linear Epitope Mapping by Native Mass Spectrometry. *Anal. Biochem.*, Vol. 395, No.1 (December 1, 2009), pp. 100-107, ISSN 0003-2697.

Machiels, J.P., van Baren, N., and Marchand, M.(2002). Peptide-Based Cancer Vaccines. *Semin Oncol.*, Vol. 29, No.5 (October, 2002), pp. 494-502, ISSN 0093-7754.

MacNamara, A., Kadolsky, U., Bangham, C.R., & Asquith, B. (2009). T-cell Epitope Prediction: Rescaling Can Mask Biological Variation between MHC Molecules. *PLoS Comput. Biol.*, Vol. 5, No. 3, (March 2009), e1000327, eISSN 1553-7358.

Mäkelä, P.H. (2000) Vaccines, Coming of Age after 200 Years. FEMS Microbiol. Rev., Vol. 24, No. 1 (January, 2000), pp. 9-20, ISSN 0168-6445.

Male, D., Brostoff, J., Roth, D. & Roitt, I. (2006). *Immunology 7th Edition*, MOSBY Elsevier, ISBN 978-0-323-05448-5.

Målen, H., Søfterland, T., & Wiker, H.G. (2008). Antigen Analysis of *Mycobacterium tuberculosis* H37Rv Culture Filtrate Proteins. *Scand. J. Immunol.*, Vol. 67, No. 3, (March, 2008), pp. 245-252, ISSN 0300-9475.

Meinke, A., Henics, T., Hanner, M., Minh, D.B., & Nagy, E. (2005) Antigenome Technology: a Novel Approach for the Selection of Bacterial Vaccine Candidate Antigens. *Vaccine,*Vol. 23, No. 17-18, (March 18, 2005), pp. 2035-2041, ISSN: 0264-410X.

Mitsuaki, N., Shizuko, I., Satoshi, N., & Takuya, I. (1987). Peptide Synthesis by Fragment Condensation on a Soluble Polymer Support. 8. Maximum Peptide Chain Lengths of Carboxyl Component Peptides for Effective Coupling Reactions with Amino Component Peptides Anchored to Soluble and Cross-Linked Polystyrene Supports. *Macromolecules*, vol. 20, No.9, (September 1987), pp. 2306-2307, ISSN 0024-9297.

Moss, C.X., Tree, T.I., & Watts, C. (2007). Reconstruction of a Pathway of Antigen Processing and Class II MHC Peptide Capture. *EMBO J.*, Vol. 26, No.8, (April 18, 2007), pp. 2137-2147, ISSN 0261-4189.

Muhlradt, P.F., Kiess, M., Meyer, H., Sussmuth, R., & Jung, G.J. (1997) Isolation, Structure Elucidation, and Synthesis of a Macrophage Stimulatory Lipopeptide from *Mycoplasma fermentans* Acting at Picomolar Concentration. *J. Exp. Med.*, Vol. 185, No. 11, (June 2, 1997), pp. 1951-1958, ISSN 0022-1007.

Müller, M.R., Wiesmüller, K.H., Jung, G., Loop, T., Humar, M., Pfannes, S.D., Bessler, W.G., Mittenbühler, K. (2002). Lipopeptide Adjuvants: Monitoring and Comparison of P3CSK4- and LPS-induced Gene Transcription. *Int. Immunopharmacol.*, Vol. 2, No.8, (July 2002), pp. 1065-1077, ISSN 1567-5769.

Okitsu, S.L., Kienzl, U., Moehle, K., Silvie, O., Peduzzi, E., Mueller, M.S., Sauerwein, R.W., Matile, H., Zurbriggen, R., Mazier, D., Robinson, J.A., & Pluschke, G. (2007) Structure-Activity-Based Design of a Synthetic Malaria Peptide Eliciting Sporozoite Inhibitory Antibodies in a Virosomal Formulation. *Chem. Biol.*, Vol. 14, No. 5 (May 2007), pp. 577-587, ISSN 1074-5521.

Olenina, L.V., Nikolaeva, L.I., Sobolev, B.N., Blokhina, N.P., Archakov, A.I., & Kolesanova, E.F. (2002) Mapping and Characterization of B Cell Linear Epitopes in the Conservative Regions of Hepatitis C Virus Envelope Glycoproteins. *J. Viral Hepat.*, Vol. 9, No.3, (May 2002), pp. 174-182, ISSN 1352-0504.

Olenina, L.V., Kuzmina, T.I., Kuraeva, T.E., Sobolev, B.N., Kolesanova, E.F. & Archakov, A.I. (2003). Development of Laboratory Experimental Samples of Artificial Vaccine against Hepatitis C Virus. Immunogenicity of Highly Conserved Envelope Protein E2 Sites in Synthetic Constructs. *Novosti nauki i tehniki. Ser. Meditsina. Allergiya, astma i klinicheskaya immunologiya*, No. 9, pp. 51-53.

Olenina, L.V., Kuzmina, T.I., Sobolev, B.N., Kuraeva, T.E., Kolesanova, E.F. & Archakov, A.I. (2005). Identification of Glycosaminoglycan-Binding Sites within Hepatitis C Virus Envelope Glycoprotein E2. *J. Viral Hepat.*, Vol. 12, No. 6, (Novemder 2005), pp. 584-593, ISSN 1352-0504.

Palena, C., Abrams, S.I., Schlom, J., & Hodge, J.W. (2006). Cancer Vaccines: Preclinical Studies and Novel Strategies. *Adv. Cancer. Res.*, Vol. 95, pp. 115-145, ISSN 0065-230X.

Panina-Bordignon, P., Tan, A., Termijtelen, A., Demotz, S., Corradin, G., & Lanzavecchia, A.(1989). Universally Immunogenic T Cell Epitopes: Promiscuous Binding to Human MHC Class II and Promiscuous Recognition by T Cells. *Eur. J. Immunol.*, Vol. 19, No.12 (December 1989), pp. 2237-2242, ISSN 0014-2980.

Pereboeva, L.A., Pereboev, A.V., Wang, L.F., & Morris, G.E. (2000). Hepatitis C Epitopes from Phage-Displayed cDNA Libraries and Improved Diagnosis with a Chimeric Antigen. *J. Med. Virol.*, Vol. 60, No. 2 (February 2000), pp. 144-151, ISSN 0146-6615.

Perry, L.C., Jones, T.D., & Baker, M.P. (2008) New Approaches to Prediction of Immune Responses to Therapeutic Proteins during Preclinical Development. *Drugs R. D.*, Vol. 9, No.6, pp. 385-396, ISSN 1174-5886.

Rappuoli, R. (2001). Reverse vaccinology, a genome-based approach to vaccine development. *Vaccine*, Vol. 19, No. 17-19 (March 21), pp. 2688-2691, ISSN 0264-410X.

Rinnová, M., Lebl, M., Souček, M. (1999). Solid-Phase Peptide Synthesis by Fragment Condensation: Coupling in Swelling Volume. *Lett. Peptide Sci.*, Vol. 6, No. 1, (pp. 15-22, ISSN 0929-5666.

Rodriguez, L.L., Barrera, J., Kramer, E., Lubroth, J., Brown, F., & Golde, W.T. (2003). A Synthetic Peptide Containing the Consensus Sequence of the G–H Loop Region of Foot-and-Mouth Disease Virus Type-O VP1 and a Promiscuous T-helper Epitope Induces Peptide-specific Antibodies but Fails to Protect Cattle against Viral Challenge. *Vaccine*, Vol. 21, No. 25-26, (September 8, 2003), pp. 3751-3756, ISSN: 0264-410X.

Roestenberg, M., Remarque, E., de Jonge, E., Hermsen, R., Blythman, H., Leroy, O., Imoukhuede, E., Jepsen, S., Ofori-Anyinam, O., Faber, B., Kocken, C.H., Arnold, M., Walraven, V., Teelen, K., Roeffen, W., de Mast, Q., Ballou, W.R., Cohen, J., Dubois, M.C., Ascarateil, S., van der Ven, A., Thomas, A., & Sauerwein R. (2008). Safety and Immunogenicity of a Recombinant Plasmodium falciparum AMA1 Malaria Vaccine Adjuvanted with Alhydrogel™, Montanide ISA 720 or AS02. *PLoS One*, Vol. 3, No.12, (December 18, 2008), e3960,pp. 1-12, eISSN-1932-6203.

Roggen, E.L. (2006). Recent Developments with B-cell Epitope Identification for Predictive Studies. *J. Immunotoxicol.*, Vol. 3, No.3 (September 1, 2006), pp. 137-149, ISSN 1547-6901.

Sabatino, G. & Papini, A.M. (2008). Advances in Automatic, Manual and Microwave-Assisted Solid-Phase Peptide Synthesis. *Curr. Opin. Drug. Discov. Devel.*, Vol. 11, No.6, (November 2008), pp. 762-770, ISSN 1367-6733.

Scheerlinck, J.P. & Greenwood, D.L. (2008). Virus-Sized Vaccine Delivery Systems. *Drug. Discov. Today*, 2008, Vol. 13, No. 19-20, (October 2008), pp. 882-887, ISSN 1359-6446.

Scheerlinck, J.P. & Greenwood, D.L. (2006). Particulate Delivery Systems for Animal Vaccines. *Methods*, 2006, Vol. 40, No. 1, pp. 118-124, ISSN 1046-2023.

Schlaphoff, V., Klade, C.S., Jilma, B., Jelovcan, S.B., Cornberg, M., Tauber, E., Manns, M.P., & Wedemeyer, H. (2007). Functional and Phenotypic Characterization of Peptide-Vaccine-Induced HCV-Specific CD8+ T Cells in Healthy Individuals and Chronic Hepatitis C Patients. *Vaccine*, Vol. 25, No.37-38, (September 17, 2007), pp. 6793-6806, ISSN 0264-410X.

Schuler, M.M., Nastke, M.D. & Stevanovic, S. (2007) SYFPEITHI: Database for Searching and T-cell Epitope Prediction. In: *Methods Mol. Biol.* Vol. 409, No.1. *Immunoinformatics. Predicting Immunogenicity In Silico*, pp. 75-93, Flower, D.R. (Ed.), Springer, ISBN 978-1-60327-118-9.

Sesardic, D. J. (1993) Synthetic peptide vaccines. *J. Med. Microbiol.*, Vol. 39, pp. 241-242, ISSN 0022-2615.

Sieker, F., May, A., & Zacharias, M. (2009). Predicting Affinity and Specificity of Antigenic Peptide Binding to Major Histocompatibility Class I Molecules. *Curr. Protein. Pept. Sci.*, Vol. 10, No. 3, (March 2009), pp. 286-296, ISSN 1389-2037.

Singh, M., Kazzaz, J., Ugozzoli, M., Malyala, P., Chesko, J., & O'Hagan, D.T. (2006), Polylactide-co-Glycolide Microparticles with Surface Adsorbed Antigens as Vaccine Delivery Systems. *Curr. Drug. Deliv.*, vol. 3, No.1 (January 2006), pp. 115-120, ISSN 1567-2018.

Sirima, S.B., Tiono, A.B., Ouédraogo, A., Diarra, A., Ouédraogo, A.L., Yaro, J.B., Ouédraogo, E., Gansané, A., Bougouma, E.C., Konaté, A.T., Kaboré, Y., Traoré, A., Roma, C., Soulama, I., Luty, A.J., Cousens, S., & Nébié, I. (2009). Safety and Immunogenicity of the Malaria Vaccine Candidate MSP3 Long Synthetic Peptide in 12-24 Months-old Burkinabe Children. *PLoS One*, Vol. 4, No.10,e7549. Available at http://www.plosone.org/article/info%3Adoi%2F10.1371%2Fjournal.pone.0007549.

Sobolev, B.N., Olenina, L.V., Kolesanova, E.F., Poroikov, V.V., & Archakov, A.I. (2005) Computer Design of Vaccines: Approaches, Software Tools and Informational Resources. *Curr. Computer-Aided Drug Design*, Vol. 1, No.2, pp. 207-222, ISSN: 1573-4099.

Sobolev, B.N., Poroikov, V.V., Olenina, L.V., Kolesanova, E.F. & Archakov, A.I. (2000). Comparative Analysis of Amino Acid Sequences from Envelope Proteins Isolated from Different Hepatitis C Virus Variants: Possible Role of conservative and variable regions. *J. Viral Hepat.*, Vol.7, No. 4, (September 2000), pp. 368-374, ISSN 1352-0504.

Sobolev, B.N., Poroikov, V.V., Olenina, L.V., Kolesanova, E.F., & Archakov, A.I. (2003). Computer-Assiated Vaccine Design. *Biomed.Khim. (Russ).*, 2003, Vol. 49, No. 4, (July-August 2003), pp. 309-332.

Soe, S., Theisen, M., Roussilhon, C., Aye, K.S., & Druilhe, P. (2004). Association between Protection against Clinical Malaria and Antibodies to Merozoite Surface Antigens in an Area of Hyperendemicity in Myanmar: Complementarity between Responses to Merozoite Surface Protein 3 and the 220-Kilodalton Glutamate-Rich Protein. *Infect. Immun.*, vol. 72, No. 1, (January 2004), pp. 247-252, ISSN 0019-9567.

Solares, A.M., Baladron, I., Ramos T., Valenzuela, C., Borbon, Z., Fanjull, S., Gonzalez, L., Castillo, D., Esmir, J., Granadillo, M., Batte, A., Cintado, A., Ale, M., de Cossio, M.E.F., Ferrer, A., Torrens, I., Lopez-Saura, P. (2011). Safety and Immunogenicity of a Human Papillomavirus Peptide Vaccine (CIGB-228) in Women with High-Grade Cervical Intraepithelial Neoplasia: First-in-Human, Proof-of-Concept Trial. *ISRN Obstetrics and Gynecology*, Vol.2011, Article ID292951, 9 pp.

Stanekova, Z., Király, J., Stropkovská. A., Mikušková. T., Mucha. V., Kostolanský. F. & Varečková, E. (2011). Heterosubtypic Protective Immunity against Influenza A Virus Induced by Fusion Peptide of the Hemagglutinin in Comparison to Ectodomain of M2 Protein. *Acta Virol.*, Vol.55, No. 1, pp. 61-67, ISSN 0001-723X.

Strohmaier, K., Franze, R., & Adam, K.H. (1982) Location and Characterization of the Antigenic Portion of the FMDV Immunizing Protein. *J. Gen. Virol.*, Vol. 59, Pt.2, (April 1982), pp. 295-306.

Svirshchevskaya, E.V., Alekseeva, L.G., Reshetov, P.D., Phomicheva, N.N., Parphenyuk, S.A., Ilyina, A.V., Zueva, V.S., Lopatin, S.A., Levov, A.N. & Varlamov, V.P. (2009). Mucoadjuvant properties of lipo- and glycoconjugated derivatives of oligochitosans. *Eur. J. Med. Chem.*, Vol.44, No.5 , pp.2030-2037.

Takahashi, H., Takeshita, T., Morein, B., Putney, S., Germain, R.N., & Berzofsky, J.A. (1990). Induction of CD8+ Cytotoxic Cells by Immunization with Purified HIV-1 Envelope Protein in ISCOMs. *Nature*, Vol. 344, No. 6269 (April 26, 1990), pp. 873-875, ISSN 0028-0836.

Takala, S.L. & Plowe, C.V. (2009). Genetic Diversity and Malaria Vaccine Design, Testing and Efficacy: Preventing and Overcoming 'Vaccine Resistant Malaria'. *Parasite Immunol.*, Vol. 31, No. 9, (September 2009), pp. 560-573, ISSN 0141-9838.

Tam, J.P. (1988). Synthetic Peptide Vaccine Design: Synthesis and Properties of a High-Density Multiple Antigenic Peptide System. *Proc. Natl. Acad. USA*, Vol. 85, No.15, (August 1988), pp. 5409-5413, ISSN 0027-8424.

Tarradas, J., Monso, M., Muños, M., Rosell, R., Fraile, L., Frias, M.T., Domingo, M., Andreu, D., Sobrino, F. & Ganges, L. (2011). Partial Protection against Classical Swine Fever Virus Elicited by Dendrimeric Vaccine Candidate Peptides in Domestic Pigs. *Vaccine*, Vol 29, No. 26, (June10, 2011), pp.4422-4429, ISSN 0264-410X.

Tedeschi, G., Taverna, F., Negri, A., Piccinini, R., Nonnis, S., Ronchi, S., & Zecconi, A. (2009) Serological Proteome Analysis of *Staphylococcus aureus* Isolated from Sub-clinical Mastitis. *Vet. Microbiol.*, Vol. 134, No. 3-4, (March 2, 2009), pp. 388-391, 0378-1135.

Tester, I., Smyk-Pearson, S., Wang, P., Wertheimer, A., Yao, E., Lewinsohn, D.M., Tavis, J.E., & Rosen, H.R. (2005) Immune Evasion versus Recovery after Acute Hepatitis C Virus Infection from a Shared Source. *J. Exp Med*, Vol. 201, No. 11 (June 6, 2005), pp. 1725-1731, ISSN 0022-1007.

*The Methodical Recommendations 1/4.2.588-96,(*1998). Information-Editorial Center, Ministry of Public Health, Moscow, Russia.

The Sanitary Rules 3.3.2.015-94 (1995). Approved by State Sanitary and Epidemiologic Inspection, on 12.08.94, Ministry of Public Health of Russian Federation, Moscow, Russia.

The Sanitary Rules 3.3.2.561-96, approved by State Sanitary and Epidemiologic Inspection, on 31.10.96, Moscow: Information-Editorial Center, Ministry of Public Health, 1998.

Theisen, M., Dodoo, D., Toure-Balde, A., Soe, S., Corradin, G., Koram, K.K., Kurtzhals, J.A., Hviid, L., Theander, T., Akanmori, B., Ndiaye, M. & Druilhe, P.(2001) Selection of Glutamate-Rich Protein Long Synthetic Peptides for Vaccine Development: Antigenicity and Relationship with Clinical Protection and Immunogenicity. *Infect. Immun.,* Vol. 69, No. 9, (September 2001), pp. 11-17, ISSN 0019-9567.

Theisen, M., Soe, S., Jessing, S.G., Okkels, L.M., Danielsen, S., Oeuvray, C., Druilhe, P. & Jepsen, S. (2000) Identification of a Major B-Cell Epitope of the *Plasmodium falciparum* Glutamate-Rich Protein (GLURP), Targeted by Human Antibodies Mediating Parasite Killing. *Vaccine,* Vol. 19, No. 2-3 (September 15, 2000), pp.204-212, ISSN 0264-410X.

Thompson, F.M., Porter, D.W., Okitsu, S.L., Westerfeld, N., Vogel, D., Todryk, S., Poulton, I., Correa, S., Hutchings, C., Berthoud, T., Dunachie, S., Andrews, L., Williams, J.L., Sinden, R., Gilbert, S.C., Pluschke, G., Zurbriggen, R., Hill, A.V. Evidence of Blood Stage Efficacy with a Virosomal Malaria Vaccine in a Phase IIa Clinical Trial. *PLoS One,*Vol. 3 No. 1 (January 30, 2008). Available at http://www.plosone.org/article/info%3Adoi%2F10.1371%2Fjournal.pone.0001493 .

Tian, F., Yang, L., Lv, F., Yang, Q., & Zhou, P. (2009). In silico Quantitative Prediction of Peptides Binding Affinity to Human MHC Molecule: an Intuitive Quantitative Structure-Activity Relationship Approach. *Amino Acids,* Vol. 36, No.3, (March 2009), pp. 535-354, ISSN 1438-2199.

Torresi, J., Stock, O.M., Fischer, A.E., Grollo, L., Drummer, H., Boo, I., Zeng, W., Earnest-Silveira, L., & Jackson, D.C. (2007). A Self-Adjuvanting Multiepitope Immunogen that Induces a Broadly Cross-Reactive Antibody to Hepatitis C Virus. *Hepatology,* Vol. 45, No. 4, (April 2007), pp. 911-920, ISSN 0270-9139.

Tribbick, G. (2002) Multipin Peptide Libraries for Antibody and Receptor Epitope Screening and Characterization. *J. Immunol. Meth.,* Vol. 267, No. 1, (September 1, 2002), pp. 27-35, ISSN 0022-1759.

Uchaikin, V.G. & Shamsheva, O.V. (2001) Vaktsinoprofilaktika (Vaccine Prophylaxis), Moscow: Geotar-Med, 2001.

Urdaneta, M., Prata, A., Struchiner, C.J., Tosta, C.E., Tauil, P., & Boulos, M. (1998). Evaluation of SPf66 Malaria Vaccine Efficacy in Brazil. *Am. J. Trop. Med. Hyg.,* Vol. 58, No. 3, (March 1998), pp. 378-385, ISSN 0002-9637.

Van Regenmortel, M.H. & Muller, S. (1999). *Synthetic Peptides as Antigens,* Elsevier Science, Amsterdam, ISBN 0-444-82176-7.

Vogel, F.R., & Alving, C.R. (2002). Progress in immunologic adjuvant development: 1982 – 2002, In: *The Jordan Report, 20th Anniversary. Accelerated Development of Vaccines*, C. P.Heilman, P.McInnis, & S. Landry (Eds.), pp. 39-43, NIH/NIAID (USA).

Voisset, C. & Dubuisson, J. (2004). Functional Hepatitis C Virus Envelope Glycoproteins. Biol. Cell, Vol. 96, No. 6, pp. 413-420, ISSN 0248-4900.

Volpina, O.M., Gelfanov, V.M., Yarov, A.V., Surovoy, A.Yu., Chepurkin, A V., & Ivanov, V.T. (1993). New Virus-Specific T-Helper Epitopes of Foot-and-Mouth Disease Viral VP1 Protein. *FEBS Lett.*, vol. 333, No. 1-2, (October 25, 1993), pp. 175-178, ISSN 0014-5793.

Volpina, O.M., Surovoi A.Y., Zhmak, M.N., Kuprianova, M.A., Koroev, D.O., Toloknov, A.S., & Ivanov, V.T. (1999). A Peptide Construct Containing B-Cell and T-Cell Epitopes from the Foot-and-Mouth Disease Viral VP1 Protein Induces Efficient Antiviral Protection. *Vaccine*, vol. 17, No. 6, (February, 12, 1999), pp. 1375-1380, ISSN 0264-410X.

Vytvytska, O., Nagy, E., Blüggel, M., Meyer, H.E., Kurzbauer, R., Huber, L.A., & Klade, C.S. (2002). Identification of Vaccine Candidate Antigens of *Staphylococcus aureus* by Serological Proteome Analysis. *Proteomics*, Vol. 2, No.5, (May, 2002), pp. 580-590, ISSN 1615-9853.

Walker, J., Ghosh, S., Pagnon, J., Colantoni, C., Newbold, A., Zeng, W., Jackson, D.C. (2007). Totally Synthetic Peptide-Based Immunocontraceptive Vaccines Show Activity in Dogs of Different Breeds . *Vaccine*, Vol. 25, No.41, (October 10, 2007), pp. 7111-7119, ISSN 0264-410X.

Wang, T.T., Tan, G.S., Hai, R., Pica, N., Ngai, L., Ekiert, D.C., Wilson, I.A., Garsia-Sastre, A., Moran, T.M. & Palese, P. (2010). Vaccination with a Synthetic Peptide from the Influenza Virus Hemagglutinin Provides Protection against Distinct Viral Subtypes. *Proc. Natl. Acad. Sci. USA*, Vol. 107, No. 44, (November 2, 2010), pp.18979-18984, ISSN 0027-8424.

Wiwanitkit, V. (2009). Predicted Epitopes of Malarial Merozoite Surface Protein 1 by Bioinformatics Method: a Clue for Further Vaccine Development. *J. Microbiol. Immunol. Infect.*, Vol. 42, No. 1, (February 2009), pp. 19-21, ISSN 1684-1182.

Worm, M., Lee, H.H., Kleine-Tebbe, J., Hafner, R.P., Laidler, P., Healey, D., Buhot, C., Verhoef, A., Maillère, B., Kay, A.B. & Larché, M. (2011). Development and Preliminary Clinical evaluation of a Peptide Immunotherapy Vaccine for Cqt Allergy. J. Allergy Clin. Immunol. , Vol. 127, No. 1, (January 2011), pp. 89-97, ISSN 0091-6749.

Wulf, M., Hoehn, P., & Trinder, P. (2009). Identification and Validation of T-cell Epitopes Using the IFN-gamma ELISPOT Assay. In: *Methods Mol. Biol.* Vol. 524, No. 4. *Epitope Mapping Protocols*, M. Schutkowski & Reineke, U. (Eds.), pp. 361-367, Humana Press, ISBN 978-1-59745-450-6_32.

Yutani S., Komatsu, N. Shichijo, S., Yoshida, K., Hiroko Takedatsu, H., Minoru Itou, M., Kuromatu, R.,Ide, T., Tanaka, M., Sata, M., Yamada, A. & Itoh, K. (2009). Phase I Clinical Study of a Peptide Vaccination for Hepatitis C Virus-Infected Patients with Different Human Leukocyte Antigen-Class I-A Alleles. Cancer Sci., Vol. 100, No. 10, (October 13, 2009), pp.1935-1942, ISSN 1349-7006.

Zeng, W., Ghosh, S., Lau, Y.F., Brown, L.E., & Jackson, D.C. (2002). Highly Immunogenic and Totally Synthetic Lipopeptides as Self-Adjuvanting Immunocontraceptive Vaccines. *J. Immunol.*, Vol. 169, No. 9, (November 1, 2002),pp. 4905-4912, ISSN 0022-1767.

Zeng, W., Jackson, D.C., Murray, J., Rose, K., & Brown, L.E. (2000). Totally Synthetic Lipid-Containing Polyoxime Peptide Constructs are Potent Immunogens. *Vaccine*, Vol. 18, No. 11-12, (January 6, 2000), pp. 1031-1039, ISSN 0264-410X.

Zhu, Q., Oei, Y., Mendel, D.B., Garrett, E.N., Patawaran, M.B., Hollenbach, P.W., Aukerman, S.L., & Weiner, A.J. (2006). Novel Robust Hepatitis C Virus Mouse Efficacy Model. *Antimicrob. Agents Chemother.*, Vol. 50, No.10, (October 2006), pp. 3260-3268, ISSN 0066-4804.

11

Studies on the Association of Meningitis and Mumps Virus Vaccination

Alejandra Lara-Sampablo[1,2], Nora Rosas-Murrieta[2],
Irma Herrera-Camacho[2], Verónica Vallejo-Ruiz[1],
Gerardo Santos-López[1] and Julio Reyes-Leyva[1]*

[1]*Laboratorio de Biología Molecular y Virología, Centro de Investigación Biomédica de
Oriente, Instituto Mexicano del Seguro Social, Metepec, Puebla;*
[2]*Centro de Química, Instituto de Ciencias, Benemérita Universidad Autónoma de Puebla,
Puebla,
México*

1. Introduction

Mumps is an acute viral infection caused by a member of the *Rubulavirus* genus in the *Paramyxoviridae* family. Although it is mostly a childhood disease, with peak incidence occurring among those aged 5–9 years, mumps virus (MuV) may also affect teenagers. MuV is known to affect the salivary glands causing parotid swelling; however, it can also produce an acute systemic infection involving glandular, lymphoid and nervous tissues, leading to some important complications such as pancreatitis, oophoritis orchitis, mastitis, nephritis and thyroiditis. The main central nervous system (CNS) complication of mumps virus infection is aseptic meningitis (in up to 15% of cases); it is also associated rarely with encephalitis, hydrocephalus and sensorineural deafness (affecting approximately 5/100 000 mumps patients) (Carbone & Rubin, 2007; Hviid et al., 2008; Plotkin & Rubin, 2007; World Health Organization [WHO], 2007).

Massive vaccination programs have decreased the incidence of MuV infection worldwide, before the introduction of live attenuated mumps virus vaccines, mumps was the main cause of virus-induced disease in the CNS of children; indeed, the annual incidence of mumps in the absence of immunization was in the range of 100–1000 cases/100 000 people. Although vaccination programs have decreased the incidence of mumps virus infection, outbreaks have not been completely eliminated (WHO, 2007). The main problems associated with MuV vaccination are lack of protection due to vaccine failure and presentation of secondary adverse complications due to the use of relatively virulent vaccine strains; indeed, L-Zagreb, Leningrad-3 and Urabe AM9 strains have been associated with post-vaccinal aseptic meningitis (Brown et al., 1991; Dourado et al., 2000; Galazka et al., 1999; Goh, 1999). The unacceptably high rate of vaccine associated meningitis and parotitis cases has resulted in vaccine withdrawal and public resistance to mumps vaccination (Schmitt et al., 1993). In consequence, mumps epidemics have re-emerged, and the incidence is rising in several countries (Choi, 2010; Dayan et al., 2008).

2. Wild-type mumps virus natural infection and CNS involvement

2.1 Mumps virus

Mumps virus (MuV) is a member of the *Rubulavirus* genus of the *Paramyxoviridae* family. Mumps virions are pleomorphic particles ranging from 100 to 600 nm in size, consisting of a helical ribonucleocapsid surrounded by a host cell-derived lipid envelope. Full-length genome is a non-segmented, single-stranded RNA of negative polarity that consists of 15,384 nucleotides containing 7 genes that code for the nucleoprotein (NP), phosphoprotein (P), matrix (M), fusion (F), small hydrophobic (SH), hemagglutinin-neuraminidase (HN), and large (L) proteins. The genomic organization of the virus from 3′ to 5′ ends is NP-P-M-F-SH-HN-L (Lamb & Parks, 2007; Pringle, 1997).

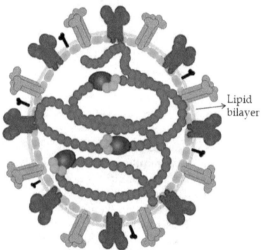

Viral protein	Biological activity	Viral protein	Biological activity
Nucleoprotein (NP)	Protects genomic RNA from cellular proteases; determines helical structure of capsid	Small hydrophobic (SH)	Unknown function. This protein has been involved in evasion of the host anti-viral response
Phosphoprotein (P)	Forms part of the transcriptase complex.	Fusion (F)	Virus-to-cell and cell-to-cell fusion
Large (L)	Forms part of the transcriptase complex	Hemagglutinin-Neuraminidase (HN)	Viral attachment and entry. Prevention of self-agglutination
Matrix (M)	Virion assembly		

Fig. 1. Schematic diagram of mumps virus (not drawn to scale). On the surface of the viral membrane 3 glycoproteins are anchored: HN, F and SH. The M protein is located inside of the viral envelope. In the center of the virion is the ribonucleoprotein complex formed by the nucleocapside (NP:RNA) and viral RNA polymerase (P:L). Information based on the references: Carbone & Rubin, 2007; Santos-López et al., 2004.

A schematic diagram of the virion and functions of viral proteins are shown in figure 1. On the surface of viral particles and infected cells are projected two glycoproteins, F and HN, which are transmembrane glycoproteins of types I and II, respectively. HN glycoprotein is responsible for mumps virus attachment; it binds to sialic acid-containing cell receptors. Its neuraminidase (sialidase) activity releases the sialic acid residues from viral progeny to prevent self-aggregation during budding; HN glycoprotein also activates the F glycoprotein, which promotes the fusion between viral and cell membranes (Carbone & Rubin, 2007; Lamb & Parks, 2007).

SH is an integral membrane protein without well-known properties; despite this, SH protein has been reported to block the TNFα mediated apoptotic signaling pathway; therefore it has been involved in evasion of the host anti-viral response (Wilson et al., 2006), so it has been proposed as a virulence factor, however, this issue is still controversial (T. Malik et al., 2011; Woznik et al., 2010). Likewise, the sequence of the mumps virus SH gene varies greatly from strain to strain and has therefore been used in molecular epidemiological studies to group mumps virus strains (Orvell et al., 1997).

Inside the envelope lies a helical nucleocapsid core containing the RNA genome and the NP, P, and L proteins, which are involved in virus replication. NP protein is an RNA-binding protein that coats and protects full-length viral (-) sense genomic and (+) sense antigenomic RNAs to form the helical nucleocapsid template (Carbone & Rubin, 2007; Lamb & Parks, 2007). Each NP protein interact with 6 nucleotides of the viral genome, therefore a full-length genome polyhexameric may be required for efficient viral replication (process known as, Rule of Six) (Kolakofsky et al., 1998, 2005; Vulliemoz & Roux, 2001). P and L proteins form an enzymatic complex with RNA-dependent RNA polymerase activity; where L protein has the catalytic domain for RNA polymerization, whereas P protein functions as a cofactor for L protein and is able to bind the ribonucleoprotein complex (RNA-NP) (Kingston et al., 2004; Lamb & Parks, 2007).

M protein resides between the envelope and the nucleocapside core; this is the most abundant protein in the virion, and it serves to physically link the ribonucleocapsid with the host cell membrane to promote the viral assembly process (Carbone & Rubin, 2007; Lamb & Parks, 2007).

Two nonstructural proteins, V and I, are encoded by the P gene and are synthesized as a result of co-transcriptional editing of messenger RNA (mRNA) (Carbone & Rubin, 2007; Paterson & Lamb, 1990). In this process the viral polymerase moves repeatedly (process known as, stuttering) in a region known as "editing site" of the P gene, which is rich in citidine nucleotides (3'CCCCCC 5') inserting some non-template guanidine (G) nucleotides in the nascent transcript (Hausmann et al., 1999; Paterson & Lamb, 1990; Vidal et al., 1990). This editing mechanism involves the production of mRNAs whose ORFs are altered by insertion of G residues (Figure 2); so, the translation of full-transcript (unedited) encodes a V protein, which plays a role in circumventing the interferon (IFN) mediated antiviral responses by blocking IFN signaling and limiting IFN production (Didcock et al., 1999a, 1999b; Fujii et al., 1999; Rodriguez et al., 2003; N. H. Rosas-Murrieta et al., 2010); while, mRNAs generated by inserting 2 and 4 G residues encode a P and I proteins respectively. The generated proteins have the same N-terminus, but differ in their C-terminus (Lamb & Parks, 2007).

P (V/P/I) gene

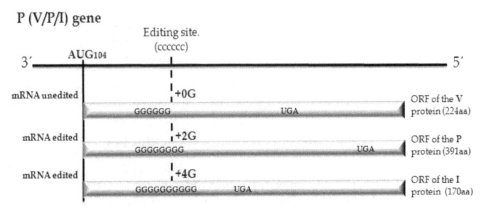

Fig. 2. Schematic representation of mumps virus P gene and mRNA editing mechanism (not drawn to scale). By a stuttering mechanism in the editing site of P gene, the viral polymerase introduces non-template G residues in the nascent transcript, which generates mRNAs with different ORFs, so, the translation of full-transcript (unedited) encodes a V protein, while mRNAs generated by inserting 2 and 4 G residues encode P and I proteins respectively. AUG and UGA sequence indicate the start and stop codons, respectively. Information based on the references: Hausmann et al., 1999; Lamb & Parks, 2007; Paterson & Lamb, 1990; Vidal et al., 1990.

2.2 Viral pathogenesis and invasion central nervous system

Natural infection with mumps virus is restricted to humans and is transmitted via the respiratory mucosa by direct contact, droplet spread or contaminated fomites. The incubation period is about 15 to 24 days (average 19 days). Infected patients become most contagious 1 to 2 days before onset of clinical symptoms and continue for several days afterwards (Hviid et al., 2008). Mumps virus initially infects the upper-respiratory-tract mucosa where it undergo a first replication cycle and then the progeny viruses spread to local lymph nodes where they undergo a second replication followed by a systemic spread with involvement of glandular, nervous and other target organs (figure 3) (Carbone & Rubin, 2007; Enders, 1996; Plotkin & Rubin, 2007).

The main clinical manifestation of mumps is parotid swelling. However, parotitis is not a primary or necessary step of mumps virus infection. Mumps virus can also infect urinary tract, genital organs, pancreas, kidney and central nervous system (CNS). It is not yet well-known how mumps virus spreads to the CNS, however, studies in newborn hamster model suggest that virus spreads by passage of infected mononuclear cells across the epithelium to epithelial cells of the choroid plexus (Fleischer & Kreth, 1982; Wolinsky et al., 1976). Alternatively, direct spread of virus is possible. At this site virus is replicated and released persistently from ependymal and choroidal cells, followed by deeper spread into the brain parenchyma causing encephalitis and several neurological complications. There are few data on the histopathology of the brain in mumps encephalitis (since death is rare). The data show the characteristic picture of a parainfectious process, characterized by perivenous demyelinisation and perivascular infiltration with mononuclear cells (Hviid et al., 2008).

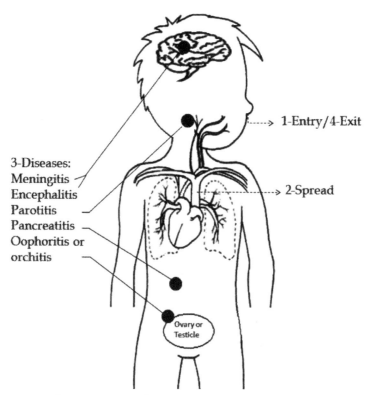

Fig. 3. Pathogenesis of mumps virus infection. Mumps virus is acquired trough the upper-respiratory-tract mucosa (1); where it undergo a first replication, after that new viruses spread (2) to local lymph nodes followed by a systemic spread with involvement of glandular and nervous tissues causing various diseases (3); finally virus is transmitted to another person through droplets or fomites (4). Based on the reference, Enders, 1996.

2.3 Aseptic meningitis and other neurological complications of mumps

Infection of the CNS is the most common extra-salivary gland manifestation of mumps virus infection, being aseptic meningitis the most frequent complication. Although the disease is usually mild should not be underestimated, mumps meningitis affects to 10%-15% of individuals infected by MuV, which is characterized by the sudden onset of fever with signs and symptoms of meningeal involvement as evidenced by changes in cerebrospinal fluid properties, including pleocytosis in absence of bacteria (Bonnet et al., 2006; Plotkin & Rubin, 2007).

Another less frequent but more serious complication of mumps virus infection is encephalitis (0.02-0.3% cases), which can lead to permanent neurologic damage including paralysis, seizures, hydrocephalus and even cause death. Likewise mumps virus infection is a major cause of sensorineural deafness in childhood and affects five per 100,000 patients (Bonnet et al., 2006; Hviid et al., 2008; Plotkin & Rubin, 2007; WHO, 2007).

3. Mumps vaccination

Safe and efficacious vaccines against mumps - based on live, attenuated viral strains – have been available since the 1960s. In most regions of the world the annual incidence of mumps in absence of vaccination ranges from 100 to 1000 per 100 000 of the general population (WHO, 2007). In 2010, the World Health Organization indicated that 61% of countries (figure 4) have incorporated mumps vaccination into their national immunization programs, in most cases using combined measles–mumps–rubella (MMR) vaccine (WHO, 2010).

Countries Using Mumps Vaccine in National Immunization Schedule, 2009

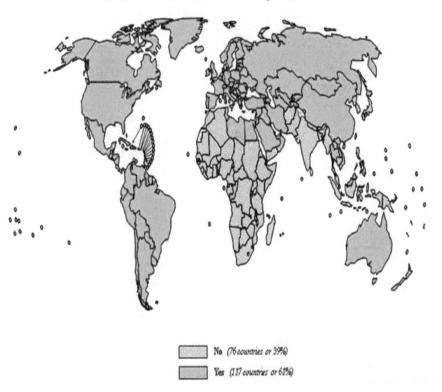

No *(76 countries or 39%)*

Yes *(117 countries or 61%)*

Fig. 4. Countries that have incorporated mumps vaccination in their national immunization programs. Yellow and gray indicate the countries immunized (61%) and unimmunized (39%) respectively. Source: WHO/IVB database, 193 WHO Member States, Data as of July 2010. Date of slide: 19 August 2010.

3.1 Effects of vaccination on epidemic mumps

Use of mumps vaccine (usually administered in measles-mumps-rubella or measles-mumps-rubella-varicella vaccines) is the best way to prevent mumps. Mumps immunization has been effective at controlling epidemic mumps infection and complications associated with it has been drastically reduced,. This is the reason why the WHO defined viral mumps as a disease preventable by vaccination (vaccine-preventable) (WHO, 2007). In countries where there is no vaccination against mumps, its incidence remains high, with epidemic peaks every 2–5 years and those aged 5-9 years consistently being the most affected. In the pre-vaccine era, mumps was a common infectious disease with a high annual incidence, usually >100 per 100 000 population (Dayan et al., 2008; Galazka et al., 1999). It was a very common disease in U.S. children, with as many as 300,000 cases reported every year. After the introduction of mumps virus vaccine in United States in 1967, cases dropped by 98%, from 152,209 cases in 1968 to 2982 cases in 1985. Since 1989, the incidence of mumps has declined, with 266 reported cases in 2001. This decrease is probably due to the fact that children have received a second dose of mumps vaccine (part of the two-dose schedule for measles, mumps, rubella or MMR). Studies have shown that the effectiveness of mumps vaccine ranges from 73% to 91% after 1 dose vaccines and from 79% to 95% after 2 doses. However, we can not let our guard down against viral mumps (Centers for Disease Control and Prevention [CDC], 2010a).

Despite mumps epidemics have decreased from the incorporation of mumps vaccine, in the late 1980s, mumps outbreaks have occurred in both unvaccinated and vaccinated adolescents and young adults. From October 1988 to April 1989 a mumps epidemic was reported in Douglas County, Kansas; of the 269 cases, 208 (77.3%) occurred among primary and secondary school students, of whom 203 (97.6%) had documentation of mumps vaccination. These data suggested that both mumps vaccine failure and the lack of vaccination have contributed to the relative resurgence of mumps. Therefore a change in immunization policy was recommended to two-dose schedule of measles-mumps-rubella vaccine, which should help reduce the occurrence of mumps outbreaks in highly vaccinated populations (Hersh et al., 1991). The widespread use of a second dose of mumps vaccine among U.S. schoolchildren beginning in 1990 was followed by low reports of mumps cases; which was established at 2010 elimination goal, however, various mumps outbreaks have been reported in several countries at different years (Brockhoff et al., 2010; CDC, 2010b; Cheek et al., 1995; Dayan et al., 2008; Dayan & Rubin, 2008; Park et al., 2007; Vandermeulen et al., 2009; Vandermeulen et al., 2004). These reports have suggested that secondary vaccine failure played an important role in mumps outbreaks, thus a more effective mumps vaccine or changes in vaccine policies may be considered to prevent future outbreaks.

3.2 Vaccine strains: preparation, attenuation, induced immune

Mumps vaccines are available in the form of live attenuated virus and may be given alone or in combination with measles and rubella vaccines, according to recommendations from the World Health Organization (WHO, 2007). Mumps viruses are attenuated by adaption in embryonated chicken eggs, chicken or quail embryo fibroblasts or human diploid cells. Through these processes virus mutants are selected because of their increased ability to replicate under new culture conditions but with a reduced capacity to produce disease but stimulating immunity in the natural host (Brown & Wright, 1998; Plotkin & Rubin, 2007).

There are more than 10 strains of mumps virus used as vaccines (Table 1), which induce different levels of seroconversion (80-99%) and protective efficacy (70-95%). Nowadays, the most often used vaccine strains are Jeryl Lynn, RIT 4385, Urabe-AM9, L-Zagreb and Leningrad-3 (Bonnet et al., 2006). The first live attenuated mumps virus vaccine, Jeryl Lynn

B (introduced in the U.S.A in 1967), represents an ideal vaccine because it induces neutralizing antibodies in 95%-98% of vaccinees and few side effects have been associated with its application (Carbone & Rubin, 2007). The Jeryl Lynn strain was attenuated by passage in embryonated hen's eggs and chicken embryo cell culture (Plotkin & Rubin, 2007). The RIT 4385 mumps vaccine was derived from a Jeryl Lynn clone (JL-1) by passage through chicken embryo fibroblast cultures. Comparative studies of the RIT 4385 and Jeryl–Lynn vaccines showed similar seroconversion rates (96-98% for RIT 4385 and 97% for Jeryl Lynn) although the geometric mean titre was significantly higher among recipients of the Jeryl–Lynn vaccine (Crovari et al., 2000; Kanra et al., 2000; Lim et al., 2007). The Urabe Am9 strain was developed by the Biken Institute in Japan from an isolate obtained from the saliva of a mumps patient. Urabe Am9 strain preparations are produced either in the amnion of embryonated hen's eggs or in chicken embryo cell cultures. Seroconversion rates in children aged 12-20 months range from 92-100%. The Rubini mumps vaccine virus was derived from a mumps isolate obtained from the urine of a child in Switzerland in 1974. Comparative efficacy of Rubini, Jeryl-Lynn and Urabe strain mumps vaccine were 80.7, 54.4 and -55.3%, respectively. Thus, Rubini vaccine was discontinued due to poor efficacy (Goh, 1999; Ong et al., 2005). The Leningrad-3 strain was developed in the 1950s in guinea pig kidney cell cultures, with further passages in Japanese quail embryo cultures. The Leningrad-3 vaccine strain has achieved seroconversion rates of 89–98% in children aged 1–7 years and protective efficacy ranged from 92% to 99%. The Leningrad-3 mumps virus was further attenuated in Croatia by adaptation and passages on chicken embryo fibroblast cell cultures. The new mumps strain, designated L-Zagreb, is used in Croatia and India (Bonnet et al., 2006; Plotkin & Rubin, 2007; WHO, 2007).

Vaccine strain	Cell substrate	Sero-conversión	Protective efficacy	Manufacturer	Main area of distribution
Jeryl-Lynn	CWE	80-100%	72.8- 91%	Merck	Worldwide
RIT 4385	CWE	96-98.1%		GlaxoSmithKline	Worldwide
Leningrad- 3	QEF	89-90%	92-99%	Bacterial Medicine Institute, Moscow	Russia
Leningrad-Zagreb	CEF	89-98%	92-99%	Institute of Immunology of Zagreb	Yugoslavia
Urabe AM9	EHE CEF	92-100%	54.4%- 93%	Sanofi Pasteur Biken	Worldwide Japan
Rubini	HDCS	N I	0-33%	Swiss Serum Institute	Discontinued
Hoshino	CEF	N I	N I	Kitasato Institute	Japan
Torii	CEF	N I	N I	Takeda Chemicals	Japan
Miyahara	CEF	N I	N I	Chem-Sero Therapeutic Research Institute	Japan
NL M-46	CEF	N I	N I	Chiba	Japan
S-12	HDCS	N I	N I	Razi State Serum and Vaccine Institute	Iran

NI, No Information; CEF, chicken embryo fibroblasts; HEF, human embryo fibroblasts; QEF, quail embryo fibroblasts; EHE, embryonated hen's eggs; HDCS, human diploid cells.
Information based on the following references: Bonnet et al., 2006; Dayan & Rubin, 2008; Dourado et al., 2000; Galazka et al., 1999; Lim et al., 2007; Peltola et al., 2007; Plotkin & Rubin, 2007; WHO, 2007.

Table 1. Live attenuated mumps vaccine stains.

4. Adverse reactions

In general, adverse reactions to mumps vaccination are rare and mild. Apart from slight soreness and swelling at the injection site, local reactions, low-grade fewer, parotitis, and rashes are the most common adverse events. Occasionally, orchitis and sensorineural deafness have been observed after mumps virus vaccination (WHO, 2007).

In a comparative study of the Jeryl Lynn, Urabe, and Leningrad-Zagreb strains in MMR combination vaccines, the frequency of parotitis in vaccinated children was 0-5%, 1-3%, and 3-1%, respectively, compared with 0-2% in unvaccinated controls (Hviid et al., 2008).

A recent study reported adverse reactions following immunization with MMR vaccine that contain the live attenuated mumps virus Hoshino strain; Parotitis was the most frequent event occurring in 1.8% of recipients, followed by fever and convulsions (0.03%), convulsions (0,16%), encephalopathy (0,004%), and anaphylactic reactions (0,004%) in children vaccinated at 12 months and at 4 to 6 years of age (Esteghamati et al., 2011).

4.1 Post vaccine meningitis

One of the most frequent side effects associated with mumps virus vaccine is aseptic meningitis which is also the most frequent complication of naturally acquired mumps infection (Table 2). In November 2006, the Global Advisory Committee on Vaccine Safety (GACVS) reviewed adverse events following mumps vaccination with special reference to the risk of vaccine associated aseptic meningitis (WHO, 2007). Cases of aseptic meningitis and estimates of incidence rates have been reported following the use of the Urabe Am9, Leningrad–Zagreb, Hoshino, Torii and Miyahara strains from various surveillance systems and epidemiological studies. The reported rate of aseptic meningitis that occurs after vaccination ranges widely, from approximately 1 in 1.8 million doses for the Jeryl Lynn strain to as high as 1 in 1000 for the Leningrad-3 strain (Bonnet et al., 2006). However, due to the variability of the methods used in the different studies, no clear conclusion can be drawn on the differences in risk for this complication among these strains.

Urabe AM9 strain was introduced in Canada and UK in 1986 as part of the MMR vaccine. In September 1992, the Urabe AM9-strain was withdrawn from the market worldwide following data indicating a higher rate of vaccination-related cases of meningitis (Schmitt et al., 1993). Despite this, Urabe AM9 strain continued in use several years later in some developing countries including but not limited to Mexico and Brasil (Dourado et al., 2000; Santos-López et al., 2006).

The first reports suggesting a relationship between MMR vaccine (which contained mumps virus strain Urabe AM9, measles virus strain Schwarz and rubella virus strain RA 27/3) and aseptic meningitis showed an estimated incidence of 1/62,000 administered doses (Furesz & Contreras, 1990). Reports of meningitis in patients immunized with Urabe AM9 strain range from 1/233,000 to 16.6/10,000 administered doses (Kimura et al., 1996; Schmitt et al., 1993). An outbreak of aseptic meningitis following the mass immunization campaign with an Urabe-containing vaccine was reported, with an estimated risk of aseptic meningitis 1 per 14,000 doses. This study confirms a link between measles-mumps-rubella vaccination and aseptic meningitis (Dourado et al., 2000). Likewise, no serious adverse effects have been

Vaccine strain	Genetic heterogeneity	Cases of aseptic meningitis/dose administered	Estimated cases of meningitis/100,000 dose	Reference
Jeryl-Lynn	Composed of two distinct viral strains: JL1 and JL2 (Amexis et al., 2002)	0.1/100,000 to 2/500,000	0,1 to 0,4	Bonnet et al., 2006; Makela et al., 2002
Urabe AM9	Composed of quasispecies mix, (Sauder et al., 2006)	1/233,000 to 16.6/10,000	0,4 to 166	Dourado et al., 2000; Furesz & Contreras, 1990; Kimura et al., 1996; Miller et al., 2007; Rebiere & Galy-Eyraud, 1995; Schmitt et al., 1993; Sugiura & Yamada, 1991
Leningrad-3	Composed more than one viral variant (Boriskin et al., 1992)	2/10,000 to 1/1000	20 to 100	Cizman et al., 1989; Plotkin & Rubin, 2007; WHO, 2007
Leningrad-Zagreb	Composed of two major variants: A and B. (Kosutic-Gulija et al., 2008)	1/19,247 to 1/ 3,390	5,1 to 29,5	Arruda & Kondageski, 2001; da Cunha et al., 2002; da Silveira et al., 2002; Phadke et al., 2004
RIT 4385	One strain, clone JL1 (Tillieux et al., 2009)	1/525,312	0,19	Bonnet et al., 2006; Schlipkoter et al., 2002

Table 2. Genetic heterogeneity and Incidence of postvaccine aseptic meningitis.

related to vaccination with RIT 4385 mumps virus strain (Lim et al., 2007). Little epidemiological information is available for other vaccines. Leningrad-Zagreb strain-containing vaccines have been associated with a high rate of aseptic meningitis (da Cunha et al., 2002; da Silveira et al., 2002); however, other reports indicate no evidence to link Leningrad-Zagreb strain with aseptic meningitis (Kulkarni et al., 2005; Sharma et al., 2010). Although high rates of aseptic meningitis ((1/1000 vaccine recipients) have been reported for vaccines containing Leningrad-3 mumps virus strain the evidence confirming causal association is limited (Cizman et al., 1989).

5. Virulence and attenuation of mumps virus strains

Problems with attenuated virus vaccines generally reflect under- or over-attenuation or lack of efficacy respectively. Different studies have attempted to establish molecular markers allow discrimination between an attenuated strain and a virulent strain, nevertheless, the genetic basis for attenuation are still not completed known for any of the mumps vaccines. Likewise the lack the laboratory studies that assure the absence of residual neurotoxicity in mumps vaccine has been a serious problem, as demonstrated by the occurrence of aseptic meningitis in recipients of certain vaccine strains. Thus, some vaccines found to be neuroattenuated in monkeys were later found to be neurovirulent in humans when administered in large numbers (Rubin & Afzal, 2011).

5.1 Genetic characterization of post vaccination virus isolates (Helvetica, 9pt, bold)

The first reports suggesting a relationship between Urabe AM9 strain with the occurrence of aseptic meningitis, suffer however of a lack of molecular markers to discriminate between vaccine- (attenuated) and wild-type strains of the virus, making it difficult to differentiate whether the patient had an infection caused by vaccine or wild type virus. Several laboratories were able to differentiate Urabe AM9 strain from wild-type isolates of mumps virus by RT-PCR and partial sequence analysis of the P, SH, F and HN genes, confirming that mumps virus isolates from post-vaccination meningitis correspond to Urabe AM9 strain, establishing a causal association of virus strain with post-vaccination meningitis (Brown et al., 1991; Forsey et al., 1990; Yamada et al., 1990).

Analysis of cDNA sequences of several isolates from vaccine-associated meningitis and parotitis cases demonstrated that Urabe AM9 strain consisted of a mixture of virus variants that could be distinguished based on the sequence of the hemagglutinin-neuraminidase gene (HN) at nt 1,081 (nt 7,616 of the genome). Viruses containing an A residue at nt 1081 and encoding a lysine at amino acid position 335 were isolated from cases of post-vaccination parotitis or meningitis whereas viruses containing a G residue at nt 1081 that codes for a glutamic acid (aa 335) were not associated with post-vaccination disease, suggesting A_{1081} (K^{335}) was a marker of neurovirulence and G_{1081} (E^{335}) was a marker of attenuation (Brown et al., 1996). The identification of an A residue at position 1081 in the HN gene sequenced from samples of either patients with post-vaccination meningitis (Afzal et al., 1998; Wright et al., 2000) and patients infected with the wild-type strain (Cusi et al., 1998), supported the previous hypothesis.

However, this hypothesis was questioned by other researchers, reporting that some UrabeAM9 vaccine lots encoding K^{355} did not lead to adverse events in vaccinees (Amexis et al., 2001; Mori et al., 1997). Moreover, K^{335} was also found in the HN glycoprotein of the Jeryl Lynn vaccine strain, a widely used vaccine not associated with aseptic meningitis (Mori et al., 1997). Nonetheless, Jeryl Lynn strain differs from Urabe AM9 at more than 900 nucleotides, so its safety is likely determined by a number of other genetic changes.

By comparison of the HN gene sequences of several Urabe AM9 vaccine derived isolates, Afzal et al., showed that those sequences differed at several other sites (M89V; N464K; N498D), complicating the interpretation of the initial findings (Afzal et al., 1998). Moreover, heterogeneity at position 464 in the HN glycoprotein (Asn464/Lys) was also reported from sequence analysis of Urabe AM9 vaccine virus and post-vaccination meningitis isolates (Afzal et al., 1998; Amexis et al., 2001; Wright et al., 2000). Further, it was shown that Urabe-AM9 strain is constituted by several virus quasispecies that differ in distinct sites all along their genome, with several amino acids changes in the NP, P, L (involved in replication/transcription), F and HN proteins (involved in the recognition, fusion and release of virus in infected cells), as well as in the intergenic region NP-P (Shah et al., 2009). Sauder et al., showed that genetic heterogeneity at the specific genome sites have a profound effect on the neurovirulent phenotype of Urabe-AM9 strain (Sauder et al., 2006), suggesting there is not a unique genetic marker responsible for virus attenuation, rather the combination of mutations may be necessary for an adequate viral attenuation (Amexis et al., 2001; Sauder et al., 2006; Shah et al., 2009).

Different vaccine strains exhibit high degree of nucleotide heterogeneity (table 2) across their entire genome making it impossible to determine which genetic change is associated with neurovirulence or neuroattenuation. At respect, the Jeryl Lynn strain contains a mixture of two substrains (JL1 and JL2) that presented 414 nucleotide differences (2.69%), leading to 87 amino acid substitutions (1.67%). Subsequent passage of Jeryl Lynn strain in Vero or CEF cell cultures resulted in rapid selection of the major component JL1, while growth in embryonated chicken eggs (ECE) favored accumulation of the minor component JL2 (Afzal et al., 1993; Amexis et al., 2002; Chambers et al., 2009). Meanwhile, Leningrad-3 strain was characterized as heterogenic on the basis of plaque morphology and with several ambiguities in P and F genes (Boriskin et al., 1992). L-Zagreb vaccine strain was developed by further subcultivation of Leningrad-3 mumps vaccine strain in primary culture of chicken embryo fibroblast (CEF) and its heterogeneity was identified throughout the entire genome (Kosutic-Gulija et al., 2008).

5.2 Structural, functional and antigenic analysis of mumps virus proteins

Mumps vaccine strains, including L-Zagreb, Leningrad-3 and Urabe AM9, have been associated with a high incidence of post-vaccination aseptic meningitis. Although several researchers have focused to study the genetic basis of mumps virus strains virulence/attenuation, there is not genetic marker that help to discriminate between a virulent strain and an attenuated strain. Previous analyses confirmed that Jeryl Lynn, Urabe-AM9, Leningrad-3 and L-Zagreb mumps virus strains are genetically heterogeneous, where each nucleotide changes may contribute to neurovirulence-neuroattenuation of the vaccine. Therefore, caution should be exercised when evaluating genetic markers because more than one nucleotide can influence the attenuation or virulence of a vaccine (Sauder et al., 2006). By other side, functional analysis of point mutations gives relevant information about the properties of a virus variant. A point mutation from guanine (G) to adenine (A) at nucleotide position 1081 in the hemagglutinin-neuraminidase (HN) gene has been associated with neurovirulence of Urabe AM9 mumps virus vaccine. This mutation corresponds to a glutamic acid (E) to lysine (K) change at position 335 in the HN glycoprotein. We have experimentally demonstrated that two variants of Urabe AM9 strain (HN-A_{1081} and HN-G_{1081}) differ in their replication efficiency in cell culture, where HN-A_{1081} variant was efficiently replicated in both human neuroblastoma cells (SHSY5Y) and newborn rat brain (10^5 and 10^4 PFU respectively), whereas HN-G_{1081} variant was replicated at low titers (10^2 PFU in both cases) (Santos-Lopez et al., 2006). These findings can be explained in part by differences in cell receptor binding affinity of each variant, where HN-A_{1081} variant showed highest affinity towards α2-6 linked sialic acids that are highly expressed in human nerve cells, whereas HN-G_{1081} viral variant showed higher affinity towards α2-3 linked sialic acids that are less expressed in nerve cells, however this latter variant also recognized α2-6 linked sialic acid but with lesser affinity than HNA$_{1081}$ virus (Reyes-Leyva et al., 2007). Controversially, two mumps virus that differ at position 335 (K/E) of HN protein exhibited similar growth kinetics in neuronal (SHSY5Y) and non neuronal cell lines (Vero cells) and similar neurotoxicity when tested in rats models. This suggests that amino acid 335 is not a crucial determinant of Urabe neurovirulence, nevertheless this point mutation can not be excluded as contributing to vaccine virulence (Sauder et al., 2009).

Likewise, we have performed a structure-function analysis of that amino acid substitution, suggesting that the E/K interchange does not affect the structure of the sialic acid binding motif; however, the electrostatic surface differs drastically due to an exposed short alpha helix. Consequently, this mutation may affect the accessibility of HN to substrates and membrane receptors of the host cells (Santos-Lopez et al., 2009). These results suggest that the change K335E affects the biological activity of HN glycoprotein, conferring neurotropism for HN-A$_{1081}$ viral variant as previously proposed (Brown et al., 1996; Wright et al., 2000). Amino acid 335 is located at an important domain of HN glycoprotein that involves the recognition of an antigenic site, thus all virus variants that possess a Glu at position 335 were completely neutralized, while those containing Lys escaped neutralization (Afzal et al., 1998).

Using a rat based model of mumps neurovirulence, Shah et al. demonstrated that viral variants with a Glu at position 335 of HN glycoprotein is significantly attenuated (hydrocephalus 1.37% ± 0.50) compared to a virus isolated from a patient with post-vaccination meningitis (hydrocephalus 4.70%±0.77) and compared with wild type (hydrocephalus 11.47%±1.16) which have Lys at this position (Shah et al., 2009).

The importance of amino acid 464 in the HN glycoprotein was demonstrated by mumps virus reverse genetic, which showed that N464S substitution is involved in virus replication in nerve cells (SH-SY5Y) (Ninomiya et al., 2009). Crystal structure studies of the HN glycoprotein of a closely related paramyxovirus Newcatle disease virus, indicates that amino acid position 466 may be at or near the active site of the HN protein (Crennell et al., 2000), thus the substitution around this site (464) might affect enzymatic activity of HN protein and might change the cell specificity of mumps virus. Amino acids 464-466 form a potential N-liked glycosylation site given that substitutions at this site were predicted to result in loss of N-linked glycosylation, and affect virus tropism and virulence (Rubin et al., 2003). Similarly, Malik et al., demonstrated that Ser-466Asp substitution in the HN protein resulted in decreased receptor binding and neuraminidase activity, Ala91Thr change in the fusion protein resulted in decreased fusion activity, and that Ile736Val substitution in the polymerase resulted in increased replication and transcriptional activity (Malik et al., 2007; Malik et al., 2009).

A study based on the extent of hydrocephalus induced in the rat brain after intracerebral vaccine inoculation showed that expression of the F gene of the neurovirulent Kilman strain alone was sufficient to induce significant levels of hydrocephalus, this experiment confirms the importance of surface glycoproteins in neuropathogenesis (Lemon et al., 2007). Moreover, recent studies done in the rat model demonstrated the ability of nucleoprotein/matrix protein of the Jeryl Lynn vaccine strain to significantly neuroattenuate wild-type 88-1961 strain, which is highly neurovirulent (Sauder et al., 2011)

6. Innate immune response against mumps virus infection

Innate immune response acts as a first line of defense during viral infections, through immunoregulatory mechanisms that increase own innate immune response and stimulate an adaptive immune response. After viral infection, intracellular signaling events are activated and innate cytokine expression are induced as interleukins (IL), tumor necrosis factor (TNF) and interferon (IFN) (Biron & Sen, 2007; Pestka, 2007).

Type-I IFNs (IFN-α/β) are a superfamily of cytokines that were discovered as a result of their induction by and action against virus infections. The interaction between Toll-like receptors (TLR) and pathogen-associated molecular patterns (as genomic RNA and viral proteins), triggers the activation cell signaling pathways that promote activation of some transcription factors such as IRF3 and NFκB, which are necessary to induce expression of IFN-β. Analogously, RNA helicase molecules (RIG-I and mda-5) trigger TLR-independent pathways that respond to viral nucleic acids (such as dsRNA) generated in the cytoplasm by viral replication, causing activation of IRF3 and NFκB, wich also promote the synthesis of IFN-β (Conzelmann, 2005; Honda et al., 2005; Randall & Goodbourn, 2008; Xagorari & Chlichlia, 2008).

The biological activities of IFNs are initiated by the recognition of IFN-α/β receptor (composed of the products of the IFNAR1 and IFNAR2 genes) on the cell surface, which results in the activation of a signaling pathway known as Jak/STAT pathways. This starts by activation of tysosine kinases Tyk2 and Jak1 located in the cytoplasmic tail of IFNAR1 and IFNAR2 subunits respectively (de Weerd et al., 2007; Randall & Goodbourn, 2008). Activation of the signal transduction occurs when Tyk2 phosphorylates Tyr^{466} residue on IFNAR1, creating a docking site for STAT2, which is then phosphorylates on Tyr^{690}. Phosphorylated STAT2 protein associates with STAT1, inducing its phosphorylation on Tyr^{701} by JAK1. Phosporylated Stat2 and Stat1 proteins form a stable heterodimer that creates a nuclear localization signal (NLS) that permits the transport of these dimers into the nucleus until their dephosphorylation (Randall & Goodbourn, 2008; Schindler et al., 2007). In addition, IFNAR2 subunit is acetylated at Lys399 and promotes the acetylation of IRF9, which is essential to DNA binding (Tang et al., 2007). Association of STAT1-STAT2 heterodimer with IRF9 constitutes ISGF3 (IFN-stimulated gene factor 3) a heterotrimeric transcription factor that binds to the IFN-stimulated response element (ISRE), present in the promoters of several IFN-stimulated genes (ISG). The final step of this signaling pathway is the induction of gene transcription whose expression establishes the antiviral state (Biron & Sen, 2007; Randall & Goodbourn, 2008; Schindler et al., 2007; Sen, 2001).

Numerous ISG products have been described such as Caspases, which are involved in cell death; Protein kinase R (PKR) that inhibits both cellular and viral translation, through phosphorylation of NF-κB and eIF2α factor; 2′5′-oligoadenylate synthetase (OAS) that binds to and activates the RNase L, which promotes the degradation cellular and viral RNAs; Mx protein that binds nucleocapsid-like structures, thereby restricting virus replication and assembly (Honda et al., 2005; Randall & Goodbourn, 2008).

6.1 Mumps virus and evasion of innate immune response

Several viruses have evolved strategies to circumvent the antiviral state stimulated by IFN through the expression of proteins that antagonize components of the Jak-Stat signaling pathway, such as the V protein of paramyxoviruses (Gotoh et al., 2002; Randall & Goodbourn, 2008). As mentioned, mumps virus P gene codes for three polypeptides: V, I and P. Their mRNAs are translated by use of overlapping reading frames (ORFs) via cotranscriptional insertion of nontemplated guanidine nucleotides (mRNA edition) (Lamb & Parks, 2007; Paterson & Lamb, 1990). Mumps virus V protein is a nonstructural protein that counteracts the IFN-induced antiviral response by different mechanisms. In some paramyxoviruses V protein interacts with and inhibits the activity of mda-5 (Andrejeva et al., 2004), but not RIG-I (Komatsu et al., 2007); in other viruses V inhibits interferon-mediated antiviral response through degradation of STAT proteins and thus promotes viral replication (Gotoh et al., 2002; Horvath, 2004; Randall & Goodbourn, 2008).

We have shown that two variants of Urabe AM9 vaccine strain (HN-A_{1081} and HN-G_{1081}) that were initially characterized by their difference in the HN gene nt 1081, also differ in their replication efficiency in nerve cells, where HN-A_{1081} variant preferentially infects nerve cells, whereas HN-G_{1081} variant has limited replication in this cells (Santos-Lopez et al., 2006); These results were associated with differences in the virus binding affinity towards cell receptors and enzymatic activity (Reyes-Leyva et al., 2007). Further experiments showed that differences in sensitivity to IFN determined the replication rate of Urabe AM9 mumps virus variants in nerve cells, where HN-G_{1081} variant was more sensitive to interferon (from 102.5 to 101.3 TCID50) than HN-A_{1081} variant (from 103.5 to 102.6 TCID50). Moreover HN-A_{1081} virus reduced the transcription of cellular IFN responsive genes such as STAT1, STA2, p48 and MxA in both unprimed and IFN-primed cells, whereas HN-G_{1081} virus just reduced MxA transcription. Sensitivity to IFN was associated with insertion of a non-coded glycine at position 156 in the V protein (V_{Gly}) of HN-G_{1081} virus variant, whereas resistance to IFN was associated with preservation of wild-type phenotype in the V protein (V_{WT}) of HN-A_{1081} virus variant (Rosas-Murrieta et al., 2007). Functional analysis of Gly 156 insertion suggested that V_{WT} protein may be more efficient than V_{Gly} protein to inactivate both the IFN signaling pathway and antiviral response due to differences in their finest molecular interaction with STAT proteins (Rosas-Murrieta et al., 2010).

On the other hand the activation of the JAK-STAT pathway by IFN simultaneously activates other processes regulated by IFN such as apoptosis. We studied the relationship between V protein variants of Urabe AM9 vaccine strain and IFN-α induced apoptosis. Our results indicated that V proteins decrease the levels of caspases and DNA fragmentation, suggesting that V_{WT} protein is a better modulator of apoptosis than Vgly in the vaccine strain (Rosas-Murrieta et al., 2011).

7. Conclusions

Several strains of mumps virus used as attenuated vaccines have been associated with post-vaccination meningitis. Experimental data indicates that neurovirulence is a complex issue that involves multiple components either viral or cellular. Further studies are in progress to recognize the role of these in viral attenuation and virulence.

8. References

Afzal, M.A.; Pickford, A.R.; Forsey, T.; Heath, A.B. & Minor, P.D. (1993). The Jeryl Lynn vaccine strain of mumps virus is a mixture of two distinct isolates. *J Gen Virol*, Vol.74 (Pt 5), pp.917-920, ISSN 0022-1317

Afzal, M.A.; Yates, P.J. & Minor, P.D. (1998). Nucleotide sequence at position 1081 of the hemagglutinin-neuraminidase gene in the mumps Urabe vaccine strain. *J Infect Dis*, Vol.177, No.1, pp.265-266, ISSN 0022-1899

Amexis, G.; Fineschi, N. & Chumakov, K. (2001). Correlation of genetic variability with safety of mumps vaccine Urabe AM9 strain. *Virology*, Vol.287, No.1, pp.234-241, ISSN 0042-6822

Amexis, G.; Rubin, S.; Chizhikov, V.; Pelloquin, F.; Carbone, K. & Chumakov, K. (2002). Sequence diversity of Jeryl Lynn strain of mumps virus: quantitative mutant analysis for vaccine quality control. *Virology*, Vol.300, No.2, pp.171-179, ISSN 0042-6822

Andrejeva, J.; Childs, K.S.; Young, D.F.; Carlos, T.S.; Stock, N.; Goodbourn, S. & Randall, R.E. (2004). The V proteins of paramyxoviruses bind the IFN-inducible RNA helicase, mda-5, and inhibit its activation of the IFN-beta promoter. *Proc Natl Acad Sci U S A*, Vol.101, No.49, pp.17264-17269, ISSN 0027-8424

Arruda, W.O. & Kondageski, C. (2001). Aseptic meningitis in a large MMR vaccine campaign (590,609 people) in Curitiba, Parana, Brazil, 1998. *Rev Inst Med Trop Sao Paulo*, Vol.43, No.5, pp.301-302, ISSN 0036-4665

Biron, C.A. & Sen, G. (2007). Innate responses to viral infections, In: *Fields Virology*, D.M. Knipe & P.M. Howley (Eds.), pp. 250-277, Lippincott Williams & Wilkins, ISBN 0781760607.

Bonnet, M.C.; Dutta, A.; Weinberger, C. & Plotkin, S.A. (2006). Mumps vaccine virus strains and aseptic meningitis. *Vaccine*, Vol.24, No.49-50, pp.7037-7045, ISSN 0264-410X

Boriskin, Y.S.; Yamada, A.; Kaptsova, T.I.; Skvortsova, O.I.; Sinitsyna, O.A.; Takeuchi, K.; Tanabayashi, K. & Sugiura, A. (1992). Genetic evidence for variant selection in the course of dilute passaging of mumps vaccine virus. *Res Virol*, Vol.143, No.4, pp.279-283, ISSN 0923-2516

Brockhoff, H.J.; Mollema, L.; Sonder, G.J.; Postema, C.A.; van Binnendijk, R.S.; Kohl, R.H.; de Melker, H.E. & Hahne, S.J. (2010). Mumps outbreak in a highly vaccinated student population, The Netherlands, 2004. *Vaccine*, Vol.28, No.17, pp.2932-2936, ISSM 1873-2518

Brown, E.G.; Dimock, K. & Wright, K.E. (1996). The Urabe AM9 mumps vaccine is a mixture of viruses differing at amino acid 335 of the hemagglutinin-neuraminidase gene with one form associated with disease. *J Infect Dis*, Vol.174, No.3, pp.619-622, ISSN 0022-1899

Brown, E.G.; Furesz, J.; Dimock, K.; Yarosh, W. & Contreras, G. (1991). Nucleotide sequence analysis of Urabe mumps vaccine strain that caused meningitis in vaccine recipients. *Vaccine*, Vol.9, No.11, pp.840-842, ISSN 0264-410X

Brown, E.G. & Wright, K.E. (1998). Genetic studies on a mumps vaccine strain associated with meningitis. *Rev Med Virol*, Vol.8, No.3, pp.129-142, ISSN 1099-1654

Carbone, K.M. & Rubin, S. (2007). Mumps virus, In: *Fields Virology*, D.M. Knipe & P.M. Howley (Eds.), pp. 1528-1551, Lippincott Williams & Wilkins, ISBN 0781760607.

CDC. Basics and Common Questions: What Would Happen If We Stopped Vaccinations?, Available from: http://www.cdc.gov/vaccines/vac-gen/whatifstop.htm#mumps

CDC (October 2010). Mumps outbreaks, In: *Mumps*, Available from: http://www.cdc.gov/mumps/outbreaks.html

Cizman, M.; Mozetic, M.; Radescek-Rakar, R.; Pleterski-Rigler, D. & Susec-Michieli, M. (1989). Aseptic meningitis after vaccination against measles and mumps. *Pediatr Infect Dis J*, Vol.8, No.5, pp.302-308, ISSN 0891-3668

Conzelmann, K.K. (2005). Transcriptional activation of alpha/beta interferon genes: interference by nonsegmented negative-strand RNA viruses. *J Virol*, Vol.79, No.9, pp.5241-5248, ISSN 0022-538X

Crennell, S.; Takimoto, T.; Portner, A. & Taylor, G. (2000). Crystal structure of the multifunctional paramyxovirus hemagglutinin-neuraminidase. *Nat Struct Biol,* Vol.7, No.11, pp.1068-1074, ISSN 1072-8368

Crovari, P.; Gabutti, G.; Giammanco, G.; Dentico, P.; Moiraghi, A.R.; Ponzio, F. & Soncini, R. (2000). Reactogenicity and immunogenicity of a new combined measles-mumps-rubella vaccine: results of a multicentre trial. The Cooperative Group for the Study of MMR vaccines. *Vaccine,* Vol.18, No.25, pp.2796-2803, ISSN 0264-410X

Cusi, M.G.; Santini, L.; Bianchi, S.; Valassina, M. & Valensin, P.E. (1998). Nucleotide sequence at position 1081 of the hemagglutinin-neuraminidasegene in wild-type strains of mumps virus is the most relevant marker of virulence. *J Clin Microbiol,* Vol.36, No.12, pp.3743-3744, ISSN 0095-1137

Chambers, P.; Rima, B.K. & Duprex, W.P. (2009). Molecular differences between two Jeryl Lynn mumps virus vaccine component strains, JL5 and JL2. *J Gen Virol,* Vol.90, No.Pt 12, pp.2973-2981, ISSN 1465-2099

Cheek, J.E.; Baron, R.; Atlas, H.; Wilson, D.L. & Crider, R.D., Jr. (1995). Mumps outbreak in a highly vaccinated school population. Evidence for large-scale vaccination failure. *Arch Pediatr Adolesc Med,* Vol.149, No.7, pp.774-778, ISSN 1072-4710

Choi, K.M. (2010). Reemergence of mumps. *Korean J Pediatr,* Vol.53, No.5, pp.623-628, ISSN 2092-7258.

da Cunha, S.S.; Rodrigues, L.C.; Barreto, M.L. & Dourado, I. (2002). Outbreak of aseptic meningitis and mumps after mass vaccination with MMR vaccine using the Leningrad-Zagreb mumps strain. *Vaccine,* Vol.20, No.7-8, pp.1106-1112, ISSN 0264-410X.

da Silveira, C.M.; Kmetzsch, C.I.; Mohrdieck, R.; Sperb, A.F. & Prevots, D.R. (2002). The risk of aseptic meningitis associated with the Leningrad-Zagreb mumps vaccine strain following mass vaccination with measles-mumps-rubella vaccine, Rio Grande do Sul, Brazil, 1997. *Int J Epidemiol,* Vol.31, No.5, pp.978-982, ISSN 0300-5771.

Dayan, G.H.; Quinlisk, M.P.; Parker, A.A.; Barskey, A.E.; Harris, M.L.; Schwartz, J.M.; Hunt, K.; Finley, C.G.; Leschinsky, D.P.; O'Keefe, A.L.; Clayton, J.; Kightlinger, L.K.; Dietle, E.G.; Berg, J.; Kenyon, C.L.; Goldstein, S.T.; Stokley, S.K.; Redd, S.B.; Rota, P.A.; Rota, J.; Bi, D.; Roush, S.W.; Bridges, C.B.; Santibanez, T.A.; Parashar, U.; Bellini, W.J. & Seward, J.F. (2008). Recent resurgence of mumps in the United States. *N Engl J Med,* Vol.358, No.15, pp.1580-1589, ISSN 1533-4406.

Dayan, G.H. & Rubin, S. (2008). Mumps outbreaks in vaccinated populations: are available mumps vaccines effective enough to prevent outbreaks? *Clin Infect Dis,* Vol.47, No.11, pp.1458-1467, ISSN 1537-6591

de Weerd, N.A.; Samarajiwa, S.A. & Hertzog, P.J. (2007). Type I interferon receptors: biochemistry and biological functions. *J Biol Chem,* Vol.282, No.28, pp.20053-20057, ISSN 0021-9258

Didcock, L.; Young, D.F.; Goodbourn, S. & Randall, R.E. (1999a). Sendai virus and simian virus 5 block activation of interferon-responsive genes: importance for virus pathogenesis. *J Virol,* Vol.73, No.4, pp.3125-3133, ISSN 0022-538X

Didcock, L.; Young, D.F.; Goodbourn, S. & Randall, R.E. (1999b). The V protein of simian virus 5 inhibits interferon signalling by targeting STAT1 for proteasome-mediated degradation. *J Virol,* Vol.73, No.12, pp.9928-9933, ISSN 0022-538X.

Dourado, I.; Cunha, S.; Teixeira, M.G.; Farrington, C.P.; Melo, A.; Lucena, R. & Barreto, M.L. (2000). Outbreak of aseptic meningitis associated with mass vaccination with a urabe-containing measles-mumps-rubella vaccine: implications for immunization programs. *Am J Epidemiol,* Vol.151, No.5, pp.524-530, ISSN 0002-9262

Enders, G. (1996). Paramyxoviruses, In: *Medical Microbiolog*, S. Baron (Ed), The University of Texas Medical Branch at Galveston, ISBN-10: 0-9631172-1-1, Galveston, Texas.

Esteghamati, A.; Keshtkar, A.; Heshmat, R.; Gouya, M.M.; Salar Amoli, M.; Armin, S. & Mahoney, F. (2011). Adverse reactions following immunization with MMR vaccine in children at selected provinces of Iran. *Arch Iran Med*, Vol.14, No.2, pp.91-95, ISSN 1029-2977.

Fleischer, B. & Kreth, H.W. (1982). Mumps virus replication in human lymphoid cell lines and in peripheral blood lymphocytes: preference for T cells. *Infect Immun*, Vol.35, No.1, pp.25-31, ISSN 0019-9567

Forsey, T.; Mawn, J.A.; Yates, P.J.; Bentley, M.L. & Minor, P.D. (1990). Differentiation of vaccine and wild mumps viruses using the polymerase chain reaction and dideoxynucleotide sequencing. *J Gen Virol*, Vol.71 (Pt 4), pp.987-990, ISSN 0022-1317.

Fujii, N.; Yokosawa, N. & Shirakawa, S. (1999). Suppression of interferon response gene expression in cells persistently infected with mumps virus, and restoration from its suppression by treatment with ribavirin. *Virus Res*, Vol.65, No.2, pp.175-185, ISSN 0168-1702

Furesz, J. & Contreras, G. (1990). Vaccine-related mumps meningitis--Canada. *Can Dis Wkly Rep*, Vol.16, No.50, pp.253-254, ISSN 0382-232X

Galazka, A.M.; Robertson, S.E. & Kraigher, A. (1999). Mumps and mumps vaccine: a global review. *Bull World Health Organ*, Vol.77, No.1, pp.3-14, ISSN 0042-9686.

Goh, K.T. (1999). Resurgence of mumps in Singapore caused by the Rubini mumps virus vaccine strain. *Lancet*, Vol.354, No.9187, pp.1355-1356, ISSN 0140-6736

Gotoh, B.; Komatsu, T.; Takeuchi, K. & Yokoo, J. (2002). Paramyxovirus strategies for evading the interferon response. *Rev Med Virol*, Vol.12, No.6, pp.337-357, ISSN 1052-9276

Hausmann, S.; Garcin, D.; Delenda, C. & Kolakofsky, D. (1999). The versatility of paramyxovirus RNA polymerase stuttering. *J Virol*, Vol.73, No.7, pp.5568-5576, ISSN 0022-538X

Hersh, B.S.; Fine, P.E.; Kent, W.K.; Cochi, S.L.; Kahn, L.H.; Zell, E.R.; Hays, P.L. & Wood, C.L. (1991). Mumps outbreak in a highly vaccinated population. *J Pediatr*, Vol.119, No.2, pp.187-193, ISSN 0022-3476

Honda, K.; Yanai, H.; Takaoka, A. & Taniguchi, T. (2005). Regulation of the type I IFN induction: a current view. *Int Immunol*, Vol.17, No.11, pp.1367-1378, ISSN 0953-8178

Horvath, C.M. (2004). Weapons of STAT destruction. Interferon evasion by paramyxovirus V protein. *Eur J Biochem*, Vol.271, No.23-24, pp.4621-4628, ISSN 0014-2956

Hviid, A.; Rubin, S. & Muhlemann, K. (2008). Mumps. *Lancet*, Vol.371, No.9616, pp.932-944, ISSN 1474-547X

Kanra, G.; Ceyhan, M. & Ozmert, E. (2000). Reactogenicity and immunogenicity of a new measles-mumps-rubella vaccine containing RIT 4385 mumps virus strain in healthy Turkish children. *Turk J Pediatr*, Vol.42, No.4, pp.275-277, ISSN 0041-4301.

Kimura, M.; Kuno-Sakai, H.; Yamazaki, S.; Yamada, A.; Hishiyama, M.; Kamiya, H.; Ueda, K.; Murase, T.; Hirayama, M.; Oya, A.; Nozaki, S. & Murata, R. (1996). Adverse events associated with MMR vaccines in Japan. *Acta Paediatr Jpn*, Vol.38, No.3, pp.205-211, ISSN 0374-5600.

Kingston, R.L.; Hamel, D.J.; Gay, L.S.; Dahlquist, F.W. & Matthews, B.W. (2004). Structural basis for the attachment of a paramyxoviral polymerase to its template. *Proc Natl Acad Sci U S A*, Vol.101, No.22, pp.8301-8306, ISSN 0027-8424.

Kolakofsky, D.; Pelet, T.; Garcin, D.; Hausmann, S.; Curran, J. & Roux, L. (1998). Paramyxovirus RNA synthesis and the requirement for hexamer genome length: the rule of six revisited. *J Virol*, Vol.72, No.2, pp.891-899, ISSN 0022-538X

Kolakofsky, D.; Roux, L.; Garcin, D. & Ruigrok, R.W. (2005). Paramyxovirus mRNA editing, the "rule of six" and error catastrophe: a hypothesis. *J Gen Virol*, Vol.86, No.Pt 7, pp.1869-1877, ISSN 0022-1317

Komatsu, T.; Takeuchi, K. & Gotoh, B. (2007). Bovine parainfluenza virus type 3 accessory proteins that suppress beta interferon production. *Microbes Infect*, Vol.9, No.8, pp.954-962, ISSN 1286-4579

Kosutic-Gulija, T.; Forcic, D.; Santak, M.; Ramljak, A.; Mateljak-Lukacevic, S. & Mazuran, R. (2008). Genetic heterogeneity of L-Zagreb mumps virus vaccine strain. *Virol J*, Vol.5, pp.79, ISSN 1743-422X

Kulkarni, P.S.; Phadke, M.A.; Jadhav, S.S. & Kapre, S.V. (2005). No definitive evidence for L-Zagreb mumps strain associated aseptic meningitis: a review with special reference to the da Cunha study. *Vaccine*, Vol.23, No.46-47, pp.5286-5288, ISSN 0264-410X

Lamb, R.A. & Parks, G.D. (2007). Paramyxoviridae: The viruses and their replication, In: *Fields Virology*, D.M. Knipe & P.M. Howley (Eds.), pp. 1450- 1497, Lippincott Williams & Wilkins, ISBN 0781760607.

Lemon, K.; Rima, B.K.; McQuaid, S.; Allen, I.V. & Duprex, W.P. (2007). The F gene of rodent brain-adapted mumps virus is a major determinant of neurovirulence. *J Virol*, Vol.81, No.15, pp.8293-8302, ISSN 0022-538X

Lim, F.S.; Han, H.H. & Bock, H.L. (2007). Safety, reactogenicity and immunogenicity of the live attenuated combined measles, mumps and rubella vaccine containing the RIT 4385 mumps strain in healthy Singaporean children. *Ann Acad Med Singapore*, Vol.36, No.12, pp.969-973, ISSN 0304-4602

Makela, A.; Nuorti, J.P. & Peltola, H. (2002). Neurologic disorders after measles-mumps-rubella vaccination. *Pediatrics*, Vol.110, No.5, pp.957-963, ISSN 1098-4275

Malik, T.; Shegogue, C.W.; Werner, K.; Ngo, L.; Sauder, C.; Zhang, C.; Duprex, W.P. & Rubin, S. (2011). Discrimination of mumps virus small hydrophobic gene deletion effects from gene translation effects on virus virulence. *J Virol*, Vol.85, No.12, pp.6082-6085, ISSN 1098-5514.

Malik, T.; Wolbert, C.; Mauldin, J.; Sauder, C.; Carbone, K.M. & Rubin, S.A. (2007). Functional consequences of attenuating mutations in the haemagglutinin neuraminidase, fusion and polymerase proteins of a wild-type mumps virus strain. *J Gen Virol*, Vol.88, No.Pt 9, pp.2533-2541, ISSN 0022-1317

Malik, T.H.; Wolbert, C.; Nerret, L.; Sauder, C. & Rubin, S. (2009). Single amino acid changes in the mumps virus haemagglutinin-neuraminidase and polymerase proteins are associated with neuroattenuation. *J Gen Virol*, Vol.90, No.Pt 7, pp.1741-1747, ISSN 0022-1317

Miller, E.; Andrews, N.; Stowe, J.; Grant, A.; Waight, P. & Taylor, B. (2007). Risks of convulsion and aseptic meningitis following measles-mumps-rubella vaccination in the United Kingdom. *Am J Epidemiol*, Vol.165, No.6, pp.704-709, ISSN 0002-9262.

Mori, C.; Tooriyama, T.; Imagawa, T. & Yamanishi, K. (1997). Nucleotide sequence at position 1081 of the hemagglutinin-neuraminidase gene in the mumps virus Urabe vaccine strain. *J Infect Dis*, Vol.175, No.6, pp.1548-1549, ISSN 0022-1899.

Ninomiya, K.; Kanayama, T.; Fujieda, N.; Nakayama, T.; Komase, K.; Nagata, K. & Takeuchi, K. (2009). Amino acid substitution at position 464 in the haemagglutinin-neuraminidase protein of a mumps virus Urabe strain enhanced the virus growth in neuroblastoma SH-SY5Y cells. *Vaccine*, Vol.27, No.44, pp.6160-6165, ISSN 1873-2518

Ong, G.; Goh, K.T.; Ma, S. & Chew, S.K. (2005). Comparative efficacy of Rubini, Jeryl-Lynn and Urabe mumps vaccine in an Asian population. *J Infect*, Vol.51, No.4, pp.294-298, ISSN 1532-2742

Orvell, C.; Kalantari, M. & Johansson, B. (1997). Characterization of five conserved genotypes of the mumps virus small hydrophobic (SH) protein gene. *J Gen Virol*, Vol.78 (Pt 1), pp.91-95, ISSN 0022-1317

Park, D.W.; Nam, M.H.; Kim, J.Y.; Kim, H.J.; Sohn, J.W.; Cho, Y.; Song, K.J. & Kim, M.J. (2007). Mumps outbreak in a highly vaccinated school population: assessment of secondary vaccine failure using IgG avidity measurements. *Vaccine*, Vol.25, No.24, pp.4665-4670, ISSN 0264-410X

Paterson, R.G. & Lamb, R.A. (1990). RNA editing by G-nucleotide insertion in mumps virus P-gene mRNA transcripts. *J Virol*, Vol.64, No.9, pp.4137-4145, ISSN 0022-538X

Peltola, H.; Kulkarni, P.S.; Kapre, S.V.; Paunio, M.; Jadhav, S.S. & Dhere, R.M. (2007). Mumps outbreaks in Canada and the United States: time for new thinking on mumps vaccines. *Clin Infect Dis*, Vol.45, No.4, pp.459-466, ISSN 1537-6591

Pestka, S. (2007). The interferons: 50 years after their discovery, there is much more to learn. *J Biol Chem*, Vol.282, No.28, pp.20047-20051, ISSN 0021-9258

Phadke, M.A.; Patki, P.S.; Kulkarni, P.S.; Jadhav, S.S. & Kapre, S.V. (2004). Pharmacovigilance on MMR vaccine containing L-Zagreb mumps strain. *Vaccine*, Vol.22, No.31-32, pp.4135-4136, ISSN 0264-410X.

Plotkin, S.A. & Rubin, S.A. (December 2007). Mumps vaccine In: *Vaccines*, Available from <http://www.thelancetglobalhealthnetwork.com/wp-content/uploads/2008/03/plotkins_ch020-x3611.PDF>

Pringle, C.R. (1997). The order Mononegavirales--current status. *Arch Virol*, Vol.142, No.11, pp.2321-2326, ISSN 0304-8608

Randall, R.E. & Goodbourn, S. (2008). Interferons and viruses: an interplay between induction, signalling, antiviral responses and virus countermeasures. *J Gen Virol*, Vol.89, No.Pt 1, pp.1-47, ISSN 0022-1317

Rebiere, I. & Galy-Eyraud, C. (1995). Estimation of the risk of aseptic meningitis associated with mumps vaccination, France, 1991-1993. *Int J Epidemiol*, Vol.24, No.6, pp.1223-1227, ISSN 0300-5771.

Reyes-Leyva, J.; Banos, R.; Borraz-Arguello, M.; Santos-Lopez, G.; Rosas, N.; Alvarado, G.; Herrera, I.; Vallejo, V. & Tapia-Ramirez, J. (2007). Amino acid change 335 E to K affects the sialic-acid-binding and neuraminidase activities of Urabe AM9 mumps virus hemagglutinin-neuraminidase glycoprotein. *Microbes Infect*, Vol.9, No.2, pp.234-240, ISSN 1286-4579

Rodriguez, J.J.; Wang, L.F. & Horvath, C.M. (2003). Hendra virus V protein inhibits interferon signaling by preventing STAT1 and STAT2 nuclear accumulation. *J Virol*, Vol.77, No.21, pp.11842-11845, ISSN 0022-538X

Rosas-Murrieta, N.; Herrera-Camacho, I.; Vallejo-Ruiz, V.; Millan-Perez-Pena, L.; Cruz, C.; Tapia-Ramirez, J.; Santos-Lopez, G. & Reyes-Leyva, J. (2007). Differential sensitivity to interferon influences the replication and transcription of Urabe AM9 mumps virus variants in nerve cells. *Microbes Infect*, Vol.9, No.7, pp.864-872, ISSN 1286-4579.

Rosas-Murrieta, N.H.; Herrera-Camacho, I.; Palma-Ocampo, H.; Santos-Lopez, G. & Reyes-Leyva, J. (2010). Interaction of mumps virus V protein variants with STAT1-STAT2 heterodimer: experimental and theoretical studies. *Virol J*, Vol.7, pp.263, ISSN 1743-422X.

Rosas-Murrieta, N.H.; Santos-Lopez, G.; Reyes-Leyva, J.; Jurado, F.S. & Herrera-Camacho, I. (2011). Modulation of apoptosis by V protein mumps virus. *Virol J*, Vol.8, pp.224, ISSN 1743-422X

Rubin, S.A. & Afzal, M.A. (2011). Neurovirulence safety testing of mumps vaccines--historical perspective and current status. *Vaccine*, Vol.29, No.16, pp.2850-2855, ISSN 1873-2518

Rubin, S.A.; Amexis, G.; Pletnikov, M.; Li, Z.; Vanderzanden, J.; Mauldin, J.; Sauder, C.; Malik, T.; Chumakov, K. & Carbone, K.M. (2003). Changes in mumps virus gene sequence associated with variability in neurovirulent phenotype. *J Virol*, Vol.77, No.21, pp.11616-11624, ISSN 0022-538X

Santos-Lopez, G.; Cruz, C.; Pazos, N.; Vallejo, V.; Reyes-Leyva, J. & Tapia-Ramirez, J. (2006). Two clones obtained from Urabe AM9 mumps virus vaccine differ in their replicative efficiency in neuroblastoma cells. *Microbes Infect*, Vol.8, No.2, pp.332-339, ISSN 1286-4579

Santos-López, G.; Hernández, J.; Borraz-Argüello, M.T.; Ramírez -Mendoza, H.; Vallejo, V. & Reyes-Leyva, J. (2004). Estructura, función e implicaciones patológicas de las proteínas del Rubulavirus porcino. *Arch. med. vet. [online]*, Vol.36, No.2, pp.119-136, ISSN 0301-732X.

Santos-Lopez, G.; Scior, T.; Borraz-Arguello Mdel, T.; Vallejo-Ruiz, V.; Herrera-Camacho, I.; Tapia-Ramirez, J. & Reyes-Leyva, J. (2009). Structure-function analysis of two variants of mumps virus hemagglutinin-neuraminidase protein. *Braz J Infect Dis*, Vol.13, No.1, pp.24-34, ISSN 1678-4391

Sauder, C.J.; Vandenburgh, K.M.; Iskow, R.C.; Malik, T.; Carbone, K.M. & Rubin, S.A. (2006). Changes in mumps virus neurovirulence phenotype associated with quasispecies heterogeneity. *Virology*, Vol.350, No.1, pp.48-57, ISSN 0042-6822

Sauder, C.J.; Zhang, C.X.; Link, M.A.; Duprex, W.P.; Carbone, K.M. & Rubin, S.A. (2009). Presence of lysine at aa 335 of the hemagglutinin-neuraminidase protein of mumps virus vaccine strain Urabe AM9 is not a requirement for neurovirulence. *Vaccine*, Vol.27, No.42, pp.5822-5829, ISSN 1873-2518.

Sauder, C.J.; Zhang, C.X.; Ngo, L.; Werner, K.; Lemon, K.; Duprex, W.P.; Malik, T.; Carbone, K. & Rubin, S.A. (2011). Gene-specific contributions to mumps virus neurovirulence and neuroattenuation. *J Virol*, Vol.85, No.14, pp.7059-7069, ISSN 1098-5514.

Schindler, C.; Levy, D.E. & Decker, T. (2007). JAK-STAT signaling: from interferons to cytokines. *J Biol Chem*, Vol.282, No.28, pp.20059-20063, ISSN 0021-9258

Schlipkoter, U.; Muhlberger, N.; von Kries, R. & Weil, J. (2002). Surveillance of measles-mumps-rubella vaccine-associated aseptic meningitis in Germany. *Infection*, Vol.30, No.6, pp.351-355, ISSN 0300-8126.

Schmitt, H.J.; Just, M. & Neiss, A. (1993). Withdrawal of a mumps vaccine: reasons and impacts. *Eur J Pediatr*, Vol.152, No.5, pp.387-388, ISSN 0340-6199

Sen, G.C. (2001). Viruses and interferons. *Annu Rev Microbiol*, Vol.55, pp.255-281, ISSN 0066-4227

Shah, D.; Vidal, S.; Link, M.A.; Rubin, S.A. & Wright, K.E. (2009). Identification of genetic mutations associated with attenuation and changes in tropism of Urabe mumps virus. *J Med Virol*, Vol.81, No.1, pp.130-138, ISSN 1096-9071.

Sharma, H.J.; Oun, S.A.; Bakr, S.S.; Kapre, S.V.; Jadhav, S.S.; Dhere, R.M. & Bhardwaj, S. (2010). No demonstrable association between the Leningrad-Zagreb mumps vaccine strain and aseptic meningitis in a large clinical trial in Egypt. *Clin Microbiol Infect*, Vol.16, No.4, pp.347-352, ISSN 1469-0691.

Sugiura, A. & Yamada, A. (1991). Aseptic meningitis as a complication of mumps vaccination. *Pediatr Infect Dis J*, Vol.10, No.3, pp.209-213, ISSN 0891-3668

Tang, X.; Gao, J.S.; Guan, Y.J.; McLane, K.E.; Yuan, Z.L.; Ramratnam, B. & Chin, Y.E. (2007). Acetylation-dependent signal transduction for type I interferon receptor. *Cell*, Vol.131, No.1, pp.93-105, ISSN 0092-8674

Tillieux, S.L.; Halsey, W.S.; Sathe, G.M. & Vassilev, V. (2009). Comparative analysis of the complete nucleotide sequences of measles, mumps, and rubella strain genomes contained in Priorix-Tetra and ProQuad live attenuated combined vaccines. *Vaccine*, Vol.27, No.16, pp.2265-2273, ISSN 0264-410X

Vandermeulen, C.; Leroux-Roels, G. & Hoppenbrouwers, K. (2009). Mumps outbreaks in highly vaccinated populations: What makes good even better? *Hum Vaccin*, Vol.5, No.7, pp.494-496, ISSN 1554-8619

Vandermeulen, C.; Roelants, M.; Vermoere, M.; Roseeuw, K.; Goubau, P. & Hoppenbrouwers, K. (2004). Outbreak of mumps in a vaccinated child population: a question of vaccine failure? *Vaccine*, Vol.22, No.21-22, pp.2713-2716, ISSN 0264-410X

Vidal, S.; Curran, J. & Kolakofsky, D. (1990). A stuttering model for paramyxovirus P mRNA editing. *EMBO J*, Vol.9, No.6, pp.2017-2022, ISSN 0261-4189

Vulliemoz, D. & Roux, L. (2001). "Rule of six": how does the Sendai virus RNA polymerase keep count? *J Virol*, Vol.75, No.10, pp.4506-4518, ISSN 0022-538X

WHO (February 2007). Mumps virus vaccines, In: *Weekly Epidemiological Record (WER)* Available from: http://www.who.int/wer/2007/wer8207/en/index.html

WHO (December 2010). Mumps, In: *Immunization surveillance, assessment and monitoring*, Available from:
http://www.who.int/immunization_monitoring/diseases/mumps/en/index.html

Wilson, R.L.; Fuentes, S.M.; Wang, P.; Taddeo, E.C.; Klatt, A.; Henderson, A.J. & He, B. (2006). Function of small hydrophobic proteins of paramyxovirus. *J Virol*, Vol.80, No.4, pp.1700-1709, ISSN 0022-538X.

Wolinsky, J.S.; Klassen, T. & Baringer, J.R. (1976). Persistence of neuroadapted mumps virus in brains of newborn hamsters after intraperitoneal inoculation. *J Infect Dis*, Vol.133, No.3, pp.260-267, ISSN 0022-1899.

Woznik, M.; Rodner, C.; Lemon, K.; Rima, B.; Mankertz, A. & Finsterbusch, T. (2010). Mumps virus small hydrophobic protein targets ataxin-1 ubiquitin-like interacting protein (ubiquilin 4). *J Gen Virol*, Vol.91, No.Pt 11, pp.2773-2781, ISSN 1465-2099.

Wright, K.E.; Dimock, K. & Brown, E.G. (2000). Biological characteristics of genetic variants of Urabe AM9 mumps vaccine virus. *Virus Res*, Vol.67, No.1, pp.49-57, ISSN 0168-1702

Xagorari, A. & Chlichlia, K. (2008). Toll-like receptors and viruses: induction of innate antiviral immune responses. *Open Microbiol J*, Vol.2, pp.49-59, ISSN 1874-2858.

Yamada, A.; Takeuchi, K.; Tanabayashi, K.; Hishiyama, M.; Takahashi, Y. & Sugiura, A. (1990). Differentiation of the mumps vaccine strains from the wild viruses by the nucleotide sequences of the P gene. *Vaccine*, Vol.8, No.6, pp.553-557, ISSN 0264-410X.

Permissions

The contributors of this book come from diverse backgrounds, making this book a truly international effort. This book will bring forth new frontiers with its revolutionizing research information and detailed analysis of the nascent developments around the world.

We would like to thank Dr. Priti Kumar Roy, for lending her expertise to make the book truly unique. She has played a crucial role in the development of this book. Without her invaluable contribution this book wouldn't have been possible. She has made vital efforts to compile up to date information on the varied aspects of this subject to make this book a valuable addition to the collection of many professionals and students.

This book was conceptualized with the vision of imparting up-to-date information and advanced data in this field. To ensure the same, a matchless editorial board was set up. Every individual on the board went through rigorous rounds of assessment to prove their worth. After which they invested a large part of their time researching and compiling the most relevant data for our readers. Conferences and sessions were held from time to time between the editorial board and the contributing authors to present the data in the most comprehensible form. The editorial team has worked tirelessly to provide valuable and valid information to help people across the globe.

Every chapter published in this book has been scrutinized by our experts. Their significance has been extensively debated. The topics covered herein carry significant findings which will fuel the growth of the discipline. They may even be implemented as practical applications or may be referred to as a beginning point for another development. Chapters in this book were first published by InTech; hereby published with permission under the Creative Commons Attribution License or equivalent.

The editorial board has been involved in producing this book since its inception. They have spent rigorous hours researching and exploring the diverse topics which have resulted in the successful publishing of this book. They have passed on their knowledge of decades through this book. To expedite this challenging task, the publisher supported the team at every step. A small team of assistant editors was also appointed to further simplify the editing procedure and attain best results for the readers.

Our editorial team has been hand-picked from every corner of the world. Their multi-ethnicity adds dynamic inputs to the discussions which result in innovative outcomes. These outcomes are then further discussed with the researchers and contributors who give their valuable feedback and opinion regarding the same. The feedback is then collaborated with the researches and they are edited in a comprehensive manner to aid the understanding of the subject.

Apart from the editorial board, the designing team has also invested a significant amount of their time in understanding the subject and creating the most relevant covers. They scrutinized every image to scout for the most suitable representation of the subject and create an appropriate cover for the book.

The publishing team has been involved in this book since its early stages. They were actively engaged in every process, be it collecting the data, connecting with the contributors or procuring relevant information. The team has been an ardent support to the editorial, designing and production team. Their endless efforts to recruit the best for this project, has resulted in the accomplishment of this book. They are a veteran in the field of academics and their pool of knowledge is as vast as their experience in printing. Their expertise and guidance has proved useful at every step. Their uncompromising quality standards have made this book an exceptional effort. Their encouragement from time to time has been an inspiration for everyone.

The publisher and the editorial board hope that this book will prove to be a valuable piece of knowledge for researchers, students, practitioners and scholars across the globe.

List of Contributors

Farrukh Jamal and Sangram Singh
Department of Biochemistry, Dr. Ram Manohar Lohia Avadh University, Faizabad, U.P. , India

Tabish Qidwai
Department of Biotechnology, Faculty of Engineering and Technology, R.B.S. College, Agra, U.P., India

Lu-Yu Hwang and Carolyn Z. Grimes
Center for Infectious Diseases, Division of Epidemiology and Center For Infectious Diseases, School of Public Health, USA
University of Texas Health Science Center at Houston, Houston, Texas, USA

Xin Pan
Animal Biosafety Level 3 Laboratory, Second Military Medical University, Shanghai, China

Nigel J. Silman
Research & Development, Health Protection Agency Porton, Porton Down, Salisbury, UK

Isaac K. Quaye
University of Botswana School of Medicine, Faculty of Medicine and Health Sciences Gaborone, Botswana

Priti Kumar Roy, Sonia Chowdhury and Amarnath Chatterjee
Centre for Mathematical Biology and Ecology, Department of Mathematics, Jadavpur University, Kolkata, India

Sutapa Biswas Majee
NSHM College of Pharmaceutical Technology, NSHM Knowledge Campus, Kolkata, India

Hiromi Takahashi-Omoe
National Institute of Science and Technology Policy (NISTEP), japan

Katsuhiko Omoe
Iwate University, Japan

Hiromi Takahashi-Omoe
National Institute of Science and Technology Policy (NISTEP), japan

Katsuhiko Omoe
Iwate University, Japan

Irina Shubina, Natalia Anisimova, Elena Gromova, Irina   Chikileva and Mikhail Kiselevsky
NN Blokhin Russian Cancer Research Center, Russia

Jon Florholmen and Rasmus Goll
Research group of Gastroenterology and Nutrition, Institute of Clinical Medicine, University of Tromsø, Tromsø, Department of Medical Gastroenterology, University Hospital North Norway, Tromsø, Norway

Alexandr A. Moisa and Ekaterina F. Kolesanova
Institute of Biomedical Chemistry, Russian Academy of Medical Sciences, Moscow, Russia

Alejandra Lara-Sampablo
Laboratorio de Biología Molecular y Virología, Centro de Investigación Biomédica de Oriente, Instituto Mexicano del Seguro Social, Metepec, Puebla, México
Centro de Química, Instituto de Ciencias, Benemérita Universidad Autónoma de Puebla, Puebla, México

Verónica Vallejo-Ruiz, Gerardo Santos-López and Julio Reyes-Leyva
Laboratorio de Biología Molecular y Virología, Centro de Investigación Biomédica de Oriente, Instituto Mexicano del Seguro Social, Metepec, Puebla, México

Nora Rosas-Murrieta and Irma Herrera-Camacho
Centro de Química, Instituto de Ciencias, Benemérita Universidad Autónoma de Puebla, Puebla, México

Printed in the USA
CPSIA information can be obtained
at www.ICGtesting.com
JSHW011425221024
72173JS00004B/671

9 781632 422446